Systems Radiology and Personalized Medicine

Systems Radiology and Personalized Medicine

Editors

Wouter Foppen
Nelleke Tolboom
Pim A. de Jong

MDPI • Basel • Beijing • Wuhan • Barcelona • Belgrade • Manchester • Tokyo • Cluj • Tianjin

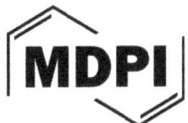

Editors
Wouter Foppen
Radiology and Nuclear Medicine
University Medical
Center Utrecht
Utrecht
The Netherlands

Nelleke Tolboom
Radiology and Nuclear Medicine
University Medical
Center Utrecht
Utrecht
The Netherlands

Pim A. de Jong
Radiology and Nuclear Medicine
University Medical
Center Utrecht
Utrecht
The Netherlands

Editorial Office
MDPI
St. Alban-Anlage 66
4052 Basel, Switzerland

This is a reprint of articles from the Special Issue published online in the open access journal *Journal of Personalized Medicine* (ISSN 2075-4426) (available at: www.mdpi.com/journal/jpm/special_issues/systems_radiology).

For citation purposes, cite each article independently as indicated on the article page online and as indicated below:

LastName, A.A.; LastName, B.B.; LastName, C.C. Article Title. *Journal Name* **Year**, *Volume Number*, Page Range.

ISBN 978-3-0365-2110-7 (Hbk)
ISBN 978-3-0365-2109-1 (PDF)

© 2021 by the authors. Articles in this book are Open Access and distributed under the Creative Commons Attribution (CC BY) license, which allows users to download, copy and build upon published articles, as long as the author and publisher are properly credited, which ensures maximum dissemination and a wider impact of our publications.

The book as a whole is distributed by MDPI under the terms and conditions of the Creative Commons license CC BY-NC-ND.

Contents

Wouter Foppen, Nelleke Tolboom and Pim A. de Jong
Systems Radiology and Personalized Medicine
Reprinted from: *Journal of Personalized Medicine* 2021, 11, 769, doi:10.3390/jpm11080769 1

Ling Lin, Xuhui Zhou, Ilona A. Dekkers and Hildo J. Lamb
Cardiorenal Syndrome: Emerging Role of Medical Imaging for Clinical Diagnosis and Management
Reprinted from: *Journal of Personalized Medicine* 2021, 11, 734, doi:10.3390/jpm11080734 5

Jordy P. Pijl, Thomas C. Kwee, Riemer H. J. A. Slart and Andor W. J. M. Glaudemans
PET/CT Imaging for Personalized Management of Infectious Diseases
Reprinted from: *Journal of Personalized Medicine* 2021, 11, 133, doi:10.3390/jpm11020133 27

Atia Samim, Godelieve A.M. Tytgat, Gitta Bleeker, Sylvia T.M. Wenker, Kristell L.S. Chatalic, Alex J. Poot, Nelleke Tolboom, Max M. van Noesel, Marnix G.E.H. Lam and Bart de Keizer
Nuclear Medicine Imaging in Neuroblastoma: Current Status and New Developments
Reprinted from: *Journal of Personalized Medicine* 2021, 11, 270, doi:10.3390/jpm11040270 43

Pieter H. Nienhuis, Gijs D. van Praagh, Andor W. J. M. Glaudemans, Elisabeth Brouwer and Riemer H. J. A. Slart
A Review on the Value of Imaging in Differentiating between Large Vessel Vasculitis and Atherosclerosis
Reprinted from: *Journal of Personalized Medicine* 2021, 11, 236, doi:10.3390/jpm11030236 65

Ui Yun Lee and Hyo Sung Kwak
Analysis of Morphological-Hemodynamic Risk Factors for Aneurysm Rupture Including a Newly Introduced Total Volume Ratio
Reprinted from: *Journal of Personalized Medicine* 2021, 11, 744, doi:10.3390/jpm11080744 79

Louise C. D. Konijn, Richard A. P. Takx, Willem P. Th. M. Mali, Hugo T. C. Veger and Hendrik van Overhagen
Different Lower Extremity Arterial Calcification Patterns in Patients with Chronic Limb-Threatening Ischemia Compared with Asymptomatic Controls
Reprinted from: *Journal of Personalized Medicine* 2021, 11, 493, doi:10.3390/jpm11060493 93

Yuan-Hsi Tseng, Chien-Wei Chen, Min Yi Wong, Teng-Yao Yang, Bor-Shyh Lin, Hua Ting and Yao-Kuang Huang
Discriminating Reflux from Non-Reflux Diseases of Superficial Veins in Legs by Novel Non-Contrast MR with QFlow Technique
Reprinted from: *Journal of Personalized Medicine* 2021, 11, 242, doi:10.3390/jpm11040242 109

Willem Paul Gielis, Harrie Weinans, Frank J. Nap, Frank W. Roemer and Wouter Foppen
Scoring Osteoarthritis Reliably in Large Joints and the Spine Using Whole-Body CT: OsteoArthritis Computed Tomography-Score (OACT-Score)
Reprinted from: *Journal of Personalized Medicine* 2020, 11, 5, doi:10.3390/jpm11010005 121

Netanja I. Harlianto, Jan Westerink, Wouter Foppen, Marjolein E. Hol, Rianne Wittenberg, Pieternella H. van der Veen, Bram van Ginneken, Jonneke S. Kuperus, Jorrit-Jan Verlaan, Pim A. de Jong, Firdaus A. A. Mohamed Hoesein and on behalf of the UCC-SMART-Study Group
Visceral Adipose Tissue and Different Measures of Adiposity in Different Severities of Diffuse Idiopathic Skeletal Hyperostosis
Reprinted from: *Journal of Personalized Medicine* **2021**, *11*, 663, doi:10.3390/jpm11070663 . . . . . . **135**

Ki-Sun Lee, Jae Young Kim, Eun-tae Jeon, Won Suk Choi, Nan Hee Kim and Ki Yeol Lee
Evaluation of Scalability and Degree of Fine-Tuning of Deep Convolutional Neural Networks for COVID-19 Screening on Chest X-ray Images Using Explainable Deep-Learning Algorithm
Reprinted from: *Journal of Personalized Medicine* **2020**, *10*, 213, doi:10.3390/jpm10040213 . . . . . . **147**

Daan J. de Jong, Wouter B. Veldhuis, Frank J. Wessels, Bob de Vos, Pim Moeskops and Madeleine Kok
Towards Personalised Contrast Injection: Artificial-Intelligence-Derived Body Composition and Liver Enhancement in Computed Tomography
Reprinted from: *Journal of Personalized Medicine* **2021**, *11*, 159, doi:10.3390/jpm11030159 . . . . . . **161**

Editorial
Systems Radiology and Personalized Medicine

Wouter Foppen , Nelleke Tolboom and Pim A. de Jong *

Department of Radiology and Nuclear Medicine, University Medical Center Utrecht,
3584 CX Utrecht, The Netherlands; w.foppen@umcutrecht.nl (W.F.); n.tolboom@umcutrecht.nl (N.T.)
* Correspondence: p.dejong-8@umcutrecht.nl

Medicine has evolved into a high level of specialization using the very detailed imaging of organs. This has impressively solved a multitude of acute health-related problems linked to single-organ diseases. Many diseases and pathophysiological processes, however, involve more than one organ. An organ-based approach is challenging when considering disease prevention and caring for elderly patients, or those with systemic chronic diseases or multiple co-morbidities. In addition, medical imaging provides more than a pretty picture. Much of the data are now revealed by quantitate algorithms with or without artificial intelligence. This Special Issue on "Systems Radiology and Personalized Medicine" includes reviews and original studies that show the strengths and weaknesses of structural and functional whole-body imaging for personalized medicine.

Cardiorenal syndrome is an example where physiological processes include more than one organ. Cardiac and renal functions may interact, in which the dysfunction of one organ may influence the function of the other. In the review on cardiorenal syndrome by Lin et al., imaging strategies are discussed in order to evaluate the cardiac and renal structure, function, and to characterize tissue using ultrasonography, computed tomography (CT), magnetic resonance imaging (MRI), and nuclear imaging techniques [1].

Nuclear molecular imaging techniques enable whole-body imaging and (patho)physiological processes, for example, in infectious diseases and oncology. Bloodstream infections of unknown origin, early spondylodiscitis, and vascular graft infections can be difficult to detect using standard diagnostics. Infectious diseases may be assessed by positron emission tomography (PET) CT by visualizing higher glucose metabolism using the glucose analog 2-Deoxy-2-[fluorine-18] fluoro-D-glucose (FDG) PET/CT. Common applications of FDG-PET/CT in the evaluation of infectious diseases are described by Pijl et al. [2]. In oncology, nuclear medicine is essential for staging and following up various types of cancer. In children, the most common extra-cranial solid malignancy is neuroblastoma, which can occur in the sympathetic trunk or in the adrenal medulla; about half of these children have metastatic disease at the time of diagnosis. Samim et al. reviewed the standard nuclear imaging technique (meta-[^{123}I]iodobenzylguanidine ([^{123}I]mIBG) whole-body scintigraphy) for the staging and response assessment of neuroblastoma, as well as new tracers and imaging techniques for neuroblastoma [3].

Vascular pathologies can occur anywhere through the body and include a wide spectrum of diseases. Imaging plays an important role in differentiating vascular pathologies which may have similar characteristics but a different etiology and thus require different treatment. For differentiation between large-vessel vasculitis and atherosclerosis, Nienhuis et al. reviewed the evidence of various imaging techniques [4]. Cerebral aneurysms may rupture, leading to morbidity and mortality. The size of the aneurysm is one of the risk factors for rupture, although other factors including morphological and hemodynamic risk factors may contribute to a better prediction of potential ruptures. Lee et al. evaluated a series of ruptured and unruptured cerebral aneurysms using cerebral angiography, and identified morphological and hemodynamic factors associated with aneurysm rupture which may be tested in larger prospective studies [5]. Peripheral artery disease and venous diseases of the legs have a huge medical and economic impact because they may eventually lead to critical limb ischemia and amputation, and deep vein thrombosis, which may cause subsequent pulmonary embolism. Imaging may be used to differentiate different patterns or causes of these diseases. Arterial calcification patterns on CT can be evaluated, for example, because these are different in patients with critical limb ischemia compared to patients without peripheral artery disease [6], and MRI flow techniques may be used to differentiate between reflux and non-reflux venous diseases [7].

Musculoskeletal diseases could severely affect patients' mobility and well-being, of which osteoarthritis is a leading cause of disability. Multiple joints are often affected by osteoarthritis, and this may hamper interpretation of the contribution of a specific joint in patients' quality of life, physical performance, or biochemical markers. Gielis et al. developed and tested the reproducibility of the OsteoArthritis Computed Tomography-Score in order to assess osteoarthritis burden throughout the body in large joints and the spine [8]. Abnormal new bone formation was observed in patients with diffuse idiopathic skeletal hyperostosis (DISH), especially in the spine near the anterior longitudinal ligament, resulting in an increased risk of spinal fractures. Although the exact pathophysiology is unknown, DISH is associated with obesity; Harlianto et al. reported the relationship between DISH and visceral adipose tissue based on data from over 4000 patients [9].

Artificial intelligence (AI) can have multiple applications in personalized medical imaging, ranging from personalized and faster scanning to aiding diagnosis and prognosis. The performance of AI in image reading and diagnosis is widely studied and expected to change the radiology workflow in the near future. In the past 1.5 years, COVID-19 has had a huge impact on healthcare worldwide, and numerous imaging studies using X-rays and CT for the evaluation of COVID-19 have been published in 2020–2021. Lee et al. report their findings on their evaluation of convolutional neural networks for COVID-19 screening on chest X-rays [10]. An important aspect of diagnostic imaging is the acquisition of the image during the study procedure. Adequate contrast enhancement is essential in abdominal CT studies, to ensure the accurate detection and characterization of liver lesions, for example. Patient-related factors such as height, weight, and cardiac output have an influence on the degree of contrast enhancement. De Jong et al. studied the relationship between liver enhancement and body composition assessed by an artificial intelligence algorithm. Their data and observation that lean body weight is more strongly associated with liver enhancement than total body weight and body mass index suggest that the use of an artificial intelligence body-composition-based algorithm may result in a reduction in variability in liver enhancement as well as lowering the amount of contrast media [11].

We now live in an era moving again towards a more holistic form of medicine. This movement is, in part, driven by population aging in several countries, by a multitude of novel therapeutic options, and by the impressive ability to combine systems biology, systems medicine and systems radiology data. In this Special Issue, some insight is provided to the broad range of possibilities that have already entered clinical medicine or will gain impact and create value in the near future.

Conflicts of Interest: The authors declare no conflict of interest.

References

1. Lin, L.; Zhou, X.; Dekkers, I.A.; Lamb, H.J. Cardiorenal Syndrome: Emerging Role of Medical Imaging for Clinical Diagnosis and Management. *J. Pers. Med.* **2021**, *11*, 734. [CrossRef]
2. Pijl, J.P.; Kwee, T.C.; Slart, R.H.J.A.; Glaudemans, A.W.J.M. PET/CT Imaging for Personalized Management of Infectious Diseases. *J. Pers. Med.* **2021**, *11*, 133. [CrossRef] [PubMed]
3. Samim, A.; Tytgat, G.A.M.; Bleeker, G.; Wenker, S.T.M.; Chatalic, K.L.S.; Poot, A.J.; Tolboom, N.; van Noesel, M.M.; Lam, M.G.E.H.; de Keizer, B. Nuclear Medicine Imaging in Neuroblastoma: Current Status and New Developments. *J. Pers. Med.* **2021**, *11*, 270. [CrossRef] [PubMed]
4. Nienhuis, P.H.; van Praagh, G.D.; Glaudemans, A.W.J.M.; Brouwer, E.; Slart, R.H.J.A. A Review on the Value of Imaging in Differentiating between Large Vessel Vasculitis and Atherosclerosis. *J. Pers. Med.* **2021**, *11*, 236. [CrossRef] [PubMed]
5. Lee, U.Y.; Kwak, H.S. Analysis of Morphological-Hemodynamic Risk Factors for Aneurysm Rupture Including a Newly Introduced Total Volume Ratio. *J. Pers. Med.* **2021**, *11*, 744. [CrossRef]

6. Konijn, L.C.D.; Takx, R.A.P.; Mali, W.P.T.M.; Veger, H.T.C.; van Overhagen, H. Different Lower Extremity Arterial Calcification Patterns in Patients with Chronic Limb-Threatening Ischemia Compared with Asymptomatic Controls. *J. Pers. Med.* **2021**, *11*, 493. [CrossRef] [PubMed]
7. Tseng, Y.-H.; Chen, C.-W.; Wong, M.Y.; Yang, T.-Y.; Lin, B.-S.; Ting, H.; Huang, Y.-K. Discriminating Reflux from Non-Reflux Diseases of Superficial Veins in Legs by Novel Non-Contrast MR with QFlow Technique. *J. Pers. Med.* **2021**, *11*, 242. [CrossRef] [PubMed]
8. Gielis, W.P.; Weinans, H.; Nap, F.J.; Roemer, F.W.; Foppen, W. Scoring Osteoarthritis Reliably in Large Joints and the Spine Using Whole-Body CT: OsteoArthritis Computed Tomography-Score (OACT-Score). *J. Pers. Med.* **2021**, *11*, 5. [CrossRef]
9. Harlianto, N.I.; Westerink, J.; Foppen, W.; Hol, M.E.; Wittenberg, R.; van der Veen, P.H.; van Ginneken, B.; Kuperus, J.S.; Verlaan, J.-J.; de Jong, P.A.; et al. Visceral Adipose Tissue and Different Measures of Adiposity in Different Severities of Diffuse Idiopathic Skeletal Hyperostosis. *J. Pers. Med.* **2021**, *11*, 663. [CrossRef]
10. Lee, K.-S.; Kim, J.Y.; Jeon, E.-T.; Choi, W.S.; Kim, N.H.; Lee, K.Y. Evaluation of Scalability and Degree of Fine-Tuning of Deep Convolutional Neural Networks for COVID-19 Screening on Chest X-ray Images Using Explainable Deep-Learning Algorithm. *J. Pers. Med.* **2020**, *10*, 213. [CrossRef] [PubMed]
11. de Jong, D.J.; Veldhuis, W.B.; Wessels, F.J.; de Vos, B.; Moeskops, P.; Kok, M. Towards Personalised Contrast Injection: Artificial-Intelligence-Derived Body Composition and Liver Enhancement in Computed Tomography. *J. Pers. Med.* **2021**, *11*, 159. [CrossRef] [PubMed]

Cardiorenal Syndrome: Emerging Role of Medical Imaging for Clinical Diagnosis and Management

Ling Lin [1], Xuhui Zhou [2,*], Ilona A. Dekkers [1] and Hildo J. Lamb [1]

1. Cardiovascular Imaging Group (CVIG), Department of Radiology, Leiden University Medical Center, 2333 ZA Leiden, The Netherlands; l.lin@lumc.nl (L.L.); i.a.dekkers@lumc.nl (I.A.D.); h.j.lamb@lumc.nl (H.J.L.)
2. Department of Radiology, The Eighth Affiliated Hospital of Sun Yat-sen University, Shenzhen 510833, China
* Correspondence: zhouxuh@mail.sysu.edu.cn; Tel.: +86-755-83982222

Abstract: Cardiorenal syndrome (CRS) concerns the interconnection between heart and kidneys in which the dysfunction of one organ leads to abnormalities of the other. The main clinical challenges associated with cardiorenal syndrome are the lack of tools for early diagnosis, prognosis, and evaluation of therapeutic effects. Ultrasound, computed tomography, nuclear medicine, and magnetic resonance imaging are increasingly used for clinical management of cardiovascular and renal diseases. In the last decade, rapid development of imaging techniques provides a number of promising biomarkers for functional evaluation and tissue characterization. This review summarizes the applicability as well as the future technological potential of each imaging modality in the assessment of CRS. Furthermore, opportunities for a comprehensive imaging approach for the evaluation of CRS are defined.

Keywords: cardiorenal syndrome; imaging biomarker; tissue characterization

1. Introduction

Cardiorenal syndrome (CRS) is an umbrella term describing the interactions between concomitant cardiac and renal dysfunctions, in which acute or chronic dysfunction of one organ may induce or precipitate dysfunction of the other [1]. CRS has been associated with increased morbidity and poor clinical outcomes, leading to high economic and societal burden [2]. The estimated incidence of acute kidney injury is 24–45% in acute decompensated heart failure and 9–19% in acute coronary syndrome [3]. The prevalence of impaired renal function is high in chronic cardiovascular diseases, and around 40–60% in chronic heart failure [4]. The combination of renal dysfunction with chronic heart failure is predictive of adverse clinical outcomes [5]. Nearly 50% of deaths in all age groups of patients with chronic kidney disease (CKD) can be attributed to cardiovascular causes [6]. CRS is also frequently observed in acute or chronic systemic conditions, such as sepsis and diabetes mellitus, and is associated with worse outcomes [7].

Despite the existing literature on the classification and management of CRS, the clinical diagnosis and treatment evaluation remains difficult due to the lack of clinical practice guidelines [8]. This has led to increased research interests, including studies focused on the early diagnosis and clinical management of CRS. The potential value of imaging biomarkers for the early detection of cardiac abnormalities in CRS has been underlined in the scientific statement from the American Heart Association [8]. Ultrasonography is currently the first-line imaging modality for structural and functional assessment of the heart, and structural assessment of the kidneys. Computed tomography (CT), nuclear imaging, and magnetic resonance imaging (MRI) have been widely used for various purposes in clinical management of cardiovascular diseases and kidney diseases. Recent technological advancements in medical imaging provides a number of promising biomarkers for the diagnosis and prognosis of CRS, and opportunities for personalized medicine. In this review, we will summarize the cardiovascular and renal imaging techniques related to CRS and the potential utility of these techniques for the diagnosis and follow-up of acute and chronic CRS (Figure 1). Finally, comprehensive imaging protocols that can be incorporated into future research studies and clinical trials will be proposed.

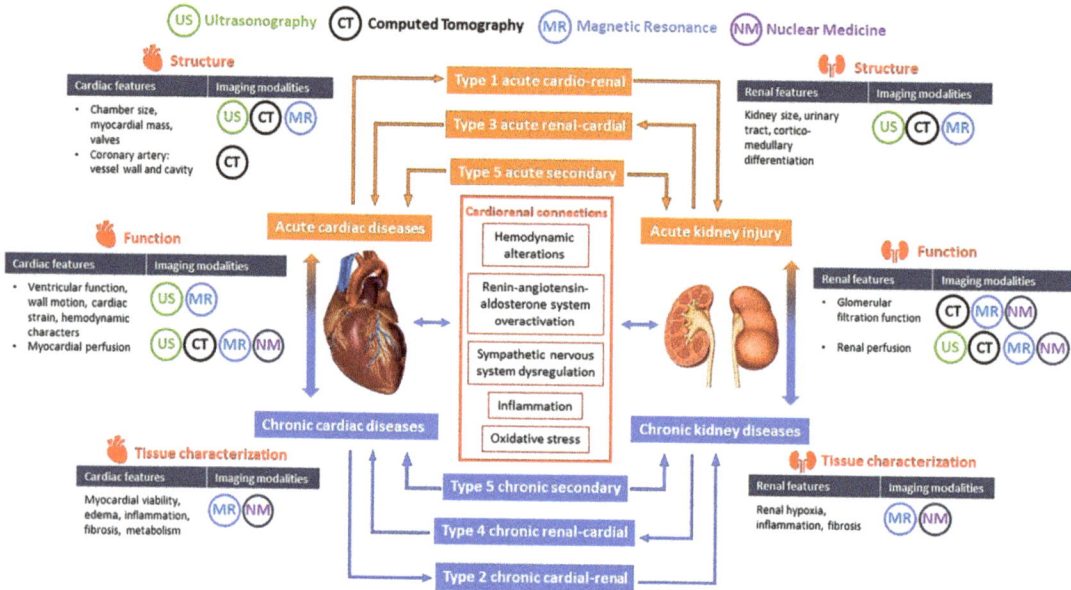

Figure 1. Overview of the contents. The heart and kidneys interact through multiple pathophysiological pathways which may lead to five subtypes of CRS. The structural, functional and tissue texture changes in the heart and kidneys can be evaluated using different imaging modalities including ultrasonography, computed tomography, magnetic resonance, and nuclear medicine.

2. Classification, Pathophysiology, and Clinical Management of CRS

2.1. Classification of CRS

Cardio-renal syndrome can be classified into five subtypes [1], with type 1 and 2 describing renal dysfunction sequent to initial acute and chronic cardiac insults, type 3 and 4 describing renocardiac syndrome after the initial insult of kidney disease, and type 5 representing secondary CRS in systemic diseases (Table 1). Although this classification simplifies the clinical concept of CRS, overlap between different subtypes and progression from one subtype to another has frequently been observed [9]. For example, it is challenging to differentiate type 2 CRS from type 4 CRS as chronic heart diseases and chronic kidney diseases frequently co-exist [10,11]. Moreover, the development of CRS is often complicated by several interconnected conditions, such as diabetes, hypertension, atherosclerosis, endothelial cell dysfunction, chronic inflammation, and anemia, rendering difficulties in defining the temporal progression patterns of CRS [8]. An alternative classification of CRS was proposed by Hatamizadeh et al. based on clinical manifestations rather than the organ that initiated the process [12], but has not received wide acceptance.

Table 1. Classification of cardiorenal syndrome.

Classification	Timing	Descriptions	Examples
Type 1 (acute cardiorenal)	Acute	Heart failure causing AKI	Acute decompensated heart failure resulting in AKI, acute ischemic heart disease, valvulopathy or arrhythmia causing cardiogenic shock and AKI
Type 2 (chronic cardiorenal)	Chronic	Chronic heart disease causing CKD	Chronic heart failure causing CKD
Type 3 (acute renocardiac)	Acute	AKI leading to acute cardiac dysfunction	AKI due to glomerulonephritis or urinary tract obstruction causing acute heart failure, acute coronary syndrome or arrhythmia
Type 4 (chronic renocardiac)	Chronic	CKD leading to chronic cardiac abnormalities	CKD-associated cardiomyopathy
Type 5 (secondary)	Acute or Chronic	Systemic diseases causing acute or chronic dysfunction of heat and kidneys	AKI and acute heart failure induced by sepsis or critical conditions, CKD and cardiac abnormalities in diabetes mellitus, cirrhosis, amyloidosis, vasculitis, etc.

AKI, acute kidney injury; CKD, chronic kidney disease.

2.2. Pathophysiology of CRS

The exact pathophysiological mechanisms of each type of CRS have not been fully elucidated. Previously, decreased cardiac output and arterial underfilling induced neurohumoral activations were believed to be the sole pathogenesis of CRS [13]. However, studies in the past decades demonstrated that decreased arterial flow does not fully explain the worsening renal function in CRS (60–63). Elevated central venous pressure has closer association with the reduction of renal perfusion than decreased cardiac output (61). Moreover, increasing evidence indicates that multiple pathophysiological processes contribute to the evolution of CRS [14]. Hemodynamic alterations, renin–angiotensin–aldosterone system (RAAS), sympathetic nervous system, inflammatory, and oxidative stress are considered as key connectors between heart and kidneys [15,16]. Other contributing factors such as biochemical perturbations, immune responses, atherosclerosis and anemia–inflammation–bone mineral axis, can also accelerate the development of CRS, especially in chronic heart failure and CKD [8,15,17]. These pathways are interconnected and exhibit varied clinical importance across different subtypes of CRS [3,18].

Hemodynamic alterations, especially right-sided heart dysfunction, is believed to be of critical importance in the development of acute CRS (type 1 and type 3) [19]. In type 1 CRS, increased central venous pressure results in renal venous congestion, which may lead to impaired glomerular filtration, tissue hypoxia and renal fibrogenesis. These pathological changes induce or aggravate renal dysfunction, which in return exacerbates fluid overload leading to further deterioration of cardiac function [4,15]. In type 3 CRS, acute heart injury can be caused by excessive cytokines due to AKI, and by indirect mechanisms including neurohumoral activation, electrolytes disturbances, uremia, and acidemia [20,21].

Non-hemodynamic pathways play a more critical role in chronic CRS (type 2 and type 4). Activation of RAAS and stimulation of sympathetic nervous system are features of both heart failure and CKD. Persistent activation of RAAS leads to peripheral vasoconstriction, exacerbated fluid overload, and sympathetic nervous system overactivation [16,22]. Sympathetic overactivation in return can stimulate RAAS via renin release, resulting in a vicious circle [16]. Chronically increased release of aldosterone is the major deleterious component of RAAS and has been associated with both myocardial and renal interstitial fibrosis [23]. Increased oxidative stress due to chronic RAAS activation has also been associated with renal injury and fluid retention [24]. Inflammation cascade can be triggered by and potentiate the other cardiorenal connectors, including the overactivation of RAAS and sympathetic nervous system, and increased oxidative stress. Systemic inflammation is associated with myocardial and renal dysfunction and interstitial fibrosis [19,25].

Fibrosis has been considered as a key driver in the pathophysiology of chronic CRS [18]. Fibrogenic responses have short-term adaptive features in the early phases of cardiac and renal diseases. However, when it progresses chronically, fibrosis can lead to myocardial and renal parenchymal scarring, cellular dysfunction and ultimately organ failure [26]. Fibrosis of heart and kidneys has also been found in a number of CRS risk factors, including aging, hypertension, diabetes mellitus, and obesity [27]. Based on these findings, a new pragmatic and dynamic cardiorenal integrative concept of CRS has been proposed, in which patients may be categorized according to the predominant pathophysiological mechanism, rather than clinical presentation [18]. This strategy has the potential to facilitate clinical interventions for CRS in the future.

2.3. Current Difficulties in Diagnosis and Management of CRS

In most circumstances, the complex interconnected pathways between heart and kidneys have already been activated by the time clinical manifestations are detectable. Both heart and kidneys have substantial functional reserve, which makes it difficult to prevent or reverse the adverse impacts of CRS at an early phase. While all types of CRSs are faced with difficulties in early diagnosis and prognosis, the dominant clinical challenges distinguish between acute CRS and chronic CRS (Table 2).

Table 2. Current difficulties in diagnosis and management of cardiorenal syndrome.

Main Challenges in All Types of CRS	
• Early diagnosis and prognosis • Preventing or reversing the adverse impacts of CRS • Difficulties in distinguishing CRS from other cardiovascular and renal comorbidities	
Specific Difficulties in Acute and Chronic CRS	
Acute CRS	Chronic CRS
• Current diagnostic criteria hinders early detection of AKI • Difficult to differentiate between true kidney injury and pseudo-worsening of kidney function • Lack of sensitive tools to assess treatment effects and to track the progression from AKI to CKD	• Lack of overt symptoms of cardiovascular diseases in CKD • Lack of sensitive tools to identify and monitor the progression of cardiovascular involvement when conventional assessments remain normal • Standard treatment is less effective in reducing cardiovascular mortality in CKD patients than in the general population.

The main challenges in acute CRS are related to AKI (Table 2). Currently, AKI is diagnosed based on serum creatinine (SCr) level and oliguria [28]. However, SCr cannot detect early kidney dysfunction, since it remains within normal range before half the kidney function is lost, resulting in a lag between kidney insult and the elevation of SCr [29]. On the other hand, pseudo-worsening of kidney function may occur due to hemodynamic changes in patients with heart failure, which is difficult to be differentiated from true kidney injury [30]. Apart from the inability to prevent or early identify AKI, the lack of sensitive tools to track the progression from AKI to CKD also challenges the clinical management of AKI. It has been reported that AKI is independently associated with higher rates of incident CKD [31]. Moreover, kidney dysfunction may decrease the efficiency of diuretics in patients with heart failure, resulting in diuretic resistance and worsening of congestion, which in return deteriorates the heart and kidney functions [19]. Strategies to prevent AKI or early interventions in the course of AKI remain to be investigated to reduce the risk of future adverse renal and cardiac outcomes. In addition, there is a demanding need of guidance on cardiac- and reno-protective therapies in acute CRS.

In chronic CRS, however, the main difficulties lie in the cardiac aspect (Table 2). Patients with CKD suffer from a high risk of cardiovascular diseases that is disproportionate to the risk expected in general population [32]. In early-stage CKD, the risk of cardiovascular death far exceeds the risk of progressing to dialysis [33]. Previous studies suggested that subtle alterations in cardiac structure and function could occur very early in the progression of CKD, even when SCr is still within the normal range [34]. In addition, nonatheromatous processes appear to predominate the progression of cardiovascular disease in CKD, which could explain the lower effect of standard treatment on decreasing cardiovascular mortality in CKD patients than in general population [35]. Early detection of cardiovascular abnormality in CKD is challenging due to lack of overt symptoms and preserved left ventricular systolic function [36].

Despite the amount of effort in research studies of novel serum and urinary biomarkers, it remains unclear whether and to what extent these biomarkers can be involved in clinical management of CRS [37]. Moreover, the global availability of biomarker technology is another obstacle upon implementing this strategy in clinical practice. Imaging techniques that provide quantitative information on blood flow, perfusion, diffusion, tissue oxygenation, and interstitial fibrosis without radiation or potential risks of contrast agents offer possibilities of noninvasive assessment of preclinical pathophysiological changes in the heart and kidneys at the early phase of CRS.

3. Cardiovascular and Renal Imaging Techniques Related to CRS

Different imaging modalities can be applied in relation to CRS that enabling comprehensive assessment of both morphology and function (Table 3). Although further validations are needed for some of these techniques, a number of promising imaging biomarkers that might be valuable for the clinical management of CRS are discussed below.

3.1. Cardiovascular Imaging Techniques

3.1.1. Transthoracic Echocardiography

Transthoracic echocardiography (TTE) is the most available non-invasive imaging technique to measure the dimensions of cardiac chambers and to estimate ventricular functions. TTE-measured left ventricular ejection fraction is the first-line tool to differentiate between heart failure with reduced ejection fraction and heart failure with reserved ejection fraction [38]. TTE can rapidly identify wall motion abnormalities, valvular diseases and pericardial effusion. Various hemodynamic markers can be estimated by Doppler imaging, such as mitral inflow and mitral annulus motion, left atrial volume and pressure, left ventricular filling pressure, systolic pulmonary artery pressure, pulmonary capillary wedge pressure, and right ventricular function [39]. Myocardial strain based on speckle tracking technique can be used to quantify ventricular wall deformation, with global longitudinal strain being more sensitive to subtle impairment of ventricular systolic function than ejection fraction [40]. Fast and cost-effective as it is, TTE-derived imaging biomarkers can be limited by inadequate acoustic window, poor Doppler signals and operator-dependent variations. The utility of ultrasonic enhancing agent improves structural and functional evaluations of various cardiovascular diseases [41]. Enhanced TTE also enables the assessment of myocardial perfusion at rest or with vasodilator-induced stress [41].

3.1.2. Cardiovascular Magnetic Resonance

Over the last decade, cardiovascular magnetic resonance (CMR) has gained increasing acknowledgement in the clinical management of cardiovascular diseases [42,43]. CMR-measured biventricular volumes, systolic function and myocardial mass are gold-standard imaging biomarkers [44], particularly right ventricular geometry and function. Myocardial strain parameters can also be generated from CMR using feature/tissue tracking post-processing algorithms, free from the suboptimal acoustic window and dropouts in TTE [45] (Figure 2). Velocity encoding using phase contrast technique enables quantitative evaluation of valvular diseases and shunt evaluation by CMR. Using gadolinium-based contrast agents, myocardial perfusion and myocardial fibrosis or infiltration can be assessed and quantified. Late gadolinium enhancement is the best non-invasive technique to visualize focal fibrosis [46]. Extracellular volume fraction (ECV) calculated by pre- and post-contrast T1 relaxation time is useful for detecting diffused myocardial fibrosis [47]. However, the application of contrast-enhanced CMR in CRS is limited in patients with severely decreased renal function (eGFR < 30 mL/min/1.73 m^2), considering the potential increased risk of gadolinium retention and nephrogenic systemic fibrosis in patients with renal dysfunction [48,49], but these risks are less clear for the more modern macrocyclic contrast agents [48].

Table 3. Modalities and techniques for cardiovascular and renal imaging related to cardiorenal syndrome.

	Ultrasonography	Magnetic Resonance Imaging	Computed Tomography	Nuclear Imaging
Assessment of Heart				
Conventional	1. 2-dimentioanl measurement of cardiac chamber size, estimation of ventricular function 2. Valvular morphology and function, ventricular wall motion 3. Estimation of hemodynamic biomarkers by Doppler imaging	1. Gold-standard measurement of chamber size and volume, ventricular systolic function, myocardial mass by cine imaging 2. Moderate to severe valvular abnormalities 3. Quantification of myocardial perfusion with contrast agent and/or vasodilator 4. Quantification of myocardial fibrosis and infiltration by late gadolinium enhancement	1. Calculation of calcium score 2. Evaluation of coronary artery morphology by CT coronary angiography using contrast agent	1. SPECT myocardial perfusion imaging is the most commonly used tool to diagnose coronary artery disease in CKD 2. Absolute quantification of myocardial blood flow by PET 3. Coronary flow reserve and stress myocardial perfusion by PET
Advanced	1. 3-dimentional measurement of ventricular volumes and myocardial mass 2. Ventricular strain quantified by speckle-tracking 3. Improved structural and functional evaluation using ultrasonic enhancing agent	1. Non-contrast quantification of myocardial infiltration/deposition by T1 mapping and T2(*) mapping 2. Myocardial infiltration/deposition by extracellular volume fraction with contrast agent 3. Ventricular strain quantified by feature/tissue tracking 4. Non-contrast assessment of myocardial perfusion by dobutamine inotropic stress CMR, MR-compatible exercise stress CMR, myocardial ASL 4. Myocardial hypoxia by BOLD, diffusion by DWI, diffusion anisotropy by DTI	1. Functional imaging and myocardial perfusion using contrast agent 2. CT angiography-based fractional flow reserve of coronary arteries 3. Myocardial infiltration/deposition by extracellular volume fraction with contrast agent	1. PET quantitative analysis of myocardial glucose utilization 2. SPECT evaluation of myocardial fatty acid oxidation 3. Hybrid imaging such as SPECT-CT, PET-CT, PET-MRI can generate multiple biomarkers in one scan
Assessment of kidneys				
Conventional	1. Kidney length, estimated volume and echogenicity of cortex and medulla 2. Identify obstruction 3. Renal resistive index	1. Volumetric measurement 2. Depiction of renal cortex and medulla by conventional T1-weighted and T2-weighted imaging	1. Preferred for evaluation of kidney stones 2. Quantification of renal perfusion and GFR using contrast enhanced CT	1. Differential diagnosis of AKI (prerenal AKI or acute tubular necrosis or postrenal AKI) by renal scintigraphy 2. Measurement of GFR 3. Measurement of renal blood flow

Table 3. Cont.

	Ultrasonography	Magnetic Resonance Imaging	Computed Tomography	Nuclear Imaging
Advanced	1. Intrarenal blood flow pattern 2. Renal venous blood flow, renal venous impedance index, renal venous discontinuity 3. Ultrasonic enhancing agent to assess renal perfusion	1. Parenchymal oxygenation by BOLD 2. Noncontrast renal perfusion by ASL 3. Microstructural changes evaluated by DWI, DTI and T1/T2 mapping 4. Quantification of renal perfusion and GFR using dynamic contrast enhancement	1. Dual energy CT for tissue characterization	1. Renal SPECT-CT for assessment of GFR 2. Renal PET with novel radiotracers for faster and more accurate quantification of GFR
Radiation	None	None	Yes	Yes
Contrast agent and safety	Mirobubbles to enhance ultrasound signals; safe	Gadolinium-based contrast agents, associated with nephrogenic systemic fibrosis, not applicable in patients with AKI and ESRD	Iodinated contrast agents, increase the risk of contrast-induced nephropathy in patients with renal dysfunction	Radionuclide labeled agents, safe.
Strengths in assessment of cardiorenal syndrome	1. Most versatile, accessible and cost effective modality to evaluate the heart and kidneys simultaneously. 2. Doppler imaging may generate hemodynamic biomarkers for diagnosis, prognosis and therapeutic evaluation, especially for acute CRS. 3. Suitable for serial imaging across the natural history of CRS	1. The most promising one-stop modality to evaluate structure, function and microstructural alterations in both heart and kidneys 2. Unique ability of quantitative assessment of fibrosis in both organs. Multiparametric scan to evaluate diffused infiltration/deposition, changes in perfusion, diffusion and oxygenation of heart and kidneys. 2. With consistent scan parameters and no radiation, non-contrast MRI is ideal for longitudinal tracking of cardiac and renal pathophysiological changes	Most widely used noninvasive technique for anatomical assessment of coronary artery disease	Important modality for evaluation of myocardial perfusion in coronary artery disease in patients with CKD, without the use of toxic contrast agent.
Limitations	Can be compromised by inadequate acoustic window, poor Doppler signals and operator-dependent variations	Expensive, prolonged acquisition time, requiring high compliance of patient, complicated post-processing procedures	Not suitable for longitudinal serial evaluation due to radiation, limited utility without contras agent	Not suitable for longitudinal serial evaluation due to radiation, low spatial resolution, prolonged acquisition time, limited utility and accessibility

SPECT, Single-photon emission computed tomography; PET, positron emission tomography; CMR, cardiovascular magnetic resonance; CT, computed tomography; BOLD, blood oxygen level dependent; ASL, arterial spin labeling; DWI, diffusion weighted imaging; DTI, diffusion tensor imaging; AKI, acute kidney injury; CKD, chronic kidney disease; ESRD, end stage renal disease; GFR, glomerular filtration rate.

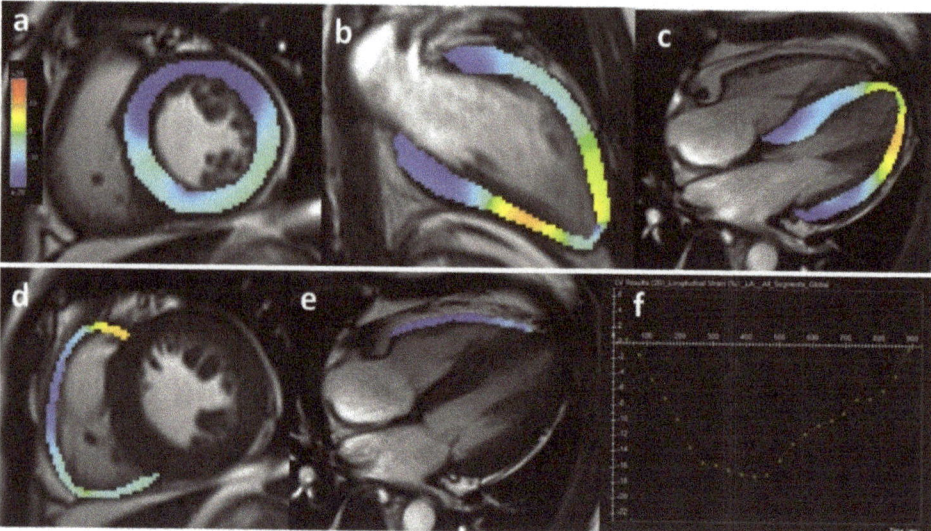

Figure 2. Example of myocardial strain analysis using MRI in a patient with CKD. Quantification of left ventricular strain (**a–c**) and right ventricular strain (**d,e**) parameter is visualized by colored overlay on cine images. (**f**) is an example of strain–time curve of the left ventricular global longitudinal strain within one cardiac cycle.

Non-contrast tissue characterization techniques including T1 mapping, T2 mapping and diffusion weighted imaging (DWI) provide unique opportunities to identify microstructural changes in myocardium (Figure 3). T1 and T2 mapping are increasingly used in clinical settings. T1 mapping quantifies the longitudinal and T2 mapping transverse magnetization relaxation times of the hydrogen nucleus proton per voxel, which can reflect the presence of fibrosis, fat, edema, and iron deposition [50]. Myocardial T1 and T2 values have been applied to detect abnormalities in myocardial tissue composition in various diseases that related to CRS—including heart failure, ischemic heart diseases, hypertensive cardiomyopathy, diabetic cardiomyopathy, and uremic cardiomyopathy [50,51]. DWI characterizes the motion of water molecules in microstructural changes, and quantifies it as apparent diffusion coefficient (ADC). Previous studies suggested that DWI was able to detect and quantify the degree of myocardial fibrosis, with the minimum amount of fibrosis larger than 20% [52–54].

3.1.3. Cardiac Computed Tomography

Computed tomography (CT) coronary angiography is the most widely used noninvasive imaging technique for anatomical assessment of coronary artery disease (CAD). CT angiography with additional perfusion imaging allows for characterization of atherosclerosis in relation to myocardial ischemia, which has great potential clinical value [55]. CT-based fractional flow reserve allows for the quantification of the impaired maximal coronary flow induced by a stenosis, which is adapted from invasive coronary pressure measurement [56]. CT can also be used to estimate myocardial ECV, and is an attractive alternative to CMR to evaluate diffused myocardial fibrosis [57]. However, major challenges of CT are the limited temporal resolution, presence of beam and scatter artefacts, radiation dose, and low contrast-to-noise ratios [58–60]. Moreover, these CT techniques rely on iodinated contrast agents, which is associated with the risk of post-contrast AKI in patients with impaired renal function [61]. Without contrast agent, CT can be used to calculate coronary artery calcium score, which is a prognostic biomarker for CAD.

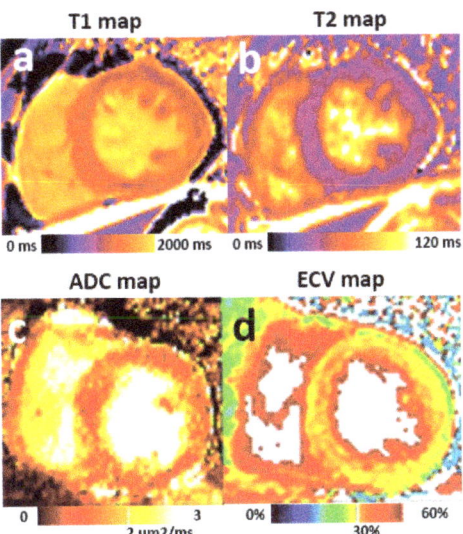

Figure 3. Myocardial tissue characterization by multiparametric MRI. Mid-cavity short-axis T1 map (**a**) and T2 map (**b**) of a patient with CKD. Myocardial T1 and T2 values can be quantified and compared with local references. ADC (**c**) and ECV (**d**) images demonstrated diffused "pepper like" hyper intensity texture in a patient with hypertrophic cardiomyopathy. Images (**c**,**d**) were adapted from published article [52] under a Creative Commons license.

3.1.4. Nuclear Cardiac Imaging

Nuclear cardiac imaging has played an important role in evaluating myocardial perfusion in ischemic heart diseases. Single-photon emission computed tomography (SPECT) is commonly employed for the diagnosis of CAD in patients with CKD [62]. However, SPECT only provides semi-quantitative assessment of myocardial perfusion, and has a wide range of sensitivity, specificity, and accuracy [63]. Quantitative positron emission tomography (PET), on the other hand, measures absolute myocardial blood flow and has shown greater prognostic value than SPECT in evaluation of patients with known or suspected CAD [64]. Currently four different tracers are used for clinical assessment of myocardial blood flow, which are ^{82}Rb, ^{13}N-ammonia, ^{15}O-water, and ^{18}F-flurpiridaz. ^{15}O-water-PET is considered the clinical reference standard for non-invasive quantification of myocardial perfusion; however, important challenges include high-cost, limited visual assessment, and the lower spatial resolution of PET compared with CT or MRI perfusion imaging [65]. Myocardial metabolism alterations such as increased glucose utility and fatty acid oxidation can also be evaluated by ^{18}F-fluoro-2-deoxyglucose [^{18}F-FDG] PET and β-Methyl-p-[123I]-iodophenyl-pentadecanoic acid SPECT [63] Hybrid imaging such as SPECT-CT, PET-CT, and PET-MRI can generate multiple imaging biomarkers by single examination.

3.2. Renal Imaging Techniques

3.2.1. Renal Ultrasonography

Renal ultrasonography is routinely used to assess renal morphology such as renal length, corticomedullary differentiation, and to identify obstruction. The usefulness of ultrasonography to identify the underlying cause of renal diseases is limited, furthermore no distinction between inflammation and fibrosis can be identified by echogenicity [66]. Renal Doppler sonography enables the quantification of renal blood flow and intrarenal hemodynamic changes, which are suggestive of renal dysfunction and/or microstructural alterations. Elevated values of renal resistive index are associated with poorer prognosis in various renal disorders and renal transplant [67]. Renal venous flow is one of the biomarkers for right-sided congestion, which is fundamental to the management of CRS Contrast-enhanced ultrasonography has showed the ability to quantify regional renal perfusion and microvascular function in rat models, and is potentially feasible for early detection and monitoring of AKI [68,69].

3.2.2. Renal Magnetic Resonance Imaging

Initial applications of renal MRI have been focused on the visualization of renal and urogenital anatomy. Conventional renal MRI sequences can be used to measure total kidney volume, which is an FDA-approved prognostic biomarker [70], with higher accuracy compared with sonography. Recent research interest has been focused on the application of sequences that provide functional (BOLD, ASL) and microstructural (DWI, DTI, T1 mapping, T2 mapping) information without the need for gadolinium-based contrast agents [71–75] (Figure 4).

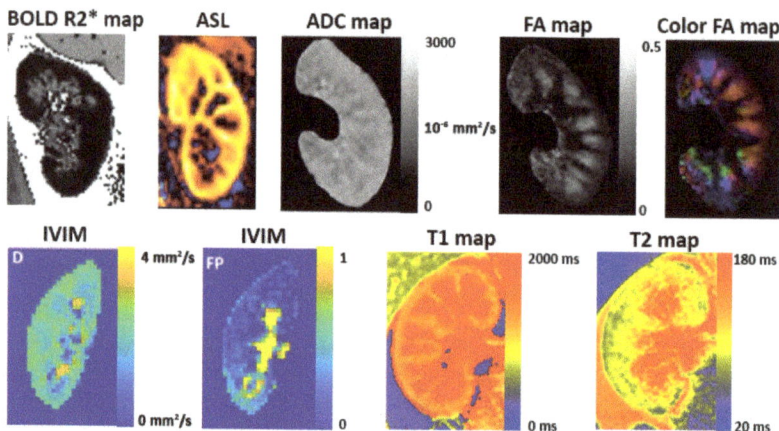

Figure 4. Multiparametric kidney MRI in healthy volunteers. BOLD R2* map is used to evaluate parenchyma oxygenation. Renal blood flow can be quantified from ASL perfusion weighted image. ADC and FA maps generated from DWI and DTI can be used to assess renal fibrosis. IVIM imaging evaluates true parenchyma diffusion by separate modeling. Renal T1 maps showing clear cortico-medullary differentiation in a healthy volunteer and T2 mapping are promising techniques to evaluate renal microstructure. The BOLD R2* map, ADC map, FA maps and IVIM images were adapted from the articles of Bane et al. [71], Adams et al. [76], and de Boer et al. [77] under Creative Commons licenses.

Renal parenchymal oxygenation is of paramount importance in the pathophysiology of AKI and CKD [78]. Blood oxygen level dependent (BOLD) imaging can demonstrate tissue oxygen level using multi-echo T2*-weighted sequence based on the paramagnetic properties of deoxyhemoglobin. The strong correlation between renal T2* (R2*) and the invasive gold-standard tissue oxygen partial pressure has been validated in rat model [79]. The outer layer of medulla has higher sensitivity to hypoxia than the cortex, which is the physiological basis of the susceptibility to hypoxia injury.

Arterial spin labeling (ASL) assesses tissue perfusion by labeling the water protons in the blood before they enter the tissue of interest, and subtracting the labeled image from a control image without labeling blood water. The signal intensity of the subtracted perfusion-weighted image is proportionate to perfusion. ASL has been widely used to calculate cerebral perfusion in various brain diseases [80]. Renal perfusion quantified by ASL has been validated by comparison with para-aminohippuric-acid clearance, which is the gold standard measurement of renal plasma flow, and with renal scintigraphy, demonstrating reproducible perfusion measurements [81,82]. High interstudy and interrater reproducibility of ASL in the quantification of cortical and medullary renal perfusion has been shown in healthy volunteers [83].

Renal DWI, diffusion tensor imaging (DTI), T1 and T2 mapping have been studied to assess interstitial fibrosis [84]. Renal cortex has higher ADC than medulla in healthy kidneys. As ADC is largely influenced by tubular flow and capillary perfusion, intravoxel incoherent motion (IVIM) is used to measure the true diffusion, alongside the pseudo-diffusion and flow fraction. DTI is a variation to DWI which measures the fractional anisotropy (FA); that is, the percentage of a tissue that displays oriented diffusion axes. Increased ADC and decreased FA can be biomarkers of fibrosis in CKD. Recent studies suggest that renal T1 mapping technique can be used to assess tissue changes in AKI and renal fibrosis in CKD in rat modal [85–87] as well as in human [88], with good reproducibility.

3.2.3. CT and Nuclear Medicine for Renal Imaging

CT and nuclear imaging are the most frequently used modalities after ultrasonography to assess renal morphology and function in clinical settings. However, the utility of renal CT in clinical management of CRS is limited due to radiation and the risk of post-contrast acute kidney injury in patients with impaired renal function (eGFR < 30 mL/min/1.73 m^2). Dual-energy CT might offer opportunities to assess renal parenchyma without contrast agent. Renal nuclear imaging such as renal scintigraphy, SPECT, and PET have been used for quantification of GFR and renal perfusion. However, they are not ideal for frequent assessments due to radiation, thus not suitable for longitudinal surveillance of CRS.

4. Application of Imaging Biomarkers in Acute CRS

4.1. Echocardiographic and CMR Biomarkers for Diagnosis and Prognosis

Echocardiography not only is essential for diagnosing cardiovascular dysfunction in acute CRS, but also provides prognostic biomarkers. In a retrospective study of 30,681 patients, at least one type of CRS was detected in 8% patients, in whom decreased left ventricular ejection fraction, increased pulmonary artery pressure and larger right ventricular diameter derived by TTE were independent risk factors of the development of CRS [9]. This study also found that acute CRS is associated with the worst prognosis in comparison with chronic CRS and no CRS [9]. In a study of 1879 critical ill patients, right ventricular dysfunction assessed by TTE was an important determinant of AKI and AKI-related mortality [89].

CMR has been increasingly used in acute cardiovascular diseases such as acute coronary syndrome and acute myocarditis, facilitating risk stratification with myocardial tissue characterization [90,91]. In the context of acute CRS, one study demonstrated an association between microvascular myocardial injury assessed by contrast-enhanced CMR and increased risk of AKI in patients with ST-elevation myocardial infarction [92]. The value of CMR in the clinical management of acute CRS is yet to be unraveled by further studies.

4.2. Kidney Sonographic Biomarkers for Prognosis

Renal resistive index and intrarenal venous flow pattern evaluated by Doppler imaging have demonstrated potential values in prognosis of acute CRS. Increased resistive index of the renal artery was found to be helpful in predicting AKI in patients after major cardiac surgery (type 1 CRS), and in patients with septic shock or in critical conditions (type 5 CRS) [93–95]. Since the key role of renal venous congestion has been recognized, intrarenal venous flow has attracted increasing interests [96–98]. The patterns of intrarenal venous flow were applied to identify renal hemodynamic disturbances in heart failure [99,100]. The discontinuous patterns of intrarenal venous flow were found to be associated with increased right atrial pressure and had independent prognostic values in patients with non-ischemic heart failure [100]. A case report observed the change of intrarenal venous flow from a monophasic to a biphasic pattern in parallel with improvement in symptoms and renal function [101]. Results of a recent clinical trial suggested that both renal arterial resistive index and intrarenal venous flow might offer guidance on the diagnosis and treatment of type 1 CRS [102].

4.3. Preclinical Kidney MRI Biomarkers of AKI

Multiparametric kidney MRI has been studied to characterize microstructural changes in AKI in recent years. Although the value of MRI biomarkers of AKI in the context of CRS remains to be investigated, there have been studies detecting the pathophysiological alterations in AKI. These techniques may facilitate early identification of AKI, which is one of the most challenging issues in clinical management of acute CRS. It has been well accepted that renal parenchymal hypoperfusion and hypoxia are closely associated with development of all forms of AKI [103]. BOLD technique by MRI has been used to evaluate intrarenal oxygenation in animal models and patients with AKI [104,105]. Renal hypoxia detected by BOLD MRI has been reported in contrast-induced AKI, renal allografts with acute tubular necrosis, sepsis-associated AKI, and other nephrotoxin-induced AKI [105]. Significantly lower perfusion of the renal cortex and medulla detected by ASL has been reported in AKI patents in comparison with healthy volunteers [106]. ASL was studied as an alternative to dynamic contrast-enhanced MRI for quantitative renal perfusion measurements in a rat model of AKI [107]. Moreover, the combination of BOLD and ASL techniques may help to achieve a better characterization of the primary cause of AKI, as the tissue oxygenation assessed by BOLD is significantly influenced by renal perfusion [108]. A study of 15 healthy volunteers demonstrated that ASL is capable of detecting renal hemodynamic change after a single-dose pharmacological intervention with captopril, highlighting the potential of ASL to provide mechanistic insights into the pharmacotherapy of kidney diseases [83]. DWI and T1 mapping techniques are potentially beneficial for the evaluation of AKI in acute CRS. Decreased ADC, alterations in IVIM parameters and diffusion anisotropy demonstrated by DTI have been shown in animal models of AKI [105]. Prolonged renal cortical T1 relaxation time and decreased corticomedullary difference was found in AKI and the cortical T1 values were positively correlated with stages of renal function [109].

5. Application of Imaging Biomarkers in Chronic CRS

5.1. Cardiac Imaging Biomarkers of CKD-Associated Cardiomyopathy

Echocardiography is currently recommended by the Kidney Disease Improving Global Outcomes (KDIGO) guidelines for all patients initiating dialysis, due to the high prevalence of underlying abnormalities among patients with CKD [110]. Characteristic cardiac changes in CKD include left ventricular (LV) hypertrophy, ventricular dilatation, cardiac dysfunction, and myocardial fibrosis [111]. However, TTE has disadvantages in identification and surveillance of LV myocardial mass and volumes in CKD. TTE tends to overestimate LV mass in comparison with CMR, and the wider intra- and inter-operator variability of TTE is disadvantageous for observation of subtle and gradual cardiac changes in CKD [112]. In addition, the impact of kidney transplantation on LV mass has been controversial, suggesting that the interventions to prevent type 4 CRS might need to be moved to earlier phase of CKD [113]. LV global longitudinal strain (GLS) is more sensitive than LV ejection fraction as a marker of subtle LV dysfunction [114–116], and is associated with an increased risk of mortality in predialysis and dialysis patients [117]. Previous studies demonstrated decreased LV-GLS and diastolic strain rates by TTE in CKD patients [114,118–121]. LV diastolic dysfunction can be diagnosed and graded by TTE, based on mitral valve annular e'/e' velocity, average E/e' ratio, left atrium volume index, and peak tricuspid regurgitation velocity [122]. However, our recent study suggests that subclinical changes in myocardial tissue composition may exist even when no systolic or diastolic dysfunction was detected by TTE in patients on peritoneal dialysis [123].

CMR has the unique value of detecting myocardial fibrosis, which was found in more than 90% of patients with CKD in a postmortem study [124]. Increased myocardial native T1 value has been observed in patients with early phase CKD and in end-stage CKD patients when compared with healthy controls [125–128]. Two previous studies revealed higher myocardial T2 values in ESRD patients than those in healthy controls [123,129]. Decreased MR-derived LV global longitudinal strain and circumferential strain were also reported in patients with early CKD and in end-stage CKD patients [123,125–128,130]. Increased native T1 value has been found to be associated with LV global strain [123,125,126]. Most recently, a study of 134 pre-dialysis patients without diabetes or myocardial ischemia showed that native myocardial T1 values and serum biomarkers of myocardial fibrosis increase with advancing CKD stages, independent of left ventricular afterload [51]. These findings suggest that myocardial fibrosis might be a pharmacological target for the treatments in CKD patients, and might improve prognosis by mitigating the effects of CRS.

CAD and myocardial infarction with non-obstructive coronary artery can be involved in both type 2 and type 4 CRS. Coexistence of CAD and CKD and with comorbidities such as diabetes often manifests in these patients as 'silent' ischemic heart disease without typical anginal chest pain. Earlier CMR study with late gadolinium enhancement showed a mixed pattern of subendocardial infarction and diffuse fibrosis in patients with advanced CKD, reflecting the dual myocardial diseases [131]. Considering the increased risk of post-contrast acute kidney injury and nephrogenic systemic fibrosis in patients with severe renal dysfunction, non-contrast imaging techniques are preferred to identify CAD in CRS. The utility of echocardiography, nuclear cardiac imaging, CMR, CT, and hybrid imaging for diagnosis of CAD in patients with CKD has been thoroughly discussed in a most recent literature review [63].

5.2. Preclinical Kidney MRI Biomarkers of CKD with Potential Value in CRS

Kidney imaging has scarcely been studied in the context of chronic CRS, since cardiovascular abnormalities are more related to mortality. However, imaging biomarkers of CKD in general may have potential value in clinical management of chronic CRS, especially in early diagnosis and monitoring disease progression.

Conventional kidney ultrasonography and MRI can hardly identify preclinical renal injury in chronic CRS. Although previous studies suggest that kidney size is associated with glomerular filtration and kidney function reserve [132], the relationship between kidney volume and function is not proportional, since the kidneys have a substantial functional reserve and homeostatic adaptive mechanisms [133]. Functional and tissue characterization MRI techniques may open new possibilities for future studies of chronic CRS. Feasibility of a multiparametric renal MRI protocol—including ASL, T1 mapping, DWI, and BOLD—for patients with CKD has been demonstrated [134]. There have been studies with histological evidences demonstrating that cortical ADC values measured by DWI correlated well with cortical fibrosis and chronic lesions [135–138]. Lower renal perfusion, significant higher cortical and medullary T1 value with reduced cortico-medullary differentiation have been observed in CKD patients compared with healthy volunteers [134,139]. The degree of cortical hypoxia indicated by decreased T2* value in BOLD was correlated with the extent of fibrosis on renal biopsy in one study [136]. However, another study failed to identify significant associations between T2* and eGFR or CKD stage in 342 patients with CKD [140]. A recent prospective study of 112 patients with CKD demonstrates that low cortical oxygenation indicated by BOLD-MRI is an independent predictor of renal function decline over the subsequent three years [141].

Type 5 chronic CRS secondary to diabetes are attracting increased attention these years, in which diabetic nephropathy has been of particular interest. Chronic hypoxia is one of the major contributors of parenchymal fibrosis and CKD in diabetes [142,143]. Lower renal ADC value and higher FA have been reported in early stage of type 2 diabetic nephropathy in comparison with healthy volunteers [144], and ADC value was correlated with urinary and serum biomarkers [145]. Decreased renal perfusion quantified by ASL was seen in patients with diabetes mellitus in comparison with healthy controls, despite normal eGFR and absence of overt albuminuria [146]. A multiparametric MRI study demonstrated significantly lower renal perfusion assessed by ASL in patients with diabetes and stage 3 CKD, and lower perfusion with lower response to furosemide in patients with progressive CKD [147].

6. Opportunities for Comprehensive Imaging Assessment of Heart and Kidneys in Future Studies

Ultrasonography remains the most versatile, accessible, and cost-effective modality for the assessment of CRS. MRI, on the other hand, is the most promising one-stop modality for the structural and functional evaluation of both heart and kidneys. Future studies aiming at finding novel biomarkers for CRS may incorporate serial ultrasonography or non-contrast MRI scans for simultaneous evaluation of heart and kidneys in their study design.

In the context of acute CRS, a combination of TTE and renal sonography can be used to assess the heart and kidneys synchronously. The evaluation of right-sided congestion and intra-renal blood flow by Doppler imaging might offer incremental diagnostic and prognostic value together with circulatory and urinary biomarkers. Quantification of global ventricular strain may have the potential of early identification of cardiac dysfunction in type 3 CRS.

The unique role of MRI in assessment of interstitial fibrosis in both the organs might complement the use of molecular biomarkers and provide new insights in the diagnosis and treatment of CRS in the future. For institutions with well-developed infrastructures for multiparametric MRI, a combined non-contrast protocol assessing the heart and kidneys in a single scan session could be considered in future studies for patients at risk of or with CRS. Myocardial T1 mapping and T2 mapping together with renal T1 mapping and DWI can provide information on the extent of fibrosis in heart and kidneys [148], which is postulated to be the key driver of chronic CRS. ASL and BOLD can reflect tissue perfusion and oxygenation in the kidneys, offering opportunities to detect preclinical hemodynamic alterations. Myocardial strain derived from CMR cine images can be used to identify early impairment of cardiac function in type 2 and type 4 CRS. With consistent scan parameters and the absence of ionizing radiation or contrast agents, non-contrast MRI is the ideal modality for longitudinal tracking of pathophysiological changes in CRS, as well as for monitoring of therapeutic response without excessive biopsies.

7. Summary

Despite endeavors to improve clinical outcome over the past decade, hospitalization rate, symptom burden, and mortality in patients with dual burden of heart and kidney diseases are still high [8]. Meanwhile the practical need for better prevention and management of CRS is imminent. CRS is a growing health, economical and societal problem as the fast increasing number of aging population lead to higher prevalence of heart and kidney diseases. Due to the multiple interconnected pathophysiological mechanisms of CRS, it is conceivable that biomarkers or interventions targeting single mechanisms are inadequate. Multi-modality and multiparametric imaging techniques have been applied for cardiovascular diseases and kidney diseases and offer opportunities for the evaluation of CRS. A consecutive and synchronous imaging strategy tracing the natural history of CRS can be encouraging for future directions. We propose a multidisciplinary approach involving cardiologists, nephrologists, and radiologists to improve the prospect of research studies and clinical management of cardiorenal syndrome in the future.

Author Contributions: Conceptualization, L.L. and H.J.L.; Writing—original draft preparation, L.L.; Writing—review and editing, I.A.D., X.Z., and H.J.L.; Supervision, X.Z.; Project administration, H.J.L. All authors have read and agreed to the published version of the manuscript.

Funding: This research received no external funding.

Institutional Review Board Statement: Not applicable.

Informed Consent Statement: Not applicable.

Conflicts of Interest: The authors declare no conflict of interest.

References

1. Ronco, C.; McCullough, P.; Anker, S.D.; Anand, I.; Aspromonte, N.; Bagshaw, S.M.; Bellomo, R.; Berl, T.; Bobek, I.; Cruz, D.N.; et al. Cardio-renal syndromes: Report from the consensus conference of the acute dialysis quality initiative. *Eur. Heart J.* 2010, *31*, 703–711. [CrossRef]
2. Bagshaw, S.M.; Cruz, D.N.; Aspromonte, N.; Daliento, L.; Ronco, F.; Sheinfeld, G.; Anker, S.D.; Anand, I.; Bellomo, R.; Berl, T.; et al. Epidemiology of cardio-renal syndromes: Workgroup statements from the 7th ADQI Consensus Conference. *Nephrol. Dial. Transplant.* 2010, *25*, 1406–1416. [CrossRef]
3. Ismail, Y.; Kasmikha, Z.; Green, H.L.; McCullough, P.A. Cardio-renal syndrome type 1: Epidemiology, pathophysiology, and treatment. *Semin. Nephrol.* 2012, *32*, 18–25. [CrossRef]
4. Deferrari, G.; Cipriani, A.; La Porta, E. Renal dysfunction in cardiovascular diseases and its consequences. *J. Nephrol.* 2020. [CrossRef] [PubMed]
5. Jois, P.; Mebazaa, A. Cardio-renal syndrome type 2: Epidemiology, pathophysiology, and treatment. *Semin. Nephrol.* 2012, *32*, 26–30. [CrossRef]
6. Shastri, S.; Sarnak, M.J. Cardiovascular disease and CKD: Core curriculum. *Am. J. Kidney Dis.* 2010, *56*, 399–417. [CrossRef] [PubMed]
7. Soni, S.S.; Ronco, C.; Pophale, R.; Bhansali, A.S.; Nagarik, A.P.; Barnela, S.R.; Saboo, S.S.; Raman, A. Cardio-renal syndrome type 5: Epidemiology, pathophysiology, and treatment. *Semin. Nephrol.* 2012, *32*, 49–56. [CrossRef] [PubMed]
8. Rangaswami, J.; Bhalla, V.; Blair, J.E.A.; Chang, T.I.; Costa, S.; Lentine, K.L.; Lerma, E.V.; Mezue, K.; Molitch, M.; Mullens, W.; et al. Cardiorenal Syndrome: Classification, Pathophysiology, Diagnosis, and Treatment Strategies: A Scientific Statement From the American Heart Association. *Circulation* 2019, *139*, e840–e878. [CrossRef]
9. Mavrakanas, T.A.; Khattak, A.; Singh, K.; Charytan, D.M. Epidemiology and Natural History of the Cardiorenal Syndromes in a Cohort with Echocardiography. *Clin. J. Am. Soc. Nephrol.* 2017, *12*, 1624–1633. [CrossRef]
10. Heywood, J.T.; Fonarow, G.C.; Costanzo, M.R.; Mathur, V.S.; Wigneswaran, J.R.; Wynne, J.; ADHERE Scientific Advisory Committee and Investigators. High prevalence of renal dysfunction and its impact on outcome in 118,465 patients hospitalized with acute decompensated heart failure: A report from the ADHERE database. *J. Card Fail.* 2007, *13*, 422–430. [CrossRef]
11. Campbell, R.C.; Sui, X.; Filippatos, G.; Love, T.E.; Wahle, C.; Sanders, P.W.; Ahmed, A. Association of chronic kidney disease with outcomes in chronic heart failure: A propensity-matched study. *Nephrol. Dial. Transplant.* 2009, *24*, 186–193. [CrossRef]
12. Hatamizadeh, P.; Fonarow, G.C.; Budoff, M.J.; Darabian, S.; Kovesdy, C.P.; Kalantar-Zadeh, K. Cardiorenal syndrome: Pathophysiology and potential targets for clinical management. *Nat. Rev. Nephrol.* 2013, *9*, 99–111. [CrossRef]
13. Schrier, R.W.; Abraham, W.T. Hormones and hemodynamics in heart failure. *N. Engl. J. Med.* 1999, *341*, 577–585. [CrossRef]
14. Rosner, M.H.; Ronco, C.; Okusa, M.D. The role of inflammation in the cardio-renal syndrome: A focus on cytokines and inflammatory mediators. *Semin. Nephrol.* 2012, *32*, 70–78. [CrossRef] [PubMed]
15. Schefold, J.C.; Filippatos, G.; Hasenfuss, G.; Anker, S.D.; von Haehling, S. Heart failure and kidney dysfunction: Epidemiology, mechanisms and management. *Nat. Rev. Nephrol.* 2016, *12*, 610–623. [CrossRef]
16. Bongartz, L.G.; Cramer, M.J.; Doevendans, P.A.; Joles, J.A.; Braam, B. The severe cardiorenal syndrome:'Guyton revisited'. *Eur. Heart J.* 2005, *26*, 11–17. [CrossRef] [PubMed]
17. Haase, M.; Mueller, C.; Damman, K.; Murray, P.T.; Kellum, J.A.; Ronco, C.; McCullough, P.A.; Acute Dialysis Quality Initiative. Pathogenesis of cardiorenal syndrome type 1 in acute decompensated heart failure: Workgroup statements from the eleventh consensus conference of the Acute Dialysis Quality Initiative (ADQI). In *ADQI Consensus on AKI Biomarkers and Cardiorenal Syndromes*; Karger Publishers: Basel, Switzerland, 2013; Volume 182, pp. 99–116.
18. Zannad, F.; Rossignol, P. Cardiorenal Syndrome Revisited. *Circulation* 2018, *138*, 929–944. [CrossRef]
19. Tabucanon, T.; Tang, W.H.W. Right Heart Failure and Cardiorenal Syndrome. *Cardiol. Clin.* 2020, *38*, 185–202. [CrossRef] [PubMed]
20. Jentzer, J.C.; Bihorac, A.; Brusca, S.B.; Del Rio-Pertuz, G.; Kashani, K.; Kazory, A.; Kellum, J.A.; Mao, M.; Moriyama, B.; Morrow, D.A.; et al. Contemporary Management of Severe Acute Kidney Injury and Refractory Cardiorenal Syndrome: JACC Council Perspectives. *J. Am. Coll. Cardiol.* 2020, *76*, 1084–1101. [CrossRef]
21. Chuasuwan, A.; Kellum, J.A. Cardio-renal syndrome type 3: Epidemiology, pathophysiology, and treatment. *Semin. Nephrol.* 2012, *32*, 31–39. [CrossRef]
22. Yogasundaram, H.; Chappell, M.C.; Braam, B.; Oudit, G.Y. Cardiorenal Syndrome and Heart Failure-Challenges and Opportunities. *Can. J. Cardiol.* 2019, *35*, 1208–1219. [CrossRef] [PubMed]
23. Hostetter, T.H.; Ibrahim, H.N. Aldosterone in chronic kidney and cardiac disease. *J. Am. Soc. Nephrol.* 2003, *14*, 2395–2401. [CrossRef]
24. Giam, B.; Kaye, D.M.; Rajapakse, N.W. Role of renal oxidative stress in the pathogenesis of the cardiorenal syndrome. *Heart Lung Circ.* 2016, *25*, 874–880. [CrossRef]
25. Hedayat, M.; Mahmoudi, M.J.; Rose, N.R.; Rezaei, N. Proinflammatory cytokines in heart failure: Double-edged swords. *Heart Fail. Rev.* 2010, *15*, 543–562. [CrossRef] [PubMed]
26. Rockey, D.C.; Bell, P.D.; Hill, J.A. Fibrosis—A common pathway to organ injury and failure. *N. Engl. J. Med.* 2015, *372*, 1138–1149. [CrossRef]

27. Travers, J.G.; Kamal, F.A.; Robbins, J.; Yutzey, K.E.; Blaxall, B.C. Cardiac Fibrosis: The Fibroblast Awakens. *Circ. Res.* **2016**, *118*, 1021–1040. [CrossRef]
28. Kellum, J.A.; Lameire, N.; Aspelin, P.; Barsoum, R.S.; Burdmann, E.A.; Goldstein, S.L.; Herzog, C.A.; Joannidis, M.; Kribben, A.; Levey, A.S. Kidney disease: Improving global outcomes (KDIGO) acute kidney injury work group. KDIGO clinical practice guideline for acute kidney injury. *Kidney Int. Suppl.* **2012**, *2*, 1–138.
29. Coca, S.; Yalavarthy, R.; Concato, J.; Parikh, C.R. Biomarkers for the diagnosis and risk stratification of acute kidney injury: A systematic review. *Kidney Int.* **2008**, *73*, 1008–1016. [CrossRef] [PubMed]
30. Damman, K.; Tang, W.W.; Testani, J.M.; McMurray, J.J. Terminology and definition of changes renal function in heart failure. *Eur. Heart J.* **2014**, *35*, 3413–3416. [CrossRef]
31. Ikizler, T.A.; Parikh, C.R.; Himmelfarb, J.; Chinchilli, V.M.; Liu, K.D.; Coca, S.G.; Garg, A.X.; Hsu, C.Y.; Siew, E.D.; Wurfel, M.M.; et al. A prospective cohort study that examined acute kidney injury and kidney outcomes, cardiovascular events and death informs on long-term clinical outcomes. *Kidney Int.* **2020**. [CrossRef]
32. House, A.A. Cardio-renal syndrome type 4: Epidemiology, pathophysiology and treatment. *Semin. Nephrol.* **2012**, *32*, 40–48. [CrossRef] [PubMed]
33. Edwards, N.C.; Moody, W.E.; Chue, C.D.; Ferro, C.J.; Townend, J.N.; Steeds, R.P. Defining the natural history of uremic cardiomyopathy in chronic kidney disease: The role of cardiovascular magnetic resonance. *JACC* **2014**, *7*, 703–714. [PubMed]
34. Consortium, C.K.D.P. Association of estimated glomerular filtration rate and albuminuria with all-cause and cardiovascular mortality in general population cohorts: A collaborative meta-analysis. *Lancet* **2010**, *375*, 2073–2081.
35. Baigent, C.; Landray, M.J.; Reith, C.; Emberson, J.; Wheeler, D.C.; Tomson, C.; Wanner, C.; Krane, V.; Cass, A.; Craig, J. The effects of lowering LDL cholesterol with simvastatin plus ezetimibe in patients with chronic kidney disease (Study of Heart and Renal Protection): A randomised placebo-controlled trial. *Lancet* **2011**, *377*, 2181–2192. [CrossRef]
36. Sosnov, J.; Lessard, D.; Goldberg, R.J.; Yarzebski, J.; Gore, J.M. Differential symptoms of acute myocardial infarction in patients with kidney disease: A community-wide perspective. *Am. J. Kidney Dis.* **2006**, *47*, 378–384. [CrossRef] [PubMed]
37. Gentile, G.; Remuzzi, G. Novel Biomarkers for Renal Diseases? None for the Moment (but One). *J. Biomol. Screen.* **2016**, *21*, 655–670. [CrossRef]
38. Ponikowski, P.; Voors, A.A.; Anker, S.D.; Bueno, H.; Cleland, J.G.; Coats, A.J.; Falk, V.; Gonzalez-Juanatey, J.R.; Harjola, V.-P.; Jankowska, E.A. 2016 ESC Guidelines for the diagnosis and treatment of acute and chronic heart failure: The Task Force for the diagnosis and treatment of acute and chronic heart failure of the European Society of Cardiology (ESC) Developed with the special contribution of the Heart Failure Association (HFA) of the ESC. *Eur. Heart J.* **2016**, *37*, 2129–2200.
39. Mitchell, C.; Rahko, P.S.; Blauwet, L.A.; Canaday, B.; Finstuen, J.A.; Foster, M.C.; Horton, K.; Ogunyankin, K.O.; Palma, R.A.; Velazquez, E.J. Guidelines for performing a comprehensive transthoracic echocardiographic examination in adults: Recommendations from the American Society of Echocardiography. *J. Am. Soc. Echocardiogr.* **2019**, *32*, 1–64. [CrossRef]
40. Pellicori, P.; Kallvikbacka-Bennett, A.; Khaleva, O.; Carubelli, V.; Costanzo, P.; Castiello, T.; Wong, K.; Zhang, J.; Cleland, J.G.; Clark, A.L. Global longitudinal strain in patients with suspected heart failure and a normal ejection fraction: Does it improve diagnosis and risk stratification? *Int. J. Cardiovasc. Imaging* **2014**, *30*, 69–79. [CrossRef]
41. Porter, T.R.; Mulvagh, S.L.; Abdelmoneim, S.S.; Becher, H.; Belcik, J.T.; Bierig, M.; Choy, J.; Gaibazzi, N.; Gillam, L.D.; Janardhanan, R. Clinical applications of ultrasonic enhancing agents in echocardiography: 2018 American Society of Echocardiography guidelines update. *J. Am. Soc. Echocardiogr.* **2018**, *31*, 241–274. [CrossRef]
42. Von Knobelsdorff-Brenkenhoff, F.; Schulz-Menger, J. Role of cardiovascular magnetic resonance in the guidelines of the European Society of Cardiology. *J. Cardiovasc. Magn. Reson.* **2015**, *18*, 6. [CrossRef]
43. Leiner, T.; Bogaert, J.; Friedrich, M.G.; Mohiaddin, R.; Muthurangu, V.; Myerson, S.; Powell, A.J.; Raman, S.V.; Pennell, D.J. SCMR Position Paper (2020) on clinical indications for cardiovascular magnetic resonance. *J. Cardiovasc. Magn. Reson.* **2020**, *22*. [CrossRef]
44. MEMBERS, W.C.; Hundley, W.G.; Bluemke, D.A.; Finn, J.P.; Flamm, S.D.; Fogel, M.A.; Friedrich, M.G.; Ho, V.B.; Jerosch-Herold, M.; Kramer, C.M. ACCF/ACR/AHA/NASCI/SCMR 2010 expert consensus document on cardiovascular magnetic resonance: A report of the American College of Cardiology Foundation Task Force on Expert Consensus Documents. *Circulation* **2010**, *121*, 2462–2508. [CrossRef] [PubMed]
45. Voigt, J.-U.; Cvijic, M. 2-and 3-dimensional myocardial strain in cardiac health and disease. *JACC* **2019**, *12*, 1849–1863. [CrossRef] [PubMed]
46. Kim, R.J.; Albert, T.S.; Wible, J.H.; Elliott, M.D.; Allen, J.C.; Lee, J.C.; Parker, M.; Napoli, A.; Judd, R.M. Performance of delayed-enhancement magnetic resonance imaging with gadoversetamide contrast for the detection and assessment of myocardial infarction: An international, multicenter, double-blinded, randomized trial. *Circulation* **2008**, *117*, 629. [CrossRef]
47. Haaf, P.; Garg, P.; Messroghli, D.R.; Broadbent, D.A.; Greenwood, J.P.; Plein, S. Cardiac T1 mapping and extracellular volume (ECV) in clinical practice: A comprehensive review. *J. Cardiovasc. Magn. Reson.* **2017**, *18*, 89. [CrossRef]
48. Dekkers, I.A.; Roos, R.; van der Molen, A.J. Gadolinium retention after administration of contrast agents based on linear chelators and the recommendations of the European Medicines Agency. *Eur. Radiol.* **2018**, *28*, 1579–1584. [CrossRef]
49. Perazella, M.A. Gadolinium-contrast toxicity in patients with kidney disease: Nephrotoxicity and nephrogenic systemic fibrosis. *Curr. Drug Saf.* **2008**, *3*, 67–75. [CrossRef]

50. Mewton, N.; Liu, C.Y.; Croisille, P.; Bluemke, D.; Lima, J.A. Assessment of myocardial fibrosis with cardiovascular magnetic resonance. *J. Am. Coll. Cardiol.* **2011**, *57*, 891–903. [CrossRef] [PubMed]
51. Hayer, M.K.; Radhakrishnan, A.; Price, A.M.; Liu, B.; Baig, S.; Weston, C.J.; Biasiolli, L.; Ferro, C.J.; Townend, J.N.; Steeds, R.P.; et al. Defining Myocardial Abnormalities Across the Stages of Chronic Kidney Disease: A Cardiac Magnetic Resonance Imaging Study. *JACC* **2020**. [CrossRef]
52. Nguyen, C.; Lu, M.; Fan, Z.; Bi, X.; Kellman, P.; Zhao, S.; Li, D. Contrast-free detection of myocardial fibrosis in hypertrophic cardiomyopathy patients with diffusion-weighted cardiovascular magnetic resonance. *J. Cardiovasc. Magn. Reson.* **2015**, *17*, 107. [CrossRef] [PubMed]
53. Ferreira, P.F.; Kilner, P.J.; McGill, L.-A.; Nielles-Vallespin, S.; Scott, A.D.; Ho, S.Y.; McCarthy, K.P.; Haba, M.M.; Ismail, T.F.; Gatehouse, P.D. In vivo cardiovascular magnetic resonance diffusion tensor imaging shows evidence of abnormal myocardial laminar orientations and mobility in hypertrophic cardiomyopathy. *J. Cardiovasc. Magn. Reson.* **2014**, *16*, 87. [CrossRef]
54. Tseng, W.Y.I.; Dou, J.; Reese, T.G.; Wedeen, V.J. Imaging myocardial fiber disarray and intramural strain hypokinesis in hypertrophic cardiomyopathy with MRI. *J. Magn. Reson. Imaging* **2006**, *23*, 1–8. [CrossRef]
55. Coenen, A.; Rossi, A.; Lubbers, M.M.; Kurata, A.; Kono, A.K.; Chelu, R.G.; Segreto, S.; Dijkshoorn, M.L.; Wragg, A.; van Geuns, R.-J.M. Integrating CT myocardial perfusion and CT-FFR in the work-up of coronary artery disease. *JACC* **2017**, *10*, 760–770. [CrossRef]
56. Al-Mallah, M.H.; Ahmed, A.M. Controversies in the Use of Fractional Flow Reserve Form Computed Tomography (FFR CT) vs. Coronary Angiography. *Curr. Cardiovasc. Imaging Rep.* **2016**, *9*, 34. [CrossRef]
57. Scully, P.R.; Bastarrika, G.; Moon, J.C.; Treibel, T.A. Myocardial Extracellular Volume Quantification by Cardiovascular Magnetic Resonance and Computed Tomography. *Curr. Cardiol. Rep.* **2018**, *20*, 15. [CrossRef]
58. Stenner, P.; Schmidt, B.; Allmendinger, T.; Flohr, T.; Kachelrie, M. Dynamic iterative beam hardening correction (DIBHC) in myocardial perfusion imaging using contrast-enhanced computed tomography. *Investig. Radiol.* **2010**, *45*, 314–323. [CrossRef]
59. Stenner, P.; Schmidt, B.; Bruder, H.; Allmendinger, T.; Haberland, U.; Flohr, T.; Kachelrieß, M. Partial scan artifact reduction (PSAR) for the assessment of cardiac perfusion in dynamic phase-correlated CT. *Med. Phys.* **2009**, *36*, 5683–5694. [CrossRef]
60. Kitagawa, K.; George, R.T.; Arbab-Zadeh, A.; Lima, J.A.; Lardo, A.C. Characterization and correction of beam-hardening artifacts during dynamic volume CT assessment of myocardial perfusion. *Radiology* **2010**, *256*, 111–118. [CrossRef] [PubMed]
61. Van der Molen, A.J.; Reimer, P.; Dekkers, I.A.; Bongartz, G.; Bellin, M.-F.; Bertolotto, M.; Clement, O.; Heinz-Peer, G.; Stacul, F.; Webb, J.A. Post-contrast acute kidney injury–part 1: Definition, clinical features, incidence, role of contrast medium and risk factors. *Eur. Radiol.* **2018**, *28*, 2845–2855. [CrossRef]
62. Cremer, P.; Hachamovitch, R.; Tamarappoo, B. Clinical decision making with myocardial perfusion imaging in patients with known or suspected coronary artery disease. *Semin. Nucl. Med.* **2014**, *44*, 320–329.
63. Dilsizian, V.; Gewirtz, H.; Marwick, T.H.; Kwong, R.Y.; Raggi, P.; Al-Mallah, M.H.; Herzog, C.A. Cardiac Imaging for Coronary Heart Disease Risk Stratification in Chronic Kidney Disease. *JACC* **2020**. [CrossRef]
64. Dilsizian, V.; Bacharach, S.L.; Beanlands, R.S.; Bergmann, S.R.; Delbeke, D.; Dorbala, S.; Gropler, R.J.; Knuuti, J.; Schelbert, H.R.; Travin, M.I. ASNC imaging guidelines/SNMMI procedure standard for positron emission tomography (PET) nuclear cardiology procedures. *J. Nucl. Cardiol.* **2016**, *23*, 1187–1226. [CrossRef]
65. Dewey, M.; Siebes, M.; Kachelrieß, M.; Kofoed, K.F.; Maurovich-Horvat, P.; Nikolaou, K.; Bai, W.; Kofler, A.; Manka, R.; Kozerke, S. Clinical quantitative cardiac imaging for the assessment of myocardial ischaemia. *Nat. Rev. Cardiol.* **2020**, *17*, 427–450. [CrossRef]
66. Grenier, N.; Merville, P.; Combe, C. Radiologic imaging of the renal parenchyma structure and function. *Nat. Rev. Nephrol.* **2016**, *12*, 348–359. [CrossRef]
67. Faubel, S.; Patel, N.U.; Lockhart, M.E.; Cadnapaphornchai, M.A. Renal relevant radiology: Use of ultrasonography in patients with AKI. *Clin. J. Am. Soc. Nephrol.* **2014**, *9*, 382–394. [CrossRef]
68. Hull, T.D.; Agarwal, A.; Hoyt, K. New Ultrasound Techniques Promise Further Advances in AKI and CKD. *J. Am. Soc. Nephrol.* **2017**, *28*, 3452–3460. [CrossRef]
69. Mahoney, M.; Sorace, A.; Warram, J.; Samuel, S.; Hoyt, K. Volumetric Contrast-Enhanced Ultrasound Imaging of Renal Perfusion. *J. Ultrasound Med.* **2014**, *33*, 1427–1437. [CrossRef]
70. US Food and Drug Administration. Qualification of Biomarker—Total Kidney Volume in Studies for Treatment of Autosomal Dominant Polycystic Kidney Disease. 2015. Available online: https://www.fda.gov/media/93105/download (accessed on 1 July 2021).
71. Bane, O.; Mendichovszky, I.A.; Milani, B.; Dekkers, I.A.; Deux, J.-F.; Eckerbom, P.; Grenier, N.; Hall, M.E.; Inoue, T.; Laustsen, C. Consensus-based technical recommendations for clinical translation of renal BOLD MRI. *Magn. Reson. Mater. Phys. Biol. Med.* **2020**, *33*, 199–215. [CrossRef]
72. Semple, S.I.; Dekkers, I.A.; de Boer, A.; Sharma, K.; Cox, E.F.; Lamb, H.J.; Buckley, D.L.; Bane, O.; Morris, D.M.; Prasad, P.V. Consensus-based technical recommendations for clinical translation of renal T1 and T2 mapping MRI. *Magn. Reson. Mater. Phys. Biol. Med.* **2020**, *33*, 163–176.
73. Ljimani, A.; Caroli, A.; Laustsen, C.; Francis, S.; Mendichovszky, I.A.; Bane, O.; Nery, F.; Sharma, K.; Pohlmann, A.; Dekkers, I.A. Consensus-based technical recommendations for clinical translation of renal diffusion-weighted MRI. *Magn. Reson. Mater. Phys. Biol. Med.* **2020**, *33*, 177–195. [CrossRef] [PubMed]

74. Mendichovszky, I.; Pullens, P.; Dekkers, I.; Nery, F.; Bane, O.; Pohlmann, A.; de Boer, A.; Ljimani, A.; Odudu, A.; Buchanan, C. Technical recommendations for clinical translation of renal MRI: A consensus project of the Cooperation in Science and Technology Action PARENCHIMA. *Magn. Reson. Mater. Phys. Biol. Med.* **2020**, *33*, 131–140. [CrossRef]
75. De Boer, A.; Villa, G.; Bane, O.; Bock, M.; Cox, E.F.; Dekkers, I.A.; Eckerbom, P.; Fernández-Seara, M.A.; Francis, S.T.; Haddock, B. Consensus-based technical recommendations for clinical translation of renal phase contrast MRI. *J. Magn. Reson. Imaging* **2020** [CrossRef]
76. Adams, L.C.; Bressem, K.K.; Scheibl, S.; Nunninger, M.; Gentsch, A.; Fahlenkamp, U.L.; Eckardt, K.U.; Hamm, B.; Makowski, M.R. Multiparametric Assessment of Changes in Renal Tissue after Kidney Transplantation with Quantitative MR Relaxometry and Diffusion-Tensor Imaging at 3 T. *J. Clin. Med.* **2020**, *9*, 1551. [CrossRef]
77. De Boer, A.; Harteveld, A.A.; Stemkens, B.; Blankestijn, P.J.; Bos, C.; Franklin, S.L.; Froeling, M.; Joles, J.A.; Verhaar, M.C.; van den Berg, N.; et al. Multiparametric Renal MRI: An Intrasubject Test–Retest Repeatability Study. *J. Magn. Reson. Imaging* **2021**, *53*, 859–873. [CrossRef] [PubMed]
78. Haase, V.H. Mechanisms of hypoxia responses in renal tissue. *J. Am. Soc. Nephrol.* **2013**, *24*, 537–541. [CrossRef] [PubMed]
79. Pohlmann, A.; Arakelyan, K.; Hentschel, J.; Cantow, K.; Flemming, B.; Ladwig, M.; Waiczies, S.; Seeliger, E.; Niendorf, T. Detailing the relation between renal T2* and renal tissue pO2 using an integrated approach of parametric magnetic resonance imaging and invasive physiological measurements. *Investig. Radiol.* **2014**, *49*, 547–560. [CrossRef] [PubMed]
80. Detre, J.A.; Rao, H.; Wang, D.J.; Chen, Y.F.; Wang, Z. Applications of arterial spin labeled MRI in the brain. *J. Magn. Reson. Imaging* **2012**, *35*, 1026–1037. [CrossRef] [PubMed]
81. Ritt, M.; Janka, R.; Schneider, M.P.; Martirosian, P.; Hornegger, J.; Bautz, W.; Uder, M.; Schmieder, R.E. Measurement of kidney perfusion by magnetic resonance imaging: Comparison of MRI with arterial spin labeling to para-aminohippuric acid plasma clearance in male subjects with metabolic syndrome. *Nephrol. Dial. Transplant.* **2010**, *25*, 1126–1133. [CrossRef]
82. Michaely, H.J.; Schoenberg, S.O.; Ittrich, C.; Dikow, R.; Bock, M.; Guenther, M. Renal disease: Value of functional magnetic resonance imaging with flow and perfusion measurements. *Investig. Radiol.* **2004**, *39*, 698–705. [CrossRef]
83. Getzin, T.; May, M.; Schmidbauer, M.; Gutberlet, M.; Martirosian, P.; Oertel, R.; Wacker, F.; Schindler, C.; Hueper, K. Usability of Functional MRI in Clinical Studies for Fast and Reliable Assessment of Renal Perfusion and Quantification of Hemodynamic Effects on the Kidney. *J. Clin. Pharm.* **2018**, *58*, 466–473. [CrossRef]
84. Jiang, K.; Ferguson, C.M.; Lerman, L.O. Noninvasive assessment of renal fibrosis by magnetic resonance imaging and ultrasound techniques. *Transl Res.* **2019**, *209*, 105–120. [CrossRef]
85. Hueper, K.; Peperhove, M.; Rong, S.; Gerstenberg, J.; Mengel, M.; Meier, M.; Gutberlet, M.; Tewes, S.; Barrmeyer, A.; Chen, R. T1-mapping for assessment of ischemia-induced acute kidney injury and prediction of chronic kidney disease in mice. *Eur. Radiol.* **2014**, *24*, 2252–2260. [CrossRef]
86. Hueper, K.; Hensen, B.; Gutberlet, M.; Chen, R.; Hartung, D.; Barrmeyer, A.; Meier, M.; Li, W.; Jang, M.-S.; Mengel, M. Kidney transplantation: Multiparametric functional magnetic resonance imaging for assessment of renal allograft pathophysiology in mice. *Investig. Radiol.* **2016**, *51*, 58–65. [CrossRef] [PubMed]
87. Tewes, S.; Gueler, F.; Chen, R.; Gutberlet, M.; Jang, M.-S.; Meier, M.; Mengel, M.; Hartung, D.; Wacker, F.; Rong, S. Functional MRI for characterization of renal perfusion impairment and edema formation due to acute kidney injury in different mouse strains. *PLoS ONE* **2017**, *12*, e0173248. [CrossRef] [PubMed]
88. Dekkers, I.A.; Paiman, E.H.M.; de Vries, A.P.J.; Lamb, H.J. Reproducibility of native T1 mapping for renal tissue characterization at 3T. *J. Magn. Reson. Imaging* **2019**, *49*, 588–596. [CrossRef] [PubMed]
89. Chen, C.; Lee, J.; Johnson, A.E.; Mark, R.G.; Celi, L.A.; Danziger, J.J.K.i.r. Right ventricular function, peripheral edema, and acute kidney injury in critical illness. *Kidney Int. Rep.* **2017**, *2*, 1059–1065. [CrossRef]
90. Saremi, F. Cardiac MR Imaging in Acute Coronary Syndrome: Application and Image Interpretation. *Radiology* **2017**, *282*, 17–32. [CrossRef]
91. Blissett, S.; Chocron, Y.; Kovacina, B.; Afilalo, J. Diagnostic and prognostic value of cardiac magnetic resonance in acute myocarditis: A systematic review and meta-analysis. *Int. J. Cardiovasc. Imaging* **2019**, *35*, 2221–2229. [CrossRef]
92. Reinstadler, S.J.; Kronbichler, A.; Reindl, M.; Feistritzer, H.-J.; Innerhofer, V.; Mayr, A.; Klug, G.; Tiefenthaler, M.; Mayer, G.; Metzler, B. Acute kidney injury is associated with microvascular myocardial damage following myocardial infarction. *Kidney Int.* **2017**, *92*, 743–750. [CrossRef]
93. Bossard, G.; Bourgoin, P.; Corbeau, J.; Huntzinger, J.; Beydon, L. Early detection of postoperative acute kidney injury by Doppler renal resistive index in cardiac surgery with cardiopulmonary bypass. *Br. J. Anaesth.* **2011**, *107*, 891–898. [CrossRef] [PubMed]
94. Lerolle, N.; Guérot, E.; Faisy, C.; Bornstain, C.; Diehl, J.L.; Fagon, J.Y. Renal failure in septic shock: Predictive value of Doppler-based renal arterial resistive index. *Intensive Care Med.* **2006**, *32*, 1553–1559. [CrossRef]
95. Schnell, D.; Deruddre, S.; Harrois, A.; Pottecher, J.; Cosson, C.; Adoui, N.; Benhamou, D.; Vicaut, E.; Azoulay, E.; Duranteau, J. Renal resistive index better predicts the occurrence of acute kidney injury than cystatin C. *Shock* **2012**, *38*, 592–597. [CrossRef]
96. Tang, W.W.; Kitai, T. Intrarenal venous flow: A window into the congestive kidney failure phenotype of heart failure? *JACC* **2016**, *4*, 683–686.
97. Jeong, S.H.; Jung, D.C.; Kim, S.H.; Kim, S.H. Renal venous doppler ultrasonography in normal subjects and patients with diabetic nephropathy: Value of venous impedance index measurements. *J. Clin. Ultrasound* **2011**, *39*, 512–518. [CrossRef]

98. Beaubien-Souligny, W.; Benkreira, A.; Robillard, P.; Bouabdallaoui, N.; Chassé, M.; Desjardins, G.; Lamarche, Y.; White, M.; Bouchard, J.; Denault, A.J. Alterations in portal vein flow and intrarenal venous flow are associated with acute kidney injury after cardiac surgery: A prospective observational cohort study. *J. Am. Heart Assoc.* **2018**, *7*, e009961. [CrossRef] [PubMed]
99. Nijst, P.; Martens, P.; Dupont, M.; Tang, W.W.; Mullens, W. Intrarenal flow alterations during transition from euvolemia to intravascular volume expansion in heart failure patients. *JACC* **2017**, *5*, 672–681. [CrossRef]
100. Iida, N.; Seo, Y.; Sai, S.; Machino-Ohtsuka, T.; Yamamoto, M.; Ishizu, T.; Kawakami, Y.; Aonuma, K. Clinical implications of intrarenal hemodynamic evaluation by Doppler ultrasonography in heart failure. *JACC* **2016**, *4*, 674–682. [CrossRef] [PubMed]
101. De la Espriella-Juan, R.; Nunez, E.; Minana, G.; Sanchis, J.; Bayes-Genis, A.; Gonzalez, J.; Chorro, J.; Nunez, J. Intrarenal venous flow in cardiorenal syndrome: A shining light into the darkness. *ESC Heart Fail.* **2018**, *5*, 1173–1175. [CrossRef] [PubMed]
102. Cakal, B.; Ozcan, O.U.; Omaygenc, M.O.; Karaca, I.O.; Kizilirmak, F.; Gunes, H.M.; Boztosun, B. Value of Renal Vascular Doppler Sonography in Cardiorenal Syndrome Type 1. *J. Ultrasound Med.* **2020**. [CrossRef]
103. Singh, P.; Ricksten, S.E.; Bragadottir, G.; Redfors, B.; Nordquist, L. Renal oxygenation and haemodynamics in acute kidney injury and chronic kidney disease. *Clin. Exp. Pharm. Physiol.* **2013**, *40*, 138–147. [CrossRef] [PubMed]
104. Neugarten, J. Renal BOLD-MRI and assessment for renal hypoxia. *Kidney Int.* **2012**, *81*, 613–614. [CrossRef] [PubMed]
105. Zhou, H.Y.; Chen, T.W.; Zhang, X.M. Functional Magnetic Resonance Imaging in Acute Kidney Injury: Present Status. *Biomed. Res. Int.* **2016**, *2016*, 2027370. [CrossRef] [PubMed]
106. Dong, J.; Yang, L.; Su, T.; Yang, X.; Chen, B.; Zhang, J.; Wang, X.; Jiang, X. Quantitative assessment of acute kidney injury by noninvasive arterial spin labeling perfusion MRI: A pilot study. *Sci. China Life. Sci.* **2013**, *56*, 745–750. [CrossRef]
107. Zimmer, F.; Zöllner, F.G.; Hoeger, S.; Klotz, S.; Tsagogiorgas, C.; Krämer, B.K.; Schad, L.R. Quantitative renal perfusion measurements in a rat model of acute kidney injury at 3T: Testing inter-and intramethodical significance of ASL and DCE-MRI. *PLoS ONE* **2013**, *8*, e53849. [CrossRef]
108. Chen, W.B.; Liang, L.; Zhang, B.; Liu, C.L.; Liu, H.J.; Luo, H.Y.; Zeng, Q.X.; Liang, C.H.; Liu, G.S.; Zhang, S.X. To evaluate the damage of renal function in CIAKI rats at 3T: Using ASL and BOLD MRI. *BioMed. Res. Int.* **2015**, *2015*. [CrossRef] [PubMed]
109. Peperhove, M.; Jang, M.-S.; Gutberlet, M.; Hartung, D.; Tewes, S.; Warnecke, G.; Fegbeutel, C.; Haverich, A.; Gwinner, W.; Lehner, F.; et al. Assessment of acute kidney injury with T1 mapping MRI following solid organ transplantation. *Eur. Radiol.* **2018**, *28*, 44–50. [CrossRef]
110. Turakhia, M.P.; Blankestijn, P.J.; Carrero, J.-J.; Clase, C.M.; Deo, R.; Herzog, C.A.; Kasner, S.E.; Passman, R.S.; Pecoits-Filho, R.; Reinecke, H.J.E.h.j. Chronic kidney disease and arrhythmias: Conclusions from a kidney disease: Improving global outcomes (KDIGO) controversies conference. *Eur. Heart J.* **2018**, *39*, 2314–2325. [CrossRef]
111. Gansevoort, R.T.; Correa-Rotter, R.; Hemmelgarn, B.R.; Jafar, T.H.; Heerspink, H.J.; Mann, J.F.; Matsushita, K.; Wen, C.P. Chronic kidney disease and cardiovascular risk: Epidemiology, mechanisms, and prevention. *Lancet* **2013**, *382*, 339–352. [CrossRef]
112. Stewart, G.A.; Foster, J.; Cowan, M.; Rooney, E.; Mcdonagh, T.; Dargie, H.J.; Rodger, R.S.C.; Jardine, A.G. Echocardiography overestimates left ventricular mass in hemodialysis patients relative to magnetic resonance imaging. *Kidney Int.* **1999**, *56*, 2248–2253. [CrossRef]
113. Patel, R.K.; Mark, P.B.; Johnston, N.; McGregor, E.; Dargie, H.J.; Jardine, A.G. Renal transplantation is not associated with regression of left ventricular hypertrophy: A magnetic resonance study. *Clin. J. Am. Soc. Nephrol.* **2008**, *3*, 1807–1811. [CrossRef]
114. Panoulas, V.F.; Sulemane, S.; Konstantinou, K.; Bratsas, A.; Elliott, S.J.; Dawson, D.; Frankel, A.H.; Nihoyannopoulos, P. Early detection of subclinical left ventricular myocardial dysfunction in patients with chronic kidney disease. *Eur. Heart J. Cardiovasc. Imaging* **2015**, *16*, 539–548. [CrossRef] [PubMed]
115. Smiseth, O.A.; Torp, H.; Opdahl, A.; Haugaa, K.H.; Urheim, S. Myocardial strain imaging: How useful is it in clinical decision making? *Eur. Heart J.* **2015**, *37*, 1196–1207. [CrossRef] [PubMed]
116. Tops, L.F.; Delgado, V.; Marsan, N.A.; Bax, J.J. Myocardial strain to detect subtle left ventricular systolic dysfunction. *Eur. J. Heart Fail.* **2017**, *19*, 307–313. [CrossRef] [PubMed]
117. Hensen, L.C.R.; Goossens, K.; Delgado, V.; Rotmans, J.I.; Jukema, J.W.; Bax, J.J. Prognostic Implications of Left Ventricular Global Longitudinal Strain in Predialysis and Dialysis Patients. *Am. J. Cardiol.* **2017**, *120*, 500–504. [CrossRef] [PubMed]
118. Liu, Y.W.; Su, C.T.; Huang, Y.Y.; Yang, C.S.; Huang, J.W.; Yang, M.T.; Chen, J.H.; Tsai, W.C. Left ventricular systolic strain in chronic kidney disease and hemodialysis patients. *Am. J. Nephrol.* **2011**, *33*, 84–90. [CrossRef] [PubMed]
119. Wang, H.; Liu, J.; Yao, X.D.; Li, J.; Yang, Y.; Cao, T.S.; Yang, B. Multidirectional myocardial systolic function in hemodialysis patients with preserved left ventricular ejection fraction and different left ventricular geometry. *Nephrol. Dial. Transplant.* **2012**, *27*, 4422–4429. [CrossRef]
120. Pirat, B.; Bozbas, H.; Simsek, V.; Sade, L.E.; Sayin, B.; Muderrisoglu, H.; Haberal, M. Assessment of Myocardial Mechanics in Patients with End-Stage Renal Disease and Renal Transplant Recipients Using Speckle Tracking Echocardiography. *Exp. Clin. Transplant.* **2015**, *13*, 235–241. [CrossRef]
121. Yan, P.; Li, H.; Hao, C.; Shi, H.; Gu, Y.; Huang, G.; Chen, J. 2D-speckle tracking echocardiography contributes to early identification of impaired left ventricular myocardial function in patients with chronic kidney disease. *Nephron Clin. Pract.* **2011**, *118*, c232–c240. [CrossRef] [PubMed]
122. Nagueh, S.F.; Smiseth, O.A.; Appleton, C.P.; Byrd, B.F.; Dokainish, H.; Edvardsen, T.; Flachskampf, F.A.; Gillebert, T.C.; Klein, A.L.; Lancellotti, P. Recommendations for the evaluation of left ventricular diastolic function by echocardiography: An update from

the American Society of Echocardiography and the European Association of Cardiovascular Imaging. *Eur. J. Echocardiogr.* **2016**, *17*, 1321–1360.
123. Lin, L.; Xie, Q.; Zheng, M.; Zhou, X.; Dekkers, I.A.; Tao, Q.; Lamb, H.J. Identification of cardiovascular abnormalities by multiparametric magnetic resonance imaging in end-stage renal disease patients with preserved left ventricular ejection fraction. *Eur. Radiol.* **2021**. [CrossRef]
124. Mall, G.; Huther, W.; Schneider, J.; Lundin, P.; Ritz, E. Diffuse intermyocardiocytic fibrosis in uraemic patients. *Nephrol. Dial. Transplant.* **1990**, *5*, 39–44. [CrossRef] [PubMed]
125. Edwards, N.C.; Moody, W.E.; Yuan, M.; Hayer, M.K.; Ferro, C.J.; Townend, J.N.; Steeds, R.P. Diffuse interstitial fibrosis and myocardial dysfunction in early chronic kidney disease. *Am. J. Cardiol.* **2015**, *115*, 1311–1317. [CrossRef] [PubMed]
126. Graham-Brown, M.P.; March, D.S.; Churchward, D.R.; Stensel, D.J.; Singh, A.; Arnold, R.; Burton, J.O.; McCann, G.P. Novel cardiac nuclear magnetic resonance method for noninvasive assessment of myocardial fibrosis in hemodialysis patients. *Kidney Int.* **2016**, *90*, 835–844. [CrossRef] [PubMed]
127. Rutherford, E.; Talle, M.A.; Mangion, K.; Bell, E.; Rauhalammi, S.M.; Roditi, G.; McComb, C.; Radjenovic, A.; Welsh, P.; Woodward, R.; et al. Defining myocardial tissue abnormalities in end-stage renal failure with cardiac magnetic resonance imaging using native T1 mapping. *Kidney Int.* **2016**, *90*, 845–852. [CrossRef]
128. Mangion, K.; McDowell, K.; Mark, P.B.; Rutherford, E. Characterizing Cardiac Involvement in Chronic Kidney Disease Using CMR-a Systematic Review. *Curr Cardiovasc. Imaging Rep.* **2018**, *11*, 2. [CrossRef]
129. Wang, L.; Yuan, J.; Zhang, S.J.; Gao, M.; Wang, Y.C.; Wang, Y.X.; Ju, S. Myocardial T1 rho mapping of patients with end-stage renal disease and its comparison with T1 mapping and T2 mapping: A feasibility and reproducibility study. *J. Magn. Reson. Imaging* **2016**, *44*, 723–731. [CrossRef] [PubMed]
130. Odudu, A.; Eldehni, M.T.; McCann, G.P.; Horsfield, M.A.; Breidthardt, T.; McIntyre, C.W. Characterisation of cardiomyopathy by cardiac and aortic magnetic resonance in patients new to hemodialysis. *Eur. Radiol.* **2016**, *26*, 2749–2761. [CrossRef] [PubMed]
131. Schietinger, B.J.; Brammer, G.M.; Wang, H.; Christopher, J.M.; Kwon, K.W.; Mangrum, A.J.; Mangrum, J.M.; Kramer, C.M. Patterns of late gadolinium enhancement in chronic hemodialysis patients. *JACC* **2008**, *1*, 450–456. [CrossRef]
132. Widjaja, E.; Oxtoby, J.; Hale, T.; Jones, P.; Harden, P.; McCall, I. Ultrasound measured renal length versus low dose CT volume in predicting single kidney glomerular filtration rate. *Br. J. Radiol.* **2004**, *77*, 759–764. [CrossRef]
133. Piras, D.; Masala, M.; Delitala, A.; Urru, S.A.M.; Curreli, N.; Balaci, L.; Ferreli, L.P.; Loi, F.; Atzeni, A.; Cabiddu, G.; et al. Kidney size in relation to ageing, gender, renal function, birthweight and chronic kidney disease risk factors in a general population. *Nephrol. Dial. Transplant.* **2020**, *35*, 640–647. [CrossRef]
134. Cox, E.F.; Buchanan, C.E.; Bradley, C.R.; Prestwich, B.; Mahmoud, H.; Taal, M.; Selby, N.M.; Francis, S.T. Multiparametric renal magnetic resonance imaging: Validation, interventions, and alterations in chronic kidney disease. *Front. Physiol.* **2017**, *8*, 696. [CrossRef] [PubMed]
135. Zhao, J.; Wang, Z.; Liu, M.; Zhu, J.; Zhang, X.; Zhang, T.; Li, S.; Li, Y. Assessment of renal fibrosis in chronic kidney disease using diffusion-weighted MRI. *Clin. Radiol.* **2014**, *69*, 1117–1122. [CrossRef] [PubMed]
136. Inoue, T.; Kozawa, E.; Okada, H.; Inukai, K.; Watanabe, S.; Kikuta, T.; Watanabe, Y.; Takenaka, T.; Katayama, S.; Tanaka, J. Noninvasive evaluation of kidney hypoxia and fibrosis using magnetic resonance imaging. *J. Am. Soc. Nephrol.* **2011**, *22*, 1429–1434. [CrossRef]
137. Li, Q.; Li, J.; Zhang, L.; Chen, Y.; Zhang, M.; Yan, F. Diffusion-weighted imaging in assessing renal pathology of chronic kidney disease: A preliminary clinical study. *Eur. J. Radiol.* **2014**, *83*, 756–762. [CrossRef]
138. Friedli, I.; Crowe, L.A.; de Perrot, T.; Berchtold, L.; Martin, P.Y.; de Seigneux, S.; Vallée, J.P. Comparison of readout-segmented and conventional single-shot for echo-planar diffusion-weighted imaging in the assessment of kidney interstitial fibrosis. *J. Magn. Reson. Imaging* **2017**, *46*, 1631–1640. [CrossRef]
139. Gillis, K.A.; McComb, C.; Patel, R.K.; Stevens, K.K.; Schneider, M.P.; Radjenovic, A.; Morris, S.T.; Roditi, G.H.; Delles, C.; Mark, P.B. Non-contrast renal magnetic resonance imaging to assess perfusion and corticomedullary differentiation in health and chronic kidney disease. *Nephron* **2016**, *133*, 183–192. [CrossRef]
140. Michaely, H.J.; Metzger, L.; Haneder, S.; Hansmann, J.; Schoenberg, S.O.; Attenberger, U. Renal BOLD-MRI does not reflect renal function in chronic kidney disease. *Kidney Int.* **2012**, *81*, 684–689. [CrossRef]
141. Pruijm, M.; Milani, B.; Pivin, E.; Podhajska, A.; Vogt, B.; Stuber, M.; Burnier, M. Reduced cortical oxygenation predicts a progressive decline of renal function in patients with chronic kidney disease. *Kidney Int.* **2018**, *93*, 932–940. [CrossRef]
142. Miyata, T.; De Strihou, C.V.Y. Diabetic nephropathy: A disorder of oxygen metabolism? *Nat. Rev. Nephrol.* **2010**, *6*, 83. [CrossRef] [PubMed]
143. Takiyama, Y.; Haneda, M. Hypoxia in diabetic kidneys. *BioMed. Res. Int.* **2014**, *2014*, 837421. [CrossRef] [PubMed]
144. Chen, X.; Xiao, W.; Li, X.; He, J.; Huang, X.; Tan, Y. In vivo evaluation of renal function using diffusion weighted imaging and diffusion tensor imaging in type 2 diabetics with normoalbuminuria versus microalbuminuria. *Front. Med.* **2014**, *8*, 471–476. [CrossRef] [PubMed]
145. Razek, A.A.K.A.; Al-Adlany, M.A.A.A.; Alhadidy, A.M.; Atwa, M.A.; Abdou, N.E.A. Diffusion tensor imaging of the renal cortex in diabetic patients: Correlation with urinary and serum biomarkers. *Abdom. Radiol.* **2017**, *42*, 1493–1500. [CrossRef]

46. Mora-Gutiérrez, J.M.; Garcia-Fernandez, N.; Slon Roblero, M.F.; Páramo, J.A.; Escalada, F.J.; Wang, D.J.; Benito, A.; Fernández-Seara, M.A. Arterial spin labeling MRI is able to detect early hemodynamic changes in diabetic nephropathy. *J. Magn. Reson. Imaging* **2017**, *46*, 1810–1817. [CrossRef] [PubMed]
47. Prasad, P.V.; Li, L.P.; Thacker, J.M.; Li, W.; Hack, B.; Kohn, O.; Sprague, S.M. Cortical Perfusion and Tubular Function as Evaluated by Magnetic Resonance Imaging Correlates with Annual Loss in Renal Function in Moderate Chronic Kidney Disease. *Am. J. Nephrol.* **2019**, *49*, 114–124. [CrossRef] [PubMed]
48. Dekkers, I.A.; Lamb, H.J. Clinical application and technical considerations of T 1 & T 2 (*) mapping in cardiac, liver, and renal imaging. *Br. J. Radiol.* **2018**, *91*, 20170825.

PET/CT Imaging for Personalized Management of Infectious Diseases

Jordy P. Pijl [1,*], Thomas C. Kwee [1], Riemer H. J. A. Slart [1,2] and Andor W. J. M. Glaudemans [1]

1. Departments of Radiology, Nuclear Medicine and Molecular Imaging, University of Groningen, 9700RB Groningen, The Netherlands; t.c.kwee@umcg.nl (T.C.K.); r.h.j.a.slart@umcg.nl (R.H.J.A.S.); a.w.j.m.glaudemans@umcg.nl (A.W.J.M.G.)
2. Department of Biomedical Photonic Imaging, Faculty of Science and Technology, University of Twente, 7500 AE Enschede, The Netherlands
* Correspondence: j.p.pijl@umcg.nl; Tel.: +31-50-361-6161

Abstract: Positron emission tomography combined with computed tomography (PET/CT) is a nuclear imaging technique which is increasingly being used in infectious diseases. Because infection foci often consume more glucose than surrounding tissue, most infections can be diagnosed with PET/CT using 2-deoxy-2-[18F]fluoro-D-glucose (FDG), an analogue of glucose labeled with Fluorine-18. In this review, we discuss common infectious diseases in which FDG-PET/CT is currently applied including bloodstream infection of unknown origin, infective endocarditis, vascular graft infection, spondylodiscitis, and cyst infections. Next, we highlight the latest developments within the field of PET/CT, including total body PET/CT, use of novel PET radiotracers, and potential future applications of PET/CT that will likely lead to increased capabilities for patient-tailored treatment of infectious diseases.

Keywords: FDG-PET/CT; infection; bloodstream infection; endocarditis; vascular graft infection; spondylodiscitis; cyst infection; white blood cell scintigraphy; total body PET/CT; radiotracers

1. Introduction

Infectious diseases are one of the most common reasons for hospital admission worldwide [1]. Commonly diagnosed infections include pneumonia, urinary tract infection, and bloodstream infection [2]. The diagnosis of most infections is often straightforward based on history taking and physical examination, and complemented with laboratory examinations and conventional (chest) radiography when clinically indicated. Microbiologic cultures and antibiotic sensitivity tests can be performed to enable more targeted treatment with narrow-spectrum antibiotic therapy. In some patients with infectious diseases, however, the infection focus may be difficult to detect with conventional diagnostics. This is especially true in patients with implanted foreign materials and electronic devices, such as artificial valves, vascular stents, prosthetic joints, and pacemakers/ICDs [3]. Positron Emission Tomography (PET) is a functional imaging technique that utilizes properties of specific molecules labeled with positron-emitting isotopes to visualize tissues or processes of interest. PET combined with Computed Tomography (PET/CT) allows for the spatial localization of radiotracer accumulation and simultaneous visualization of anatomy and structural abnormalities. PET/CT can be used for a wide variety of diseases, including infections. The most commonly used PET tracer for evaluating infectious diseases is 2-deoxy-2-[18F]fluoro-D-glucose (FDG). FDG-PET/CT can be used to visualize glucose uptake throughout the whole body in a single noninvasive examination. White blood cells and other inflammatory cells that are drawn to infection foci have a high glucose metabolism compared to other cells. Additionally, inflammatory mediators cause a local upregulation of glucose transporters, resulting in an increased cellular FDG uptake. Therefore, infection sites are often readily visible on FDG-PET/CT, even before gross structural changes such as abscess formation have occurred [4].

PET/CT capacity and patient throughput is relatively lower than that of conventional diagnostics such as ultrasonography, CT, and even magnetic resonance imaging (MRI) in most hospitals. Because more time is necessary for patient preparation and scanning, the use of FDG-PET/CT is usually reserved for specific infections in which conventional diagnostics are of limited value for identifying the infection focus [5,6]. Nevertheless, research on the diagnostic role of FDG-PET/CT for various infectious diseases is rapidly expanding leading to more standard application of this technique in a number of infectious diseases [7,8]. In this review, we describe the most common diagnostic applications of FDG-PET/CT in infectious diseases, highlight alternative nuclear imaging techniques used for diagnosing infectious diseases, and discuss the latest developments in the field of PET/CT that will likely contribute to increased capabilities for patient-tailored treatment of infectious diseases.

2. Current Common Applications of FDG-PET/CT

2.1. Bloodstream Infection of Unknown Origin

Bloodstream infection, defined as the presence of viable bacteria or fungi in the blood, is a common reason for hospitalization [9] (Figure 1). The most important treatment for bloodstream infection consists of source control and antimicrobial treatment [10]. In patients with an unknown source of infection or with multiple potential infection foci, FDG-PET/CT has been shown to be valuable in diagnosing the infection focus and thereby enabling more targeted treatment [11]. In several large clinical studies, FDG-PET/CT was able to identify the primary infection focus in 56% to 68% of patients with bloodstream infection of unknown origin, and previously unidentified septic emboli in approximately 60% of patients with *Staphylococcus aureus* bacteremia [4,12–15]. Because timely identification of the infection focus is associated with higher survival rates and is also cost-efficient in, for example, *Staphylococcus aureus* bacteremia, the clinical use of FDG-PET/CT in bloodstream infection of unknown origin is increasing [16–18].

In addition to the identification of the primary infection focus, FDG-PET/CT is increasingly performed as a routine examination in patients with a known source of bacteremia that has a high risk of septic dissemination. Risk factors for this include bacteremia with *Staphylococcus aureus*, persisting positive blood cultures despite appropriate antibiotic treatment, the presence of foreign materials such as artificial cardiac valves or vascular stents, electronic devices, or persisting fever [4,14]. Because septic dissemination of a primary infection focus can occur throughout the body and the location of these septic infection foci may not be clinically apparent, FDG-PET/CT is usually the method of choice to examine the whole body for septic infection foci in a single procedure [4]. Additionally, the presence or absence of septic foci also has consequences for the duration of antibiotic treatment. For example, in case of *Staphylococcus aureus* bacteremia, patients are generally treated with antibiotics for two weeks in case of uncomplicated bacteremia. Dissemination of disease is a feature of complicated bacteremia which requires prolonged antibiotic treatment of four to six weeks [19]. Therefore, the results of FDG-PET/CT can be helpful in determining the appropriate duration or adaption of antibiotic treatment.

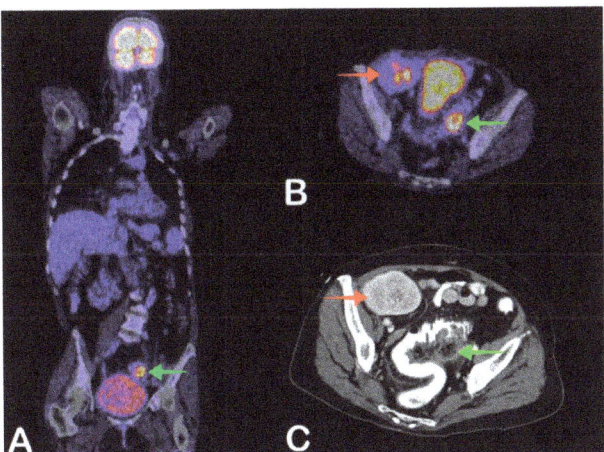

Figure 1. A 54-year-old woman was admitted to the hospital with fever. During hospitalization, she repeatedly had blood cultures positive for *Escherichia coli* and *Klebsiella pneumoniae* without localizing symptoms. Two years earlier, she had received a kidney transplant. Fused coronal2-deoxy-2-[18F]fluoro-D-glucose Positron Emission Tomography combined with Positron Tomography (FDG-PET/CT) showed increased FDG uptake at the left side of the sigmoid colon (**A**, green arrow), also shown on fused axial FDG-PET/CT (**B**, green arrow), indicative of either diverticulitis or abscess formation, as an explanation for the positive blood culture (*Escherichia coli*). Antibiotic treatment was started, but 9 days after PET/CT, the patient developed severe abdominal pain, and abdominal CT was performed. Axial CT also shows the abscess, with adjacent free intraperitoneal air, in keeping with perforated diverticulitis (**C**, green arrow). The kidney transplant in the right iliac fossa is also visible (**B** and **C**, red arrow). A laparotomic sigmoidectomy was performed, after which the patient recovered.

2.2. Fever of Unknown Origin

Fever, defined by an elevated body temperature of 38.3 degrees Celsius or higher, is a common symptom that can be caused by a large number of diseases [20] (Figure 2). The causes of fever can usually be categorized into infectious disease, noninfectious inflammatory disease, and malignant disease [21,22]. In some patients, diagnosing the cause of fever can present a diagnostic challenge. Although many different definitions are available, patients are usually considered to have fever of unknown origin when they have persistent fever for two to three weeks with no apparent cause after extensive clinical evaluation [21].

Because elevated glucose uptake occurs in many infectious, inflammatory, and malignant diseases, FDG-PET/CT can be an important aid in diagnosing the cause of the fever. A large number of studies has already been conducted to evaluate the use of FDG-PET/CT in finding the cause of fever. A recent study from 2017 described 15 retrospective studies including a total of 823 patients with fever of unknown origin and one prospective study including 48 patients [22]. In 58% of all patients, the FDG-PET/CT result was considered helpful, which was most often defined by identifying the cause of fever or guiding further therapy [22]. This is in line with a study of our own including 110 children with fever of unknown origin who underwent FDG-PET/CT, in whom the cause of fever was eventually identified in 62% [23]. In 48% of children, this was based on FDG-PET/CT. The most common causes of fever included endocarditis, systemic juvenile idiopathic arthritis, and inflammatory bowel disorder. Diseases such as Kawasaki arteritis, drug-induced fever, familial Mediterranean fever, and urinary tract infection were based on diagnostics other than FDG-PET/CT. Because FDG-PET/CT is able to identify the cause of fever in approximately half of patients with fever of unknown origin, clinicians should consider performing this technique in patients with persistent fever without apparent cause after extensive clinical evaluation. Performing FDG-PET/CT earlier on in patients with persistent fever of unknown origin may also be cost-effective, as it can lead to a faster diagnosis, reduce the number of diagnostic tests, and decrease hospitalization days [24,25].

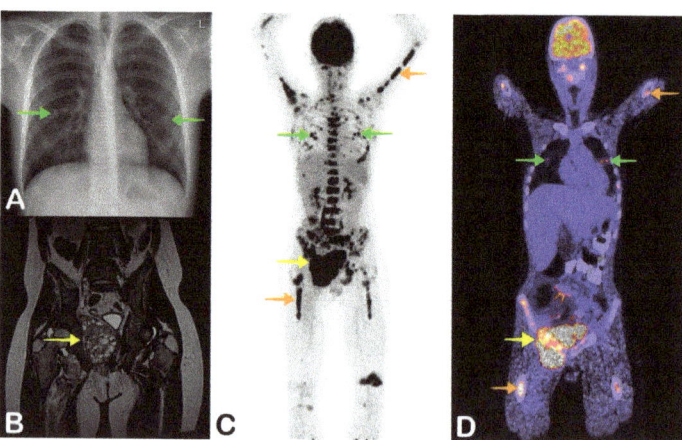

Figure 2. A 13-year-old boy presented to the hospital with a fever of three weeks, weight loss, and general malaise. He also had nonspecific pain in his legs and back and complained of nausea and vomiting. On physical examination, hepatomegaly was noticed. Laboratory testing showed normocytic anemia with a hemoglobin level of 5.2 mmol/L, leukopenia with a leukocyte count of 0.8×10^9/L, and elevated lactate dehydrogenase of 300 U/L. Abdominal ultrasonography confirmed the hepatomegaly, but showed no clear cause of the fever. A chest X-ray showed multiple pulmonary nodules (**A**, green arrows), suggestive of metastases of an unknown primary tumor. Because the patient had multiple nonguiding symptoms, FDG-PET/CT was performed. Coronal maximum intensity projection FDG-PET and fused FDG-PET/CT showed a large FDG-avid mass in the right lesser pelvis (**C** and **D**, yellow arrow), multiple pulmonary metastases (**C** and **D**, green arrows), and focally FDG avid bone marrow (**C** and **D**, orange arrows). Biopsy confirmed the diagnosis of metastasized Ewing sarcoma. MRI was performed before treatment was started, which also showed the primary site of the Ewing sarcoma in the right side of the pelvis (**B**, yellow arrow). After chemotherapy, radiotherapy, and an autologous stem cell transplant, the patient recovered and remained in complete remission for five years of follow-up.

2.3. Infective Endocarditis

Infective endocarditis is an endocardial infection with high morbidity and mortality [26] (Figure 3). Although artificial heart valves are an important risk factor for developing infective endocarditis, infective endocarditis also occurs in patients with native valves [27]. Currently, infective endocarditis is mostly diagnosed based on the modified Duke criteria. This diagnostic algorithm consists of major and minor criteria that represent common features of infective endocarditis. The sensitivity of these criteria for diagnosing infective endocarditis is approximately 72% [28]. One of the major criteria is the presence of valvular vegetations on transthoracic or transesophageal ultrasonography. However, the image quality of ultrasonography can be limited for various reasons such as the presence of artificial intracardiac material including artificial heart valves or vascular stents [29]. Because a definitive diagnosis of endocarditis has important treatment consequences such as prolonged intravenous use of antibiotics or even cardiac valve replacement, additional imaging such as FDG-PET/CT or alternatively white blood cell scintigraphy is often performed. Although FDG-PET/CT has a relatively low sensitivity of approximately 14% in patients with native valve endocarditis, it has a high sensitivity of 71–100% in patients with prosthetic valve endocarditis [30,31]. Nevertheless, FDG-PET/CT can still be valuable in native valve endocarditis for the detection of septic infection foci [30]. In current

European Society of Cardiology guidelines for the management of infective endocarditis, FDG-PET/CT is only included as a diagnostic technique in patients with suspected, but not definite, prosthetic valve endocarditis [32]. However, a recent study also mentions a role for FDG-PET/CT in patients with definite prosthetic valve endocarditis to detect silent embolism and metastatic infection [33]. In addition, performing FDG-PET/CT seems cost-effective in patients with Gram positive bacteremia and risk factors for septic dissemination, including prosthetic valves. Therefore, a wider implementation of FDG-PET/CT may be recommended in future endocarditis guidelines [18,34].

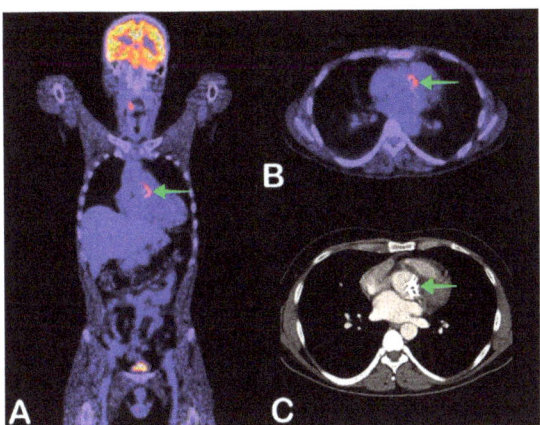

Figure 3. A 39-year-old man presented with general malaise for one week, fever of 41 degrees Celsius, and petechiae. Blood cultures were positive for *Streptococcus pneumoniae*. One year earlier, his native aortic valve was replaced with a mechanical valve. Endocarditis was strongly suspected, but transthoracic and transesophageal ultrasound did not prove valvular vegetations or other signs of infection. Fused coronal and axial FDG-PET/CT showed FDG avidity of the prosthetic aortic valve suggestive of infection (**A** and **B**, green arrow). No other infection foci were found. The aortic valve is also shown on full-dose thoracic CT (**C**, green arrow), without any anatomical signs of infection. The aortic valve was surgically replaced after which the patient recovered.

To increase the sensitivity of FDG-PET/CT for diagnosing endocarditis, adequate patient preparation is very important. Because myocardial tissue is highly glucose metabolic, patients should be kept on a low carbohydrate diet at least 24 h prior to FDG-PET/CT to suppress physiologic FDG uptake of the heart as this masks pathologic FDG uptake of the valves in case of endocarditis [35].

In patients with an infected prosthetic heart valve, choosing between conservative treatment with antibiotics instead of surgical valve replacement can be a difficult decision. In case conservative antibiotic treatment is chosen, follow-up FDG-PET/CT may be performed to assess persisting or resolved FDG avidity of the infected valve, monitor septic complications, and the potential need for surgical replacement.

2.4. Vascular Graft Infection

Approximately 1% to 5% of patients with a vascular graft develop a vascular graft infection [36] (Figure 4). This can occur shortly after vascular graft implantation (within two months of surgery) which is defined as an early infection, or after more than two months after surgery, which is defined as a late infection [36].

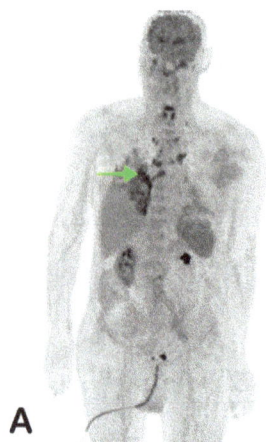
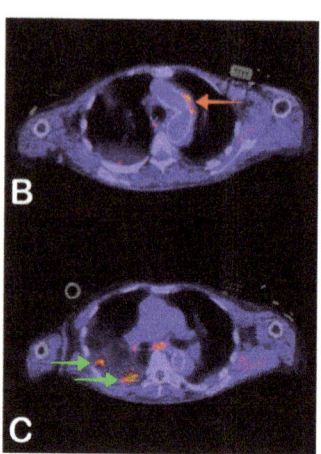

Figure 4. A 72-year-old man with a vascular graft in the aortic arch, abdominal aorta, and left common iliac artery was admitted with a fever of 38.5 degrees Celsius. Blood cultures were positive for *Enterococcus faecalis*. A clinical diagnosis of endocarditis was made based on the modified Duke criteria, although transthoracic and transesophageal ultrasound did not show signs of endocarditis. Coronal maximum-intensity projection FDG-PET showed increased FDG uptake in the right lower pulmonary lobe suggestive of infection (**A**, green arrow), and multiple metabolically active mediastinal and paratracheal lymph nodes. Fused axial FDG-PET/CT showed increased FDG uptake of the aortic arch stent suggestive of infection (**B**, red arrow), as well as FDG avid lesions suggestive of pulmonary infection (**C**, green arrows). The patient died three days after the PET/CT.

Clinical signs of vascular graft infection include fever, pain located at the vascular graft, erythema around the surgical site, and positive blood cultures. CT angiography may show periprosthetic infiltration or abscess and the formation of gas bubbles in cases of vascular graft infection. To diagnose early vascular graft infection, CT angiography is usually preferred over FDG-PET/CT because postsurgical or foreign body inflammation may also result in elevated FDG uptake around the vascular graft, resulting in false positive results [37]. In late vascular graft infections, however, FDG-PET/CT is the imaging modality of choice due to superior sensitivity (95% for FDG-PET/CT versus 67% for CT angiography), with a specificity of 85% [38,39]. Additionally, the whole body can be assessed for septic infection foci, infected lymph nodes, or another primary focus of infection in case the vascular graft infection is secondary to another infection. Although CT angiography often remains the first step imaging in suspected vascular graft infection, FDG-PET/CT is now included in the standard imaging workflow in suspected vascular graft infection and should especially be considered when CT angiography shows inconclusive results or no signs of infection, while vascular graft infection is still clinically suspected [40].

Diagnosing a vascular graft infection always has major treatment consequences. Because of biofilm formation on the vascular graft, antibiotic therapy will rarely lead to complete eradication of the pathogen. The vascular graft either has to be surgically explanted, or the patient has to be treated with lifelong antibiotics. In patients with another primary focus of infection and only secondary infection of the vascular graft, antibiotic therapy may be sufficient to eliminate the pathogen [40]. Therefore, FDG-PET/CT can present valuable information in patients with suspected vascular graft infection.

2.5. Spondylodiscitis

Spondylodiscitis, including discitis and vertebral osteomyelitis, is a spinal infection that usually presents with back or neck pain, fever, and elevated serum inflammatory markers when the onset is acute (Figure 5). Because of these nonspecific signs, additional imaging is required to diagnose spondylodiscitis. MRI is usually the first modality of choice, with a reported sensitivity of between 67% and 96% for diagnosing spondylodiscitis [41]. The sensitivity of MRI largely depends on the stage of disease, as MRI has a lower sensitivity in patients with an early infection. Early diagnosis and adequate treatment are very important for treatment outcome, as a delayed diagnosis may lead to complications such as persisting back pain or even paraplegia [42].

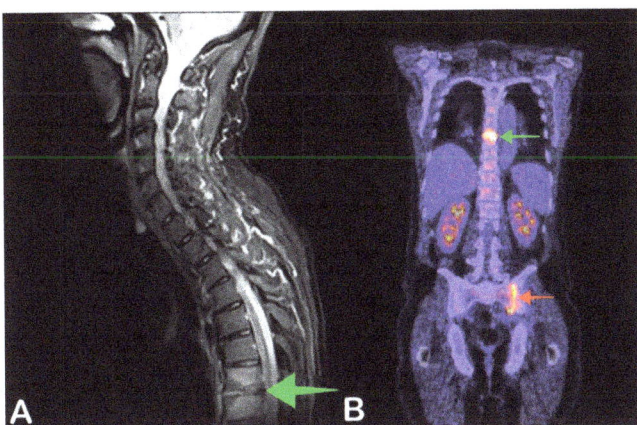

Figure 5. A 63-year-old man presented with fever and back pain. His left upper leg was also painful. Blood cultures were positive for *Staphylococcus aureus*. Sagittal fat-suppressed T2-weighted MRI showed increased signal intensity of thoracic vertebrae seven and eight, and the seventh and eighth intervertebral discs of the thoracic vertebrae–disc complex confirming the spondylodiscitis found on MRI (**B**, green arrow), but also showed increased FDG uptake at the left sacroiliac joint, indicative of sacroiliitis (**B**, red arrow). Antibiotic therapy was continued for six weeks after which the patient recovered.

Although MRI is often the modality of choice in patients with suspected spondylodiscitis, it can present important limitations in patients with foreign spinal materials (after spinal osteosynthesis, for example) causing scatter artefacts on MRI, which significantly decreases image readability. Some patients may also not be eligible for MRI due to non-MRI compatible implants or claustrophobia. In these patients, FDG-PET/CT is often used to examine patients with suspected spondylodiscitis. As FDG-PET/CT detects elevated glucose uptake associated with infection and does not rely on anatomical changes, it may also show higher sensitivity in early spondylodiscitis compared to MRI [43].

The reported sensitivity of FDG-PET/CT for diagnosing spondylodiscitis is 96%, with a specificity of 95% [41]. Because treatment for spondylodiscitis includes antibiotic treatment for at least six weeks, a definite diagnosis is very important to ensure an adequate duration of treatment, as antibiotics may be prescribed for a shorter duration and a lower dose when no infection focus is found on MRI or other diagnostics [42]. Follow-up FDG-PET/CT after a diagnosis of spondylodiscitis may also be performed to evaluate response to antibiotic treatment.

2.6. Cyst Infection

In patients with multiple abdominal cysts, including patients with autosomal dominant polycystic kidney disease (ADPKD) and polycystic liver disease (PLD), cyst infection can present a diagnostic challenge (Figure 6). Patients usually present with nonspecific signs such as abdominal pain and fever [44]. Conventional diagnostics such as ultrasonography or CT often show no signs of infection or nonspecific signs, such as cystic wall thickening [45]. The gold diagnostic standard is cyst puncture to obtain fluid that can be microbiologically cultured. However, this poses a risk of complications such as contamination of adjacent cysts or bleeding [46]. Therefore, percutaneous puncture is usually only performed in case of frank abscess formation, antibiotic treatment failure, or large infected cysts [47].

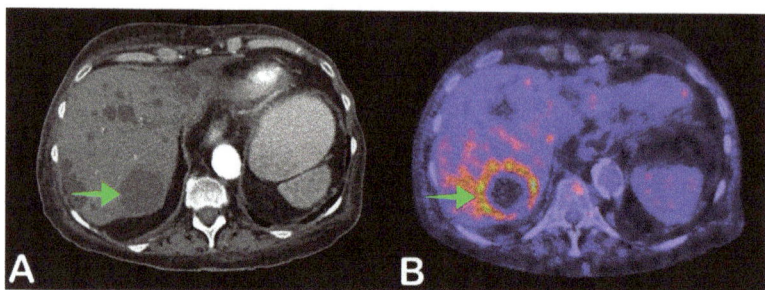

Figure 6. A 68-year-old woman presented with general malaise and night sweats for two weeks. She did not have a fever. She had received a kidney transplant 20 years earlier due to kidney failure caused by autosomal dominant polycystic kidney disease (ADPKD). Blood cultures were positive for *Escherichia coli*. Abdominal CT showed multiple liver cysts consistent with ADPKD, but no obvious signs of infection (**A**, green arrow). Fused axial FDG-PET/CT demonstrated increased FDG uptake in a large cyst in liver segment VII, suggestive of infection (**B**, green arrow). Antibiotic therapy was started with ciprofloxacin, after which the patient recovered.

Achieving a definitive diagnosis is important for treatment, as cyst infections usually require specific antibiotic treatment with lipophilic antibiotics that can penetrate cyst walls, such as fluoroquinolones. Empirical antibiotic treatment is usually not suitable for treating cyst infections [44]. FDG-PET/CT has been shown to be valuable in diagnosing cyst infection, especially in patients with multiple cysts, with a reported sensitivity of 77–100% and specificity of 75–100% in patients with ADPKD [48–51]. When cyst infection is suspected, performing FDG-PET/CT early in the diagnostic workup can lead to faster diagnosis and subsequent faster initiation of adequate antibiotic treatment.

3. Limitations of FDG-PET/CT

Because most cells metabolize glucose for ATP synthesis, physiologic FDG uptake occurs throughout the body. Therefore, FDG uptake is not specific for infection. Besides infection, FDG uptake can be locally elevated for other reasons as well [8]. For example, tumors often show increased FDG uptake, inflammatory diseases such as vasculitis or rheumatoid arthritis can cause increased FDG uptake, and postsurgical inflammation can also present challenges in diagnosing infection in patients who recently underwent a surgical procedure [52]. Additionally, foreign materials such as prosthetic joints, prosthetic heart valves, or vascular grafts often cause mild sterile inflammation and subsequent FDG uptake, affecting FDG-PET/CT's sensitivity and specificity for diagnosing infection [53]. Furthermore, not all infections can be diagnosed with FDG-PET/CT. For example, urinary tract infections may be difficult to diagnose due to renal FDG excretion.

Although conventional imaging such as CT or ultrasonography can often readily be performed, FDG-PET/CT requires adequate patient preparation. For example, patients have to fast for at least 6 h before FDG-PET/CT is performed, and refrain from carbohydrate-rich foods and (intravenous) fluids for at least 24 h when the possibility of endocarditis needs to be evaluated [7]. This can dissuade physicians from performing FDG-PET/CT in acutely ill patients, especially when FDG-PET/CT is only performed during office hours. Hospital capacity for FDG-PET/CT is usually also much lower than for stand-alone CT.

Antibiotic treatment may also negatively affect FDG-PET/CT's ability to diagnose infection. In a study of our own, longer duration of antibiotic treatment was associated with a lower chance of detecting an infection focus on FDG-PET/CT in patients with bloodstream infection [15]. However, another study from 2017 found no significant effect between duration of antibiotic treatment and diagnosing infection on FDG-PET/CT [54]. It could be hypothesized that longer antibiotic treatment may clear the infection before FDG-PET/CT is performed, but future research is needed to confirm this. Nevertheless, FDG-PET/CT should not be delayed in patients with bloodstream infection of unknown origin, especially not when there are risk factors for septic dissemination [4].

4. White Blood Cell Cintigraphy

In some patients, radiolabeled white blood cells may be used to overcome these limitations, as the accumulation of leukocytes is generally more specific for infection than increased glucose uptake. White blood cell (WBC) scintigraphy is performed on a gamma camera. A common indication for WBC scintigraphy is suspected prosthetic joint infection. However, this is also dependent on the location of the infection. For example, in patients with a prosthetic hip infection, elevated FDG uptake due to sterile inflammation is expected around the head and neck of the prosthesis, but not at other sites [55]. Extensive, heterogeneous FDG uptake along the bone prosthesis interface, especially in the middle portion of the shaft, is indicative of periprosthetic infection. White blood cell scintigraphy is sometimes also performed in patients with suspected endocarditis or vascular graft infection, especially when results from FDG-PET/CT are inconclusive but clinical suspicion of infection remains.

Several tracers can be used to radiolabel leukocytes. One of the most commonly used tracers is Technetium 99 m. Because this radioisotope does not produce positrons but gamma radiation photons, Single-Photon Emission Computed Tomography (SPECT) is used for this procedure instead of PET. PET-tracers can also be used to label leukocytes. Because labelled leukocytes require 20–24 h to be recruited to infection sites, FDG is not suitable for radiolabeling glucose due to its short half-life [56].

WBC scintigraphy also presents important limitations compared to FDG-PET/CT. The procedure is much more complex than regular FDG-PET/CT, the resolution of SPECT is inferior to the resolution of PET, and WBC scintigraphy also presents logistical challenges. First, blood has to be drawn from patients to obtain autologous leukocytes. Then, the harvested leukocytes have to be radiolabeled and reinjected into the patient, which also poses a risk of blood mix-up with other patients. Usually, two scans at two different time intervals are necessary so they can be compared to be able to accurately diagnose infection. The whole procedure usually takes two days to complete. These factors often render white blood cell scintigraphy less favorable than FDG-PET/CT.

5. Future Applications of PET/CT

5.1. Total Body PET/CT

One of the most promising current advances in PET/CT technology is the development of total body PET/CT [57]. Current PET/CT systems mostly operate with a 20 cm wide detector ring and thus a maximum of 20 cm field of view per bed position. To image the whole body, the table is shifted through the detector ring while the patient has to lie still during the entire procedure. For PET imaging of the whole body, a short field of view presents important limitations. When positron annihilation occurs, two anticollinear high energy photons are ejected in a random direction. As FDG is distributed through the whole body, only 3–5% of the high energy photons emitted hit the detector ring and are recorded, and the photons emitted outside the 20 cm field of view are not recorded. This means that less than 1% of the positron annihilation events that occur in the patient during PET scanning are recorded on current PET/CT systems [58].

The new total body PET/CT systems try to overcome this limitation by significantly extending the field of view. Total body PET/CT systems have an extended field of view of up to 200 cm instead of 20 cm. During scanning, the patient will be placed in this 200 cm tube covered by PET detectors (or slightly shorter tube length, depending on the model), which will significantly decrease photon scattering outside the field of view. For a 200 cm total body PET/CT system, this could theoretically increase sensitivity by a factor of 40 compared to whole-body scans on current PET/CT systems with similar scanning time and FDG dosage. Alternatively, it could also decrease scanning time by a factor of 40 to 15–30 s with similar sensitivity and FDG dosage, or decrease FDG dosage by a factor of 40 to 0.2 mSv (equivalent to 2 chest X-rays) while maintaining similar sensitivity and scanning time [58,59]. The ideal settings and properties of these total body PET/CT systems will be depending on the type of examination and clinical experience, but it will likely revolutionize the possibilities of PET/CT. For infectious disease, it would likely be possible to detect much smaller metastatic infection foci, increase the possibilities of follow-up PET/CT imaging to monitor treatment response, increase the number of infection-specific radiotracers that can be effectively used in PET imaging, and enable real time imaging of various organ–organ axes. Severely ill patients can be scanned very rapidly, and this will benefit intensive care patients.

5.2. Infection-Specific Radiotracers

FDG is the most widely used radiotracer for diagnosing infectious disease with PET/CT. As already mentioned, elevated FDG uptake due to infection cannot always be distinguished from elevated FDG uptake due to sterile inflammation or due to postsurgical inflammation. Therefore, many studies have been performed and are still ongoing to develop more infection-specific radiotracers [60–62]. These include radiolabeled bacteria-specific monoclonal antibodies such as antibodies against *Staphylococcus aureus* surface molecule lipoteichoic acid labeled with Zirkonium-89 [63], radiolabeled antibiotics such as ciprofloxacin or fluoropropyl-trimethoprim labeled with Fluorine-18 [64,65] radiolabeled antimicrobial peptides such as ubiquicidin labeled with Gallium-68 [66], radiolabeled molecules involved in bacteria-specific synthesis pathways such as p-aminobenzoic acid labeled with Fluorine-18 [67], and fluorodeoxysorbitol labeled with Fluorine-18 which specifically targets Enterobacteriaceae [68] (Table 1). Most of these novel tracers have only been used in vitro, in animal models, or in small human-based research settings. Nevertheless, the clinical application of bacteria or infection-specific radiotracers could present important benefits compared to current diagnostic possibilities. In patients with nonspecific signs of prosthetic joint infection, for example, being able to distinguish aseptic loosening from infection could prevent invasive procedures such as repeated biopsies (which also pose a risk of infecting the prosthesis) or unnecessary surgical replacement of the prosthesis. In cases where biopsy may pose significant risks due to the anatomic location of the lesion of interest, bacteria-specific tracers may be used to identify the specific bacterial strain and subsequently enable more specific antimicrobial treatment.

Table 1. Various examples of bacterial (novel)tracers for PET/CT.

Tracer	Isotope (Half-Life)	Ligand	Target/Substrate	Comment
89Zr-SAC55	Zirkonium-89 (78.4 h) [69]	Monoclonal antibody	*Staphylococcus aureus* surface molecule lipoteichoic acid	Promising results from animal studies, currently no human studies available [63]
18F-ciprofloxacin	Fluorine-18 (110 min) [70]	Ciprofloxacin	Bacterial DNA gyrase or topoisomerase IV	In-human studies did not indicate bacteria-specific binding [64]
18F-fluoropropyl-trimethoprim	Fluorine-18 (110 min) [70]	Trimethoprim	Bacterial dihydrofolate reductase	No in-human studies available [65]
68Ga-NOTA-UBI	Gallium-68 (68 min) [71]	Chelated ubiquicidin	Bacterial cytoplasmic membrane	Promising results in animal models, but very limited in-human experience [66]
2-18F-F-p-Aminobenzoic Acid	Fluorine-18 (110 min) [70]	p-aminobenzoic acid	Dihydropteroate synthase	Promising results from animal studies, also targets different types of bacteria [72]
2-18F-fluorodeoxysorbitol	Fluorine-18 (110 min) [70]	Sorbitol	Sorbitol-6-phosphate dehydrogenase	Promising results from animal studies, limited in-human experience. Sorbitol is not metabolized by Gram positive bacteria [73].

The half-life of the isotope used in radiotracers has various implications. For medical practices, isotopes with a short half-life, such as FDG with a half-life of 110 min, are often preferred due to lower radiation exposure [70]. In most examinations such as FDG-PET/CT, FDG quickly reaches the target cells and PET/CT is often performed one hour after FDG administration. Some radiotracers, however, require more time to reach their target cells. In case of larger molecules such as radiolabeled antibodies, it takes several days for the antibodies to reach their target cells [74]. This requires the use of isotopes with a longer half-life, but is also associated with higher radiation exposure. However, total body PET/CT could significantly decrease this radiation exposure.

Limitations of bacteria-specific radiotracers include the fact that the number of bacteria present in a low-grade infection may be too low for current PET/CT systems to detect and visualize. However, an increased sensitivity of PET/CT with novel PET/CT systems such as total body PET/CT may enable more widespread bacteria-specific PET imaging. Of interest is the fact that alternative techniques to specifically diagnose these infections are also being explored, such as in vivo imaging using fluorescently labeled vancomycin [75].

5.3. Personalized Duration of Antibiotic Treatment

Most patients with infectious diseases are treated with antibiotics or antifungals for a standardized time duration, depending on the type and extent of infection, microorganism species, and clinical response to treatment in terms of symptoms and infection parameters such as C-reactive protein and leukocyte count. In uncomplicated infections such as urinary tract infections or mild pneumonia that only require a short duration of antimicrobial treatment without important side effects, a standardized duration of antibiotic treatment can be accepted even though some of those patients may not need to be treated for the standardized duration of time.

Patients with more complicated and difficult to treat infections, such as endocarditis, vascular graft infection, or hernia mesh infection may need to receive antimicrobial treatment for an extended period ranging from multiple weeks to lifelong suppression therapy [76]. These standardized treatment durations are often based on large cohorts of patients with limited attention to patient-specific characteristics. Physicians may be hesitant to deviate from these standardized long-term treatment plans. Not all patients need such prolonged antimicrobial treatment, but guidance is needed [77]. In these patients, it would be very interesting to follow up infection activity either by using PET/CT with FDG or with more infection-specific novel radiotracers. Future research could be aimed at the relation between infectious disease activity on PET/CT and clinical response over the course of treatment, as this may also allow more patient-tailored treatment. Quantitative FDG-PET/CT follow up is already performed in oncologic diseases such as lymphoma and melanoma to monitor treatment response, but may also be beneficial in patients with chronic infection and long-term antimicrobial treatment [78]. Additionally, (follow up) PET/CT may also aid physicians in deciding to switch from intravenous to oral antibiotic treatment, or from more expensive antifungals such as anidulafungin to the cheaper but maybe less effective fluconazole [79].

It is difficult to predict the cost effectiveness of applying such a technique. PET/CT may be a relatively expensive imaging technique, but prolonged hospitalization for intravenous administration of antibiotics or the placement of peripherally inserted central catheters for intravenous antibiotic treatment at home may be more expensive. Additionally, the prolonged use of antibiotics also increases the risk of severe side effects such as *Clostridium difficile* superinfection, bone marrow suppression, or toxic levels of aminoglycosides leading to deafness or kidney failure, which are all associated with significant morbidity costs and reduced quality of life [77].

6. Conclusions

PET/CT is a valuable imaging technique that is increasingly being used in infectious diseases. Although it can accurately diagnose a number of infectious diseases, its main benefits are derived from the ability to examine the whole body for an infection focus or septic infection foci in a single procedure, the ability to diagnose early infections before significant anatomical changes have occurred, and the ability to diagnose artificial material infections such as vascular graft infection, orthopedic prostheses, electronic implantable devices, or prosthetic valve endocarditis. Technological developments in PET/CT and tracers will likely contribute to more widespread use of PET/CT in diagnosing and monitoring infectious disease, allowing more patient-tailored treatment of infectious disease in terms of treatment duration and deciding between conservative antibiotic treatment or invasive surgical procedures.

Author Contributions: Conceptualization, J.P.P., T.C.K. and A.W.J.M.G.; methodology, J.P.P., T.C.K. and A.W.J.M.G.; writing—original draft preparation, J.P.P., T.C.K., A.W.J.M.G., and R.H.J.A.S.; writing—review and editing, J.P.P., T.C.K., A.W.J.M.G., and R.H.J.A.S.; visualization, J.P.P.; supervision, T.C.K. and A.W.J.M.G.; project administration, J.P.P. All authors have read and agreed to the published version of the manuscript.

Funding: No funding was received for this study.

Institutional Review Board Statement: Due to the descriptive nature of the study, no IRB statement was required.

Informed Consent Statement: Not applicable.

Data Availability Statement: No new data were created or analyzed in this study. Data sharing is not applicable to this article.

Conflicts of Interest: All authors declare no conflict of interest.

References

1. Rudd, K.E.; Johnson, S.C.; Agesa, K.M.; Shackelford, K.A.; Tsoi, D.; Kievlan, D.R.; Colombara, D.V.; Ikuta, K.S.; Kissoon, N.; Finfer, S.; et al. Global, regional, and national sepsis incidence and mortality, 1990–2017: Analysis for the Global Burden of Disease Study. *Lancet* **2020**, *395*, 200–211. [CrossRef]
2. Bradley, S.F. Infections. *Pract. Geriatr.* **2007**, 475–494. [CrossRef]
3. Vanepps, J.S.; Younger, J.G. Implantable Device-Related Infection. *Shock* **2016**, *46*, 597–608. [CrossRef] [PubMed]
4. Vos, F.J.; Bleeker-Rovers, C.P.; Sturm, P.D.; Krabbe, P.F.M.; Van Dijk, A.P.J.; Cuijpers, M.L.H.; Adang, E.M.M.; Wanten, G.J.A.; Kullberg, B.-J.; Oyen, W.J.G. 18F-FDG PET/CT for Detection of Metastatic Infection in Gram-Positive Bacteremia. *J. Nucl. Med.* **2010**, *51*, 1234–1240. [CrossRef] [PubMed]
5. Vaidyanathan, S.; Patel, C.; Scarsbrook, A.; Chowdhury, F. FDG PET/CT in infection and inflammation—Current and emerging clinical applications. *Clin. Radiol.* **2015**, *70*, 787–800. [CrossRef]
6. Fuchs, S.; Grössmann, N.; Ferch, M.; Busse, R.; Wild, C. Evidence-based indications for the planning of PET or PET/CT capacities are needed. *Clin. Transl. Imaging* **2019**, *7*, 65–81. [CrossRef]
7. Jamar, F.; Buscombe, J.; Chiti, A.; Christian, P.E.; Delbeke, D.; Donohoe, K.J.; Israel, O.; Martin-Comin, J.; Signore, A. EANM/SNMMI Guideline for 18F-FDG Use in Inflammation and Infection. *J. Nucl. Med.* **2013**, *54*, 647–658. [CrossRef]
8. Kung, B.T.; Seraj, S.M.; Zadeh, M.Z.; Rojulpote, C.; Kothekar, E.; Ayubcha, C.; Ng, K.S.; Ng, K.K.; Au-Yong, T.K.; Werner, T.J.; et al. An update on the role of 18F-FDG-PET/CT in major infectious and inflammatory diseases. *Am. J. Nucl. Med. Mol. Imaging* **2019**, *9*, 255–273.
9. Goto, M.; Al-Hasan, M.N. Overall burden of bloodstream infection and nosocomial bloodstream infection in North America and Europe. *Clin. Microbiol. Infect.* **2013**, *19*, 501–509. [CrossRef]
10. Lagunes, L.; Encina, B.; Ramirez-Estrada, S. Current understanding in source control management in septic shock patients: A review. *Ann. Transl. Med.* **2016**, *4*, 330. [CrossRef]
11. Treglia, G. Diagnostic Performance of 18F-FDG PET/CT in Infectious and Inflammatory Diseases according to Published Meta-Analyses. *Contrast Media Mol. Imaging* **2019**, *2019*, 1–12. [CrossRef] [PubMed]
12. Tseng, J.-R.; Chen, K.-Y.; Lee, M.-H.; Huang, C.-T.; Wen, Y.-H.; Yen, T.-C. Potential Usefulness of FDG PET/CT in Patients with Sepsis of Unknown Origin. *PLoS ONE* **2013**, *8*, e66132. [CrossRef] [PubMed]
13. Brøndserud, M.B.; Pedersen, C.; Rosenvinge, F.S.; Høilund-Carlsen, P.F.; Hess, S. Clinical value of FDG-PET/CT in bacteremia of unknown origin with catalase-negative gram-positive cocci or Staphylococcus aureus. *Eur. J. Nucl. Med. Mol. Imaging* **2019**, *46*, 1351–1358. [CrossRef] [PubMed]
14. Berrevoets, M.A.; Kouijzer, I.J.; Aarntzen, E.H.; Janssen, M.J.; Wertheim, H.F.; Kullberg, B.-J.; Oyen, W.J.G.; Bleeker-Rovers, C.P.; De Geus-Oei, L.-F.; Oever, J.T. 18 F-FDG PET/CT Optimizes Treatment in Staphylococcus Aureus Bacteremia and Is Associated with Reduced Mortality. *J. Nucl. Med.* **2017**, *58*, 1504–1510. [CrossRef] [PubMed]

15. Pijl, J.; Glaudemans, A.; Slart, R.; Yakar, D.; Wouthuyzen-Bakker, M.; Kwee, T. FDG-PET/CT for Detecting an Infection Focus in Patients with a Bloodstream Infection: Factors Affecting Diagnostic Yield. *SSRN Electron. J.* **2018**, *44*, 99–106. [CrossRef]
16. Tabah, A.; Koulenti, D.; Laupland, K.B.; Misset, B.; Valles, J.; De Carvalho, F.B.; Paiva, J.A.; Çakar, N.; Ma, X.; Eggimann, P.; et al. Characteristics and determinants of outcome of hospital-acquired bloodstream infections in intensive care units: The EUROBACT International Cohort Study. *Intensiv. Care Med.* **2012**, *38*, 1930–1945. [CrossRef]
17. Hess, S.; Hansson, S.H.; Pedersen, K.T.; Basu, S.; Høilund-Carlsen, P.F. FDG-PET/CT in Infectious and Inflammatory Diseases. *PET Clin.* **2014**, *9*, 497–519. [CrossRef]
18. Vos, F.J.; Bleeker-Rovers, C.P.; Kullberg, B.J.; Adang, E.M.; Oyen, W.J.G. Cost-Effectiveness of Routine 18F-FDG PET/CT in High-Risk Patients with Gram-Positive Bacteremia. *J. Nucl. Med.* **2011**, *52*, 1673–1678. [CrossRef]
19. Holland, T.L.; Arnold, C.J.; Fowler, V.G. Clinical Management of Staphylococcus aureus Bacteremia. *JAMA* **2014**, *312*, 1330–1341. [CrossRef]
20. Petersdorf, R.G.; Beeson, P.B. Fever of unexplained origin: Report on 100 cases. *Medicine* **1961**, *40*, 1–30. [CrossRef]
21. Meller, J.; Sahlmann, C.-O.; Scheel, A.K. 18F-FDG PET and PET/CT in fever of unknown origin. *J. Nucl. Med.* **2007**, *48*, 35–45.
22. Kouijzer, I.J.; Mulders-Manders, C.M.; Bleeker-Rovers, C.P.; Oyen, W.J. Fever of Unknown Origin: The Value of FDG-PET/CT. *Semin. Nucl. Med.* **2018**, *48*, 100–107. [CrossRef]
23. Pijl, J.P.; Kwee, T.C.; Legger, G.; Peters, H.J.; Armbrust, W.; Schölvinck, E.; Glaudemans, A.W. Role of FDG-PET/CT in children with fever of unknown origin. *Eur. J. Nucl. Med. Mol. Imaging* **2020**, *47*, 1596–1604. [CrossRef]
24. Nakayo, E.B.; Vicente, A.G.; Castrejón, Á.M.S.; Narváez, J.M.; Rubio, M.T.; García, V.P.; García, J.C. Analysis of cost-effectiveness in the diagnosis of fever of unknown origin and the role of 18F-FDG PET–CT: A proposal of diagnostic algorithm. *Rev. Esp. Med. Nucl. Imagen Mol. Engl. Ed.* **2012**, *31*, 178–186. [CrossRef]
25. Balink, H.; Tan, S.S.; Veeger, N.J.G.M.; Holleman, F.; Van Eck-Smit, B.L.F.; Bennink, R.J.; Verberne, H.J. 18F-FDG PET/CT in inflammation of unknown origin: A cost-effectiveness pilot-study. *Eur. J. Nucl. Med. Mol. Imaging* **2015**, *42*, 1408–1413. [CrossRef] [PubMed]
26. McDonald, J.R. Acute Infective Endocarditis. *Infect. Dis. Clin. N. Am.* **2009**, *23*, 643–664. [CrossRef] [PubMed]
27. Rajani, R.; Klein, J.L. Infective endocarditis: A contemporary update. *Clin. Med.* **2020**, *20*, 31–35. [CrossRef] [PubMed]
28. Shrestha, N.; Shakya, S.; Hussain, S.; Pettersson, G.; Griffin, B.; Gordon, S. Sensitivity and Specificity of Duke Criteria for Diagnosis of Definite Infective Endocarditis: A Cohort Study. *Open Forum Infect. Dis.* **2017**, *4*, 550. [CrossRef]
29. Evangelista, A. Echocardiography in infective endocarditis. *Hearth* **2004**, *90*, 614–617. [CrossRef] [PubMed]
30. Chen, W.; Dilsizian, V. FDG PET/CT for the diagnosis and management of infective endocarditis: Expert consensus vs evidence-based practice. *J. Nucl. Cardiol.* **2018**, *26*, 313–315. [CrossRef]
31. Gomes, A.; Glaudemans, A.W.J.M.; Touw, D.J.; Van Melle, J.P.; Willems, T.P.; Maass, A.H.; Natour, E.; Prakken, N.H.J.; Borra, R.J.H.; Van Geel, P.P.; et al. Diagnostic value of imaging in infective endocarditis: A systematic review. *Lancet Infect. Dis.* **2017**, *17*, e1–e14. [CrossRef]
32. Habib, G.; Lancellotti, P.; Antunes, M.J.; Bongiorni, M.G.; Casalta, J.-P.; Del Zotti, F.; Dulgheru, R.; El Khoury, G.; Erba, P.A.; Iung, B.; et al. 2015 ESC Guidelines for the management of infective endocarditis. The Task Force for the Management of Infective Endocarditis of the European Society of Cardiology (ESC). Endorsed by: European Association for Cardio-Thoracic Surgery (EACTS), the European Association of Nuclear Medicine (EANM). *G. Ital. Cardiol. Rome* **2016**, *17*, 3075–3128.
33. Erba, P.A.; Pizzi, M.N.; Roque, A.; Salaun, E.; Lancellotti, P.; Tornos, P.; Habib, G. Multimodality Imaging in Infective Endocarditis. *Circulation* **2019**, *140*, 1753–1765. [CrossRef] [PubMed]
34. Bleeker-Rovers, C.P.; Vos, F.J.; Wanten, G.J.A.; Van Der Meer, J.W.M.; Corstens, F.H.M.; Kullberg, B.-J.; Oyen, W.J.G. 18F-FDG PET in detecting metastatic infectious disease. *J. Nucl. Med.* **2005**, *46*, 2014–2019. [PubMed]
35. Slart, R.H.J.A.; Glaudemans, A.W.J.M.; Gheysens, O.; Lubberink, M.; Kero, T.; Dweck, M.R.; Habib, G.; Gaemperli, O.; Saraste, A.; Gimelli, A.; et al. Procedural recommendations of cardiac PET/CT imaging: Standardization in inflammatory-, infective-, infiltrative-, and innervation (4Is)-related cardiovascular diseases: A joint collaboration of the EACVI and the EANM. *Eur. J. Nucl. Med. Mol. Imaging* **2020**, 1–24. [CrossRef] [PubMed]
36. Wilson, W.R.; Bower, T.C.; Creager, M.A.; Amin-Hanjani, S.; O'Gara, P.T.; Lockhart, P.B.; Darouiche, R.O.; Ramlawi, B.; Derdeyn, C.P.; Bolger, A.F.; et al. Vascular Graft Infections, Mycotic Aneurysms, and Endovascular Infections: A Scientific Statement from the American Heart Association. *Circulation* **2016**, *134*, e412–e460. [CrossRef]
37. Keidar, Z.; Nitecki, S. FDG-PET in Prosthetic Graft Infections. *Semin. Nucl. Med.* **2013**, *43*, 396–402. [CrossRef]
38. Keidar, Z.; Engel, A.; Hoffman, A.; Israel, O.; Nitecki, S. Prosthetic Vascular Graft Infection: The Role of 18F-FDG PET/CT. *J. Nucl. Med.* **2007**, *48*, 1230–1236. [CrossRef]
39. Saleem, B.R.; Pol, R.A.; Slart, R.H.J.A.; Reijnen, M.M.P.J.; Zeebregts, C.J. 18F-Fluorodeoxyglucose Positron Emission Tomography/CT Scanning in Diagnosing Vascular Prosthetic Graft Infection. *BioMed Res. Int.* **2014**, *2014*, 1–8. [CrossRef]
40. Chakfé, N.; Diener, H.; Lejay, A.; Assadian, O.; Berard, X.; Caillon, J.; Fourneau, I.; Glaudemans, A.W.; Koncar, I.; Lindholt, J.; et al. Editor's Choice—European Society for Vascular Surgery (ESVS) 2020 Clinical Practice Guidelines on the Management of Vascular Graft and Endograft Infections. *Eur. J. Vasc. Endovasc. Surg.* **2020**, *59*, 339–384. [CrossRef]
41. Smids, C.; Kouijzer, I.J.E.; Vos, F.J.; Sprong, T.; Hosman, A.J.F.; De Rooy, J.W.J.; Aarntzen, E.H.J.G.; De Geus-Oei, L.-F.; Oyen, W.J.G.; Bleeker-Rovers, C.P. A comparison of the diagnostic value of MRI and 18F-FDG-PET/CT in suspected spondylodiscitis. *Infection* **2017**, *45*, 41–49. [CrossRef]

42. Gouliouris, T.; Aliyu, S.H.; Brown, N.M. Spondylodiscitis: Update on diagnosis and management. *J. Antimicrob. Chemother.* **2010**, *65*, iii11–iii24. [CrossRef]
43. Altini, C.; Lavelli, V.; Niccoli-Asabella, A.; Sardaro, A.; Branca, A.; Santo, G.; Ferrari, C.; Rubini, G. Comparison of the Diagnostic Value of MRI and Whole Body 18F-FDG PET/CT in Diagnosis of Spondylodiscitis. *J. Clin. Med.* **2020**, *9*, 1581. [CrossRef]
44. Torres, V.E.; Harris, P.C.; Pirson, Y. Autosomal dominant polycystic kidney disease. *Lancet* **2007**, *369*, 1287–1301. [CrossRef]
45. Oh, J.; Shin, C.-I.; Kim, S.Y. Infected cyst in patients with autosomal dominant polycystic kidney disease: Analysis of computed tomographic and ultrasonographic imaging features. *PLoS ONE* **2018**, *13*, e0207880. [CrossRef]
46. Lantinga, M.A.; Drenth, J.P.; Gevers, T.J.G. Diagnostic criteria in renal and hepatic cyst infection. *Nephrol. Dial. Transpl.* **2014**, *30*, 744–751. [CrossRef]
47. Lantinga, M.A.; Casteleijn, N.F.; Geudens, A.; De Sévaux, R.G.; Van Assen, S.; Leliveld, A.M.; Gansevoort, R.T.; Drenth, J.P. Management of renal cyst infection in patients with autosomal dominant polycystic kidney disease: A systematic review. *Nephrol. Dial. Transpl.* **2016**, *32*, 144–150. [CrossRef] [PubMed]
48. Sallée, M.; Rafat, C.; Zahar, J.-R.; Paulmier, B.; Grünfeld, J.-P.; Knebelmann, B.; Fakhouri, F. Cyst Infections in Patients with Autosomal Dominant Polycystic Kidney Disease. *Clin. J. Am. Soc. Nephrol.* **2009**, *4*, 1183–1189. [CrossRef] [PubMed]
49. Bobot, M.; Ghez, C.; Gondouin, B.; Sallée, M.; Fournier, P.; Burtey, S.; Legris, T.; Dussol, B.; Berland, Y.; Souteyrand, P.; et al. Diagnostic performance of [18F] fluorodeoxyglucose positron emission tomography–computed tomography in cyst infection in patients with autosomal dominant polycystic kidney disease. *Clin. Microbiol. Infect.* **2016**, *22*, 71–77. [CrossRef] [PubMed]
50. Jouret, F.; Lhommel, R.; Beguin, C.; Devuyst, O.; Pirson, Y.; Hassoun, Z.; Kanaan, N. Positron-Emission Computed Tomography in Cyst Infection Diagnosis in Patients with Autosomal Dominant Polycystic Kidney Disease. *Clin. J. Am. Soc. Nephrol.* **2011**, *6*, 1644–1650. [CrossRef] [PubMed]
51. Pijl, J.P.; Glaudemans, A.W.; Slart, R.H.; Kwee, T.C. 18F-FDG PET/CT in Autosomal Dominant Polycystic Kidney Disease Patients with Suspected Cyst Infection. *J. Nucl. Med.* **2018**, *59*, 1734–1741. [CrossRef]
52. Garg, G.; Benchekroun, M.T.; Abraham, T. FDG-PET/CT in the Postoperative Period: Utility, Expected Findings, Complications, and Pitfalls. *Semin. Nucl. Med.* **2017**, *47*, 579–594. [CrossRef]
53. Gelderman, S.J.; Jutte, P.C.; Boellaard, R.; Ploegmakers, J.J.W.; García, D.V.; Kampinga, G.A.; Glaudemans, A.W.J.M.; Wouthuyzen-Bakker, M. 18F-FDG-PET uptake in non-infected total hip prostheses. *Acta Orthop.* **2018**, *89*, 634–639. [CrossRef]
54. Kagna, O.; Kurash, M.; Ghanem-Zoubi, N.; Keidar, Z.; Israel, O. Does Antibiotic Treatment Affect the Diagnostic Accuracy of 18F-FDG PET/CT Studies in Patients with Suspected Infectious Processes? *J. Nucl. Med.* **2017**, *58*, 1827–1830. [CrossRef]
55. Basu, S.; Kwee, T.C.; Saboury, B.; Garino, J.P.; Nelson, C.L.; Zhuang, H.; Parsons, M.; Chen, W.; Kumar, R.; Salavati, A.; et al. FDG PET for Diagnosing Infection in Hip and Knee Prostheses. *Clin. Nucl. Med.* **2014**, *39*, 609–615. [CrossRef]
56. Lauri, C.; Glaudemans, A.W.J.M.; Campagna, G.; Keidar, Z.; Muchnik Kurash, M.; Georga, S.; Arsos, G.; Noriega-Álvarez, E.; Argento, G.; Kwee, T.C.; et al. Comparison of White Blood Cell Scintigraphy, FDG PET/CT and MRI in Suspected Diabetic Foot Infection: Results of a Large Retrospective Multicenter Study. *J. Clin. Med.* **2020**, *9*, 1645. [CrossRef] [PubMed]
57. Vandenberghe, S.; Moskal, P.; Karp, J.S. State of the art in total body PET. *EJNMMI Phys.* **2020**, *7*, 1–33. [CrossRef] [PubMed]
58. Cherry, S.R.; Jones, T.; Karp, J.S.; Qi, J.; Moses, W.W.; Badawi, R.D. Total-Body PET: Maximizing Sensitivity to Create New Opportunities for Clinical Research and Patient Care. *J. Nucl. Med.* **2018**, *59*, 3–12. [CrossRef]
59. Diederich, S.; Lenzen, H. Radiation exposure associated with imaging of the chest: Comparison of different radiographic and computed tomography techniques. *Cancer* **2000**, *89*, 2457–2460. [CrossRef]
60. Auletta, S.; Varani, M.; Horvat, R.; Galli, F.; Signore, A.; Hess, S. PET Radiopharmaceuticals for Specific Bacteria Imaging: A Systematic Review. *J. Clin. Med.* **2019**, *8*, 197. [CrossRef] [PubMed]
61. Welling, M.M.; Hensbergen, A.W.; Bunschoten, A.; Velders, A.H.; Roestenberg, M.; Van Leeuwen, F.W.B. An update on radiotracer development for molecular imaging of bacterial infections. *Clin. Transl. Imaging* **2019**, *7*, 105–124. [CrossRef]
62. Gordon, O.; Ruiz-Bedoya, C.A.; Ordonez, A.A.; Tucker, E.W.; Jain, S.K. Molecular Imaging: A Novel Tool to Visualize Pathogenesis of Infections In Situ. *mBio* **2019**, *10*, e00317-19. [CrossRef]
63. Pickett, J.E.; Thompson, J.M.; Sadowska, A.; Tkaczyk, C.; Sellman, B.R.; Minola, A.; Corti, D.; Lanzavecchia, A.; Miller, L.S.; Thorek, D.L. Molecularly specific detection of bacterial lipoteichoic acid for diagnosis of prosthetic joint infection of the bone. *Bone Res.* **2018**, *6*, 13. [CrossRef] [PubMed]
64. Langer, O.; Brunner, M.; Zeitlinger, M.; Ziegler, S.; Dobrozemsky, G.; Lackner, E.; Joukhadar, C.; Mitterhauser, M.; Wadsak, W.; Minar, E.; et al. In vitro and in vivo evaluation of [18F]ciprofloxacin for the imaging of bacterial infections with PET. *Eur. J. Nucl. Med. Mol. Imaging* **2004**, *32*, 143–150. [CrossRef]
65. Sellmyer, M.A.; Lee, I.; Hou, C.; Weng, C.-C.; Li, S.; Lieberman, B.P.; Zeng, C.; Mankoff, D.A.; Mach, R.H. Bacterial Infection Imaging with [18F]Fluoropropyl-Trimethoprim. *Proc. Natl. Acad. Sci. USA* **2017**, *114*, 8372–8377. [CrossRef] [PubMed]
66. Ebenhan, T.; Sathekge, M.M.; Lengana, T.; Koole, M.; Gheysens, O.; Govender, T.; Zeevaart, J.R.; Lenagana, T. 68Ga-NOTA-Functionalized Ubiquicidin: Cytotoxicity, Biodistribution, Radiation Dosimetry, and First-in-Human PET/CT Imaging of Infections. *J. Nucl. Med.* **2017**, *59*, 334–339. [CrossRef] [PubMed]
67. Zhang, Z.; Ordonez, A.A.; Wang, H.; Li, Y.; Gogarty, K.R.; Weinstein, E.A.; Daryaee, F.; Merino, J.; Yoon, G.E.; Kalinda, A.S.; et al. Positron Emission Tomography Imaging with 2-[18F]F-p-Aminobenzoic Acid Detects Staphylococcus Aureus Infections and Monitors Drug Response. *ACS Infect. Dis.* **2018**, *4*, 1635–1644. [CrossRef]

8. Weinstein, E.A.; Ordonez, A.A.; Demarco, V.P.; Murawski, A.M.; Pokkali, S.; Macdonald, E.M.; Klunk, M.; Mease, R.C.; Pomper, M.G.; Jain, S.K. Imaging Enterobacteriaceae infection in vivo with 18F-fluorodeoxysorbitol positron emission tomography. *Sci. Transl. Med.* **2014**, *6*, 259ra146. [CrossRef]
9. Miller, L.; Winter, G.; Baur, B.; Witulla, B.; Solbach, C.; Reske, S.; Lindén, M. Synthesis, characterization, and biodistribution of multiple 89Zr-labeled pore-expanded mesoporous silica nanoparticles for PET. *Nanoscale* **2014**, *6*, 4928–4935. [CrossRef]
10. Rahmani, S.; Shahhoseini, S.; Mohamadi, R.; Vojdani, M. Synthesis, Quality Control and Stability Studies of 2-[18F]Fluoro-2-Deoxy-D-Glucose(18F-FDG) at Different Conditions of Temperature by Physicochemical and Microbiological Assays. *Iran. J. Pharm. Res. IJPR* **2017**, *16*, 602–610.
11. Martiniova, L.; De Palatis, L.; Etchebehere, E.; Ravizzini, G. Gallium-68 in Medical Imaging. *Curr. Radiopharm.* **2016**, *9*, 187–207. [CrossRef]
12. Ordonez, A.A.; Weinstein, E.A.; Bambarger, L.E.; Saini, V.; Chang, Y.S.; Demarco, V.P.; Klunk, M.H.; Urbanowski, M.E.; Moulton, K.L.; Murawski, A.M.; et al. A Systematic Approach for Developing Bacteria-Specific Imaging Tracers. *J. Nucl. Med.* **2016**, *58*, 144–150. [CrossRef]
13. Li, J.; Zheng, H.; Fodah, R.A.; Warawa, J.M.; Ng, C.K. Validation of 2-18F-Fluorodeoxysorbitol as a Potential Radiopharmaceutical for Imaging Bacterial Infection in the Lung. *J. Nucl. Med.* **2017**, *59*, 134–139. [CrossRef]
14. Moek, K.L.; Giesen, D.; Kok, I.C.; De Groot, D.J.A.; Jalving, M.; Fehrmann, R.S.; Hooge, M.N.L.-D.; Brouwers, A.H.; De Vries, E.G. Theranostics Using Antibodies and Antibody-Related Therapeutics. *J. Nucl. Med.* **2017**, *58*, 83S–90S. [CrossRef]
15. Schoenmakers, J.W.A.; Heuker, M.; López-Álvarez, M.; Nagengast, W.B.; Van Dam, G.M.; Van Dijl, J.M.; Jutte, P.C.; Van Oosten, M. Image-guided in situ detection of bacterial biofilms in a human prosthetic knee infection model: A feasibility study for clinical diagnosis of prosthetic joint infections. *Eur. J. Nucl. Med. Mol. Imaging* **2020**, 1–11. [CrossRef]
16. Lau, J.S.Y.; Kiss, C.; Roberts, E.; Horne, K.; Korman, T.M.; Woolley, I.J. Surveillance of life-long antibiotics: A review of antibiotic prescribing practices in an Australian Healthcare Network. *Ann. Clin. Microbiol. Antimicrob.* **2017**, *16*, 3. [CrossRef] [PubMed]
17. Lau, J.S.Y.; Korman, T.M.; Woolley, I. Life-long antimicrobial therapy: Where is the evidence? *J. Antimicrob. Chemother.* **2018**, *73*, 2601–2612. [CrossRef] [PubMed]
18. Perng, P.; Marcus, C.; Subramaniam, R.M. (18)F-FDG PET/CT and Melanoma: Staging, Immune Modulation and Mutation-Targeted Therapy Assessment, and Prognosis. *AJR Am. J. Roentgenol.* **2015**, *205*, 259–270. [CrossRef] [PubMed]
19. Mayr, A.; Aigner, M.; Lass-Flörl, C. Anidulafungin for the treatment of invasive candidiasis. *Clin. Microbiol. Infect.* **2011**, *17* (Suppl. 1), 1–12. [CrossRef]

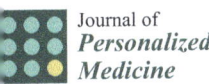

Review

Nuclear Medicine Imaging in Neuroblastoma: Current Status and New Developments

Atia Samim [1,2], Godelieve A.M. Tytgat [1], Gitta Bleeker [3], Sylvia T.M. Wenker [1,2], Kristell L.S. Chatalic [1,2], Alex J. Poot [1,2], Nelleke Tolboom [1,2], Max M. van Noesel [1], Marnix G.E.H. Lam [2] and Bart de Keizer [1,2,*]

1. Princess Maxima Center for Pediatric Oncology, Heidelberglaan 25, 3584 CS Utrecht, The Netherlands; a.samim-4@prinsesmaximacentrum.nl (A.S.); g.a.m.tytgat@prinsesmaximacentrum.nl (G.A.M.T.); S.T.M.Wenker-3@prinsesmaximacentrum.nl (S.T.M.W.); k.l.s.chatalic@umcutrecht.nl (K.L.S.C.); a.j.poot@umcutrecht.nl (A.J.P.); n.tolboom@umcutrecht.nl (N.T.); m.m.vannoesel@prinsesmaximacentrum.nl (M.M.v.N.)
2. Department of Radiology and Nuclear Medicine, University Medical Center Utrecht/Wilhelmina Children's Hospital, Heidelberglaan 100, 3584 CX Utrecht, The Netherlands; m.lam@umcutrecht.nl
3. Department of Radiology and Nuclear Medicine, Northwest Clinics, Wilhelminalaan 12, 1815 JD Alkmaar, The Netherlands; gbleeker78@gmail.com
* Correspondence: b.dekeizer@umcutrecht.nl; Tel.: +31-887-571-794

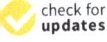

Abstract: Neuroblastoma is the most common extracranial solid malignancy in children. At diagnosis, approximately 50% of patients present with metastatic disease. These patients are at high risk for refractory or recurrent disease, which conveys a very poor prognosis. During the past decades, nuclear medicine has been essential for the staging and response assessment of neuroblastoma. Currently, the standard nuclear imaging technique is *meta*-[^{123}I]iodobenzylguanidine ([^{123}I]mIBG) whole-body scintigraphy, usually combined with single-photon emission computed tomography with computed tomography (SPECT-CT). Nevertheless, 10% of neuroblastomas are mIBG non-avid and [^{123}I]mIBG imaging has relatively low spatial resolution, resulting in limited sensitivity for smaller lesions. More accurate methods to assess full disease extent are needed in order to optimize treatment strategies. Advances in nuclear medicine have led to the introduction of radiotracers compatible for positron emission tomography (PET) imaging in neuroblastoma, such as [^{124}I]mIBG, [^{18}F]mFBG, [^{18}F]FDG, [^{68}Ga]Ga-DOTA peptides, [^{18}F]F-DOPA, and [^{11}C]mHED. PET has multiple advantages over SPECT, including a superior resolution and whole-body tomographic range. This article reviews the use, characteristics, diagnostic accuracy, advantages, and limitations of current and new tracers for nuclear medicine imaging in neuroblastoma.

Keywords: neuroblastoma; nuclear medicine; radionuclide imaging; [^{123}I]mIBG; [^{124}I]mIBG; [^{18}F]mFBG; [^{18}F]FDG; [^{68}Ga]Ga-DOTA peptides; [^{18}F]F-DOPA; [^{11}C]mHED

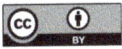

1. Introduction

1.1. Neuroblastoma

Neuroblastoma is the most common extracranial solid malignancy in children and more than 95% of patients are younger than 10 years of age. It is responsible for approximately 15% of all cancer deaths in children [1]. As an embryonic tumor derived from the sympathoadrenal lineage of the neural crest, neuroblastoma is classified as a neuroendocrine tumor. It can arise anywhere along the sympathetic trunk or adrenal medulla but most primary tumors are found in the abdomen (70%) [2]. About 50% of patients present with distant metastasis, which most commonly involves bone marrow, bone, and lymph nodes and less frequently involves the liver and skin [2,3].

Tumor stage is defined by the presurgical International Neuroblastoma Risk Group Staging System (INRGSS) [4] and the postsurgical International Neuroblastoma Staging System (INSS) [5]. Stage is the most important prognostic factor [6,7]. Other risk factors include age $\geq$ 18 months and unfavorable histopathological and/or biological features of the tumor [8].

The clinical course of disease is highly variable and ranges from spontaneous tumor regression to aggressive disease with fatal tumor progression. Despite intensive multimodality treatment, long-term survival of patients with high-risk neuroblastoma, comprising more than half of patients, is approximately 40% [9,10] and less than 20% in patients with refractory or relapsed disease [11,12].

1.2. Diagnostic Imaging

Radiological and nuclear medicine imaging are essential for the staging of neuroblastoma at diagnosis, along with the monitoring of treatment response and surveillance of any recurrent disease during follow-up. Radiological imaging of the chest, abdomen, and pelvis is required for morphological characterization of the primary tumor and to assess locoregional disease extent, such as soft tissue metastases and image-defined risk factors (IDRFs) representing the tumor's relationship to adjacent vital structures [13]. Magnetic resonance imaging (MRI) is generally preferred over contrast-enhanced computed tomography (CT) due to its lack of radiation, higher soft tissue contrast resolution, and superior visualization of intraspinal extension [14].

For the detection of metastases in neuroblastoma, meta-$[^{123}I]$iodobenzylguanidine ($[^{123}I]$mIBG) planar whole-body scintigraphy is the current standard nuclear imaging technique. The addition of single-photon emission computed tomography with computed tomography (SPECT-CT) to planar scintigraphy has become standard in gamma camera imaging. SPECT-CT increases the certainty of interpretation and anatomical localization of small focal uptake [15–17].

1.3. Advances in Nuclear Imaging

With metastatic disease being an important prognostic factor, more accurate diagnostic methods for the assessment of disease extent are needed in order to optimize treatment strategies. Neuroblastomas express various molecular targets for nuclear medicine imaging. Several new tracers have been introduced that are compatible with positron emission tomography (PET) imaging in neuroblastoma, such as $[^{124}I]$mIBG, $[^{18}F]$mFBG, $[^{18}F]$FDG, $[^{68}Ga]$Ga-DOTA peptides, $[^{18}F]$F-DOPA, and $[^{11}C]$mHED.

PET imaging has multiple advantages over SPECT imaging [18,19]. First, PET has a higher spatial resolution and tumor-to-background contrast, enabling better detection of smaller lesions and better delineation of lesions. Second, PET is more suitable for quantification of tracer uptake, measured either as the standardized uptake value (SUV) or a percentage of the injected dose per unit volume. Third, PET enables whole-body tomographic reconstruction as opposed to the limited ($\pm$40 cm axial) field-of-view of SPECT. Fourth, PET acquisition is much faster ($\pm$15 min) compared to SPECT and scintigraphy ($\pm$90 min) [18,20]. This advantage is especially important for pediatric applications because a shorter scan time reduces the number and length of sedations and motion artifacts. Lastly, most PET-radioisotopes allow for same-day tracer administration and image acquisition.

This comprehensive review discusses the use, characteristics, diagnostic accuracy, and (dis)advantages of current and new tracers in the management of neuroblastoma.

2. $[^{123}I]$mIBG

2.1. Uptake and Biodistribution

$[^{123}I]$mIBG is meta-iodobenzylguanidine (mIBG), a norepinephrine analogue, labeled with gamma-emitting iodine-123 (^{123}I). mIBG is taken up by the sympathicomedullary tissue via the norepinephrine transporter (NET), referred to as the uptake-1 system, and stored in neurosecretory granules [21]. As immature neuroblastoma cells contain few storage granules, mIBG is predominantly stored in the cytoplasm [22]. Physiological activity is seen in the liver, salivary glands, thyroid (if not blocked), nasal mucosa, gallbladder, myocardium, brown adipose tissue, adrenals, and urinary system (including the bladder). Occasionally, low diffuse activity is present in the colon, lungs, lacrimal glands, and spleen [20]. mIBG is not metabolized after administration and is almost entirely excreted by the kidneys via glomerular filtration. About 50% is excreted within the first 24 h after administration and 90% within 4 days [21].

2.2. Indication

For over 30 years, radiolabeled mIBG with either iodine-131 (^{131}I) or ^{123}I has been used as a tumor-specific agent for the imaging (and therapy) of neural crest tumors, such as neuroblastoma (including ganglioneuroblastoma), pheochromocytoma/paraganglioma, medullary thyroid carcinoma, and carcinoids [23]. The majority (90%) of neuroblastomas overexpress NET and actively accumulate mIBG [24].

For diagnostic imaging, [^{123}I]mIBG is preferred over [^{131}I]mIBG because [^{123}I]mIBG provides better image quality at a lower radiation dose. [^{123}I]mIBG has more favorable dosimetric properties compared to [^{131}I]mIBG, including shorter half-life (13 h vs. 8 days), lower energy gamma emission (159 keV vs. 364 keV), and a lack of beta emission [23]. Therefore, [^{123}I]mIBG scintigraphy is the first-line nuclear imaging used for the initial staging of neuroblastoma, monitoring of response, surveillance for recurrent disease during follow-up, and selection of eligible patients for [^{131}I]mIBG radionuclide therapy [18,25].

2.3. Preparation

Antihypertensive agents, calcium channel blockers, sympathomimetics, central nervous system stimulants, tricyclic antidepressants, antipsychotics, antihistamines, and opioid analgesics are known to interfere with mIBG uptake. It is important to avoid these drugs (at least four times the biologic half-life) prior to [^{123}I]mIBG imaging. Furthermore, thyroid-blocking medication is necessary to prevent the uptake and irradiation of the thyroid gland due to the presence of small amounts of free radioactive iodine [18].

Slow intravenous administration of [^{123}I]mIBG over 1–5 min is recommended to avoid rare adverse reactions such as hypertension, tachycardia, nausea, and pallor. Planar whole-body scintigraphy, preferably with additional SPECT-CT, is performed 20–24 h after tracer administration. For all tracers that are renally excreted, voiding prior to imaging is important to limit radiation exposure to the bladder and enable adequate evaluation of the pelvis. Due to the long acquisition times (±90 min), sedation or general anesthesia is often necessary in young children [18].

2.4. Image Interpretation

Tracer uptake beyond the normal physiological distribution, for instance, any osteomedullary uptake, should be taken into consideration as pathological uptake [20]. One unequivocal mIBG-positive lesion at a distant site is sufficient to define metastatic disease, whereas one equivocal lesion requires confirmation by another imaging modality and/or biopsy [13]. Correlation of [^{123}I]mIBG imaging with radiological imaging is important, as combined analysis has shown to increase diagnostic accuracy for lesion detection [26].

2.5. Prognostic Scoring Systems

There are two widely used semiquantitative scoring systems that provide a standardized evaluation of the involvement of body segments on mIBG scintigraphy (Figure 1): The Curie score [27] and the International Society of Pediatric Oncology Europe Neuroblastoma (SIOPEN) score [28]. Large international clinical trials have shown that both scoring systems are equally reliable as prognostic indicators with respect to outcome (overall and event-free survival) [9,28,29]. Persisting metastatic disease at the end of induction chemotherapy is of great prognostic significance. Postinduction scores (Curie > 2 and SIOPEN > 3) can identify patients with a very poor outcome who require alternative treatment strategies [9,30,31].

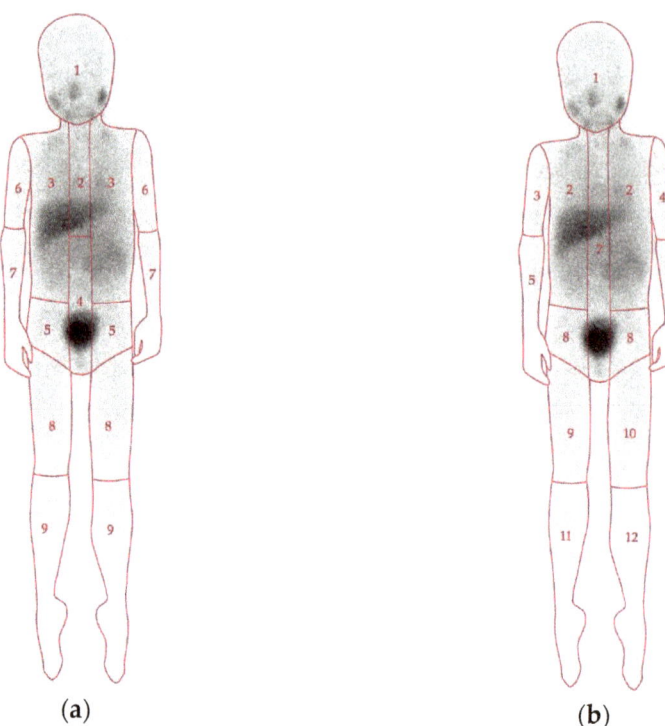

Figure 1. Scoring systems for mIBG scintigraphy. The Curie score (**a**) consists of 9 osteomedullary segments and a 10th soft tissue segment. Each segment is graded as: 0, no involvement; 1, one distinct lesion; 2, two or more distinct lesions; or 3, >50% involvement [27]. The International Society of Pediatric Oncology Europe Neuroblastoma Group (SIOPEN) score (**b**) consists of 12 osteomedullary segments. Each segment is graded as: 0, no involvement; 1, one distinct lesion; 2, two distinct lesions; 3, three distinct lesions; 4, four or more distinct lesions or <50% involvement; 5, >50% involvement; or 6, >95% diffuse involvement [28].

2.6. Diagnostic Accuracy

[^{123}I]mIBG imaging (scintigraphy and SPECT-CT) has high sensitivity and specificity (both around 90%) for neuroblastoma [24,32]. False-negative results can be a result of pharmacological interference.

However, without pharmacological interference, approximately 10% of neuroblastomas fail to accumulate mIBG [24,33,34]. This is the result of either insufficient NET expression or a modified mIBG uptake mechanism [35] of which the exact determinants are unclear. One of the possible explanations is tumor cell dedifferentiation, which has been supported to some extent by available studies [33–37]. However, this has not been confirmed. Patients with mIBG-negative disease are known to have superior outcomes compared to patients with mIBG-positive disease [30,36], and low mIBG uptake has been associated with tumors with low proliferative activity [33] Mixed patterns of both mIBG-positive and mIBG-negative disease may be present within the same patient or tumor [34]. Moreover, cases have been described of initially mIBG-positive tumors that were mIBG-negative at relapse [38,39] and vice versa [40]. Loss of mIBG uptake during treatment is of great concern because of the subsequent risk of missing any recurrent disease.

It is known that more differentiated neuroblastic tumors may likewise accumulate mIBG. Neuroblastoma lesions can mature to benign ganglioneuromas in response to chemotherapy and may remain mIBG-positive [41], although approximately 30% of ganglioneuromas are mIBG-negative [33,42]. In addition, rare benign uptake can occur in atelectasis, pneumonia, focal nodular hyperplasia, radiation injury of the liver, splenunculi, focal pyelonephritis, and vascular malformations [20]. Lastly, lesions in or close to areas of high physiological uptake may be missed. Physiological liver uptake is known to cause difficulty in identifying liver metastases.

2.7. Advantages and Limitations

Unlike MRI, [^{123}I]mIBG imaging is unaffected by posttreatment changes, which contributes to the high specificity in the assessment of treatment response. Moreover, [^{123}I]mIBG imaging can select eligible patients with mIBG-avid disease for [^{131}I]mIBG therapy [25]. However, [^{123}I]mIBG imaging has several limitations, such as limited spatial resolution, limited sensitivity for small lesions, prolonged acquisition sessions, limited tomographic field-of-view, need for pharmacological thyroid protection, and inconvenience of a 2-days schedule [18].

3. [^{124}I]mIBG

3.1. Uptake and Biodistribution

mIBG imaging is also possible with PET radioisotope iodine-124 (^{124}I). [^{124}I]mIBG has a similar uptake mechanism and biodistribution to [^{123}I]mIBG.

3.2. Indication

Only few reports have described the use of [^{124}I]mIBG imaging in neuroblastoma concerning preclinical studies [43,44] and experimental studies in a total of eleven patients with neuroblastoma [45–47]. These reports studied the role of [^{124}I]mIBG PET-CT for diagnostic imaging, as well as for dosimetric purposes before [^{131}I]mIBG therapy.

3.3. Preparation

[^{124}I]mIBG PET-CT has a similar preparation to [^{123}I]mIBG imaging. PET-CT can be performed 1 day after tracer administration but also at later timepoints because of the long physical half-life of ^{124}I (4.2 days). However, no recommended dose or optimal timing for acquisition have yet been established.

3.4. Diagnostic Accuracy

Cistaro et al. (2015) was the first to report the use of [^{124}I]mIBG PET-CT in two patients with metastatic neuroblastoma. [^{124}I]mIBG PET-CT detected more osteomedullary lesions in comparison to mIBG scintigraphy [45]. The most important limitation of diagnostic [^{124}I]mIBG imaging, especially in the pediatric population, is the high radiation exposure. The effective dose (mSv/MBq) of [^{124}I]mIBG is estimated to be approximately 20-times higher than that of [^{123}I]mIBG for a 70 kg adult, and even up to 30-times higher for children under the age of 5 years [44,48]. Beijst et al. (2017) suggested that the administered [^{124}I]mIBG activity could be limited to 10-times lower while maintaining an acceptable quality [44]. This was recently demonstrated by Aboian et al. (2020) in eight patients with neuroblastoma. With a lower dose, [^{124}I]mIBG PET-CT still detected significant more lesions as compared to [^{123}I]mIBG scintigraphy and SPECT-CT [47]. However, the effective doses of [^{124}I]mIBG were still much higher: 15.5 mSv for a 63 kg child and 19.1 mSv for a 23 kg child, as compared to those calculated for [^{123}I]mIBG: 4.7 mSv and 5.8 mSv, respectively (EANM dosage card version 01.02.2014 [49]).

3.5. Advantages and Limitations

[^{124}I]mIBG was first investigated for the purpose of dosimetry before [^{131}I]mIBG therapy [48,50], for which the additional radiation dose is neglectable [45]. The whole-body tomographic capability of PET imaging and relatively long half-life of ^{124}I, similar to ^{131}I, could provide a more personalized adjustment of administered [^{131}I]mIBG activity to normal organs and tumor tissue. The feasibility of using [^{124}I]mIBG PET for personalized dosimetry estimation for [^{131}I]mIBG therapy was demonstrated in a neuroblastoma patient by Huang et al. (2015) [46].

Apart from the high radiation exposure for diagnostic purposes, [^{124}I]mIBG has several other limitations. The complex decay scheme of ^{124}I, with a positron abundance of only 23%, results in a relatively poorer image quality, compared to fluorine-18 (^{18}F) or gallium-68 (^{68}Ga)-labeled radiotracers [51]. Moreover, cyclotron-produced [^{124}I]mIBG is not widely available for clinical use, which is accompanied by high costs and lack of experience. There is still need for pharmacological thyroid protection and the inconvenience of a 2-days imaging schedule.

4. [^{18}F]mFBG

4.1. Uptake and Biodistribution

meta-[^{18}F]Fluorobenzylguanidine ([^{18}F]mFBG) is the fluorinated analog of mIBG, labeled with PET radioisotope ^{18}F. [^{18}F]mFBG accumulates in cells via the same norepinephrine transporter uptake mechanism as [^{123}I]mIBG, with a biodistribution similar to that of [^{123}I]mIBG. However, the more hydrophilic [^{18}F]mFBG has the advantage of much faster tissue uptake and renal clearance. One hour after administration, 45% of the administered activity is already excreted, and after 3–4 h, up to 95% [52,53]. A preclinical study by Zhang et al. (2014) reported that tumor uptake of [^{18}F]mFBG was three-times higher than [^{123}I]mIBG in vivo [52].

4.2. Indication

[^{18}F]mFBG is a new experimental tracer developed for diagnostic PET imaging of NET-expressing tumors. The use of [^{18}F]mFBG has only been reported in eleven human cases, five of which were patients with neuroblastoma [53,54].

4.3. Preparation

Due to limited experience, no recommended dose or optimal timing for acquisition have been established. Acquisition 1–2 h after [^{18}F]mFBG administration has been proposed [53]. In contrast to [^{123}I]mIBG there is no need for pharmacological thyroid protection due to the absence of radioactive iodine.

4.4. Diagnostic Accuracy

Pandit-Taskar et al. (2018) conducted the first human study on [^{18}F]mFBG in five patients with neuroblastoma and five patients with pheochromocytoma/paraganglioma [53]. [^{18}F]mFBG PET-CT detected all 63 lesions detected on [^{123}I]mIBG imaging (scintigraphy and SPECT-CT) and 59 additional lesions.

4.5. Advantages and Limitations

Besides the general advantages of PET imaging compared to scintigraphy/SPECT (Figure 2), the radioisotope ^{18}F has an ideal half-life of 110 min, which allows for 1-day imaging. [^{18}F]mFBG PET-CT was found to be safe and feasible [53]. Despite the shorter physical half-life of ^{18}F and biologic half-life of [^{18}F]mFBG, radiation exposure is comparable to that of [^{123}I]mIBG, because of the high-energy ^{18}F emissions [52]. Disadvantages of cyclotron-produced [^{18}F]mFBG are the limited availability and lack of experience.

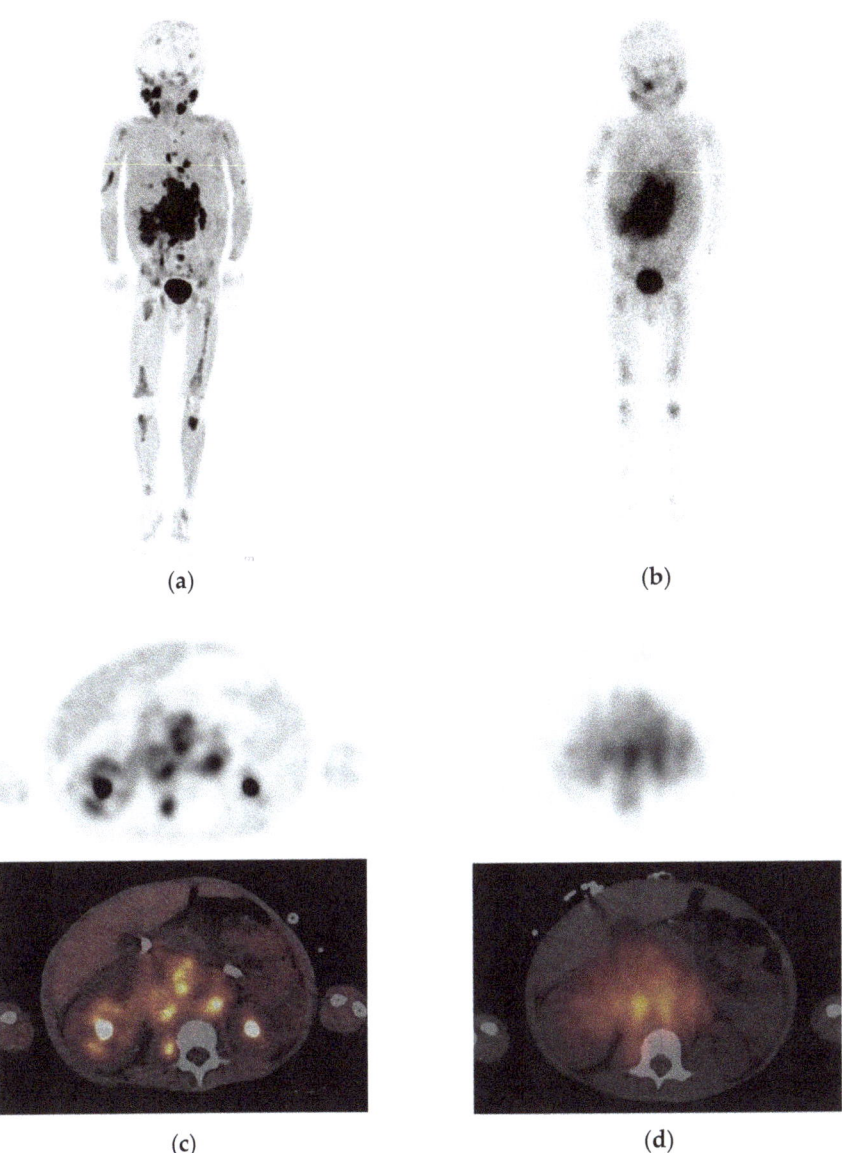

Figure 2. Example of a neuroblastoma patient with extensive metastasis who underwent [^{123}I]mIBG and [^{18}F]mFBG imaging within 1 day. These figures illustrate the superior image quality and tumor delineation of (**a**) [^{18}F]mFBG PET maximum intensity projection and (**c**) axial PET-CT due to higher spatial resolution, higher tumor-to-background contrast, and improved counting statistics compared to (**b**) [^{123}I]mIBG planar scintigraphy and (**d**) axial single-photon emission computed tomography with computed tomography (SPECT-CT).

5. [^{18}F]FDG

5.1. Uptake and Biodistribution

[^{18}F]Fluorodeoxyglucose ([^{18}F]FDG) is a glucose analogue labeled with the PET radioisotope ^{18}F. As a metabolic compound, [^{18}F]FDG uptake reflects anatomical locations with high glucose metabolism. [^{18}F]FDG is transported into the cell via passive glucose transporters and intracellularly phosphorylated by hexokinase into [^{18}F]FDG-6-phosphate. Unlike glucose-6-phosphate, [^{18}F]FDG-6-phosphate cannot be dephosphorylated or further metabolized in the glycolytic process and steadily accumulates in metabolically active cells [55].

Physiological activity is seen in the brain, salivary glands, Waldeyer's ring, myocardium, thymus, brown adipose tissue, liver, spleen, and gastrointestinal tract. [^{18}F]FDG is excreted by the kidneys. Therefore, the urinary system shows prominent activity. Physiological bone marrow activity in children is variable, but flat and symmetrical uptake is usually present in epiphyseal growth plates [56].

5.2. Indication

Malignant tissues strongly accumulate [^{18}F]FDG because of an increased glucose metabolism rate [56]. [^{18}F]FDG PET-CT is increasingly used in pediatric malignancies, including neuroblastoma. Several studies have confirmed that the majority of neuroblastoma lesions concentrate [^{18}F]FDG [57–62]. [^{18}F]FDG frequently accumulates in mIBG non-avid neuroblastoma due to a different uptake mechanism that is not dependent on NET expression [32,58], [^{18}F]FDG is the only PET-tracer that has been recommended by the current guidelines for the following two indications [18]. First, as a replacement of [^{123}I]mIBG in the evaluation of mIBG-negative or weakly mIBG-positive neuroblastoma, and second, as complementary modality when radiological imaging or clinical findings suggest more extensive disease than is revealed by [^{123}I]mIBG imaging. [^{18}F]FDG has taken over the role of technetium-99m (^{99m}Tc) skeletal scintigraphy, which has long been the second-line imaging to assess bone metastases in mIBG-negative tumors or in the case of solitary equivocal mIBG bone uptake [63,64].

5.3. Preparation

Regarding interactions with [^{18}F]FDG, there is only evidence for interaction with glucose. Fasting and discontinuing any intravenous glucose administration is recommended for at least 4 h prior to [^{18}F]FDG administration [18]. Right before administration, blood glucose levels should be below 7 mmol/L. To prevent physiological [^{18}F]FDG uptake by brown adipose tissue and peripheral muscles, it is important to let the patient rest in a warm environment. Some centers use additional premedication such as propranolol prior to [^{18}F]FDG administration [65]. Acquisition is generally started 60 min postadministration.

5.4. Diagnostic Accuracy

Overall, most studies have reported that [^{18}F]FDG PET cannot replace [^{123}I]mIBG imaging in mIBG avid neuroblastoma due to lower sensitivity and specificity, especially for osteomedullary lesions, the most frequent site of metastases [57,58,60,61,66]. This is in contrast with the study of Kushner et al. (2001) in 51 high-risk neuroblastoma patients, who suggested that, in the absence of skull lesions and after primary tumor resection, [^{18}F]FDG PET and bone marrow sampling would suffice for disease monitoring in high-risk patients [62]. There is evidence that [^{18}F]FDG may be superior in localized neuroblastoma due to better depiction of locoregional soft tissue disease [57,66]. All studies conjointly support the value of the [^{18}F]FDG PET in mIBG non-avid neuroblastoma and the complementary role in case of discrepant findings between mIBG imaging and radiological/clinical findings. Melzer et al. (2011) demonstrated the complementary role of [^{18}F]FDG PET to [^{123}I]mIBG imaging (scintigraphy and SPECT) in 19 patients with [^{123}I]mIBG non-avid tumors or discrepant findings. [^{18}F]FDG PET correctly identified 32 out of 34 discrepant lesions. In this setting, [^{18}F]FDG PET was more sensitive (78% vs. 50%) and specific (92% vs. 75%) than [^{123}I]mIBG imaging for the detection of neuroblastoma lesions [59].

It is important to realize that [^{18}F]FDG-positive and [^{123}I]mIBG-negative lesions (and vice versa) can coexist in the same patient [67–69]. When [^{123}I]mIBG uptake is absent or lost during disease course, [^{18}F]FDG may still show pathological uptake. Generally, poorly differentiated tumors tend to show high [^{18}F]FDG uptake due to high glucose metabolism [38]. On the other hand, persisting posttherapy [^{123}I]mIBG activity but normal

[^{18}F]FDG distribution is also possible [70,71]. This may indicate that the tumor has matured to a benign ganglioneuroma, which can be confirmed by biopsy [66].

By reflecting increased metabolism, [^{18}F]FDG is not a tumor-specific agent. [^{18}F]FDG can therefore accumulate in nonmalignant lesions, as often seen in infection/inflammation [56]. Misinterpretation can be minimized by correlation with radiological imaging and a complete clinical history. Nevertheless, false-positive results are relatively common. Increased bone marrow activity can be seen in physiological bone marrow hyperplasia, which can be the result of chemotherapy or granulocyte colony-stimulating factor treatment [56]. On [^{18}F]FDG PET, this is generally seen as diffuse activity, but focal activity is also possible, which may mimic metastatic bone marrow disease [57,58,60]. Therefore, [^{18}F]FDG PET imaging is less optimal for assessment of treatment response of osteomedullary lesions.

Also, not all neuroblastoma lesions show elevated [^{18}F]FDG activity, causing false-negative results of lesions with slow metabolic activity or necrosis. Furthermore, [^{18}F]FDG is associated with the impaired detection of small lesions in the bone marrow and skull because of the presence of (nearby) physiological activity [60,62,66].

5.5. Advantages and Limitations

A major advantage of [^{18}F]FDG PET-CT is that it is widely available. Moreover, several studies have reported that more prominent [^{18}F]FDG activity (SUV_{max}) of primary tumor and metastases is significantly correlated with decreased survival [60,72–75]. Therefore, [^{18}F]FDG uptake may assist in the identification of patients with poor prognosis.

6. [^{68}Ga]Ga-DOTA Peptides

6.1. Uptake and Biodistribution

Gallium-68 (^{68}Ga)-labeled DOTA-Tyr^3-octreotate (DOTATATE), DOTA-Tyr^3-octreotide (DOTATOC), and DOTA-Nal^3-octreotide (DOTANOC) are somatostatin analogues that are compatible with PET imaging. The five subtypes of somatostatin receptors (SSTR1–SSTR5) are expressed by many cells, mainly of the central and peripheral nervous system, endocrine glands, and gastrointestinal tract [76].

High physiological activity of [^{68}Ga]Ga-DOTA peptides is seen in the spleen, adrenal glands, liver, kidneys, urinary system, and pituitary, and moderate uptake in the salivary glands, thyroid, pancreas, and gastrointestinal tract. Uptake in the pancreas is often heterogenous and low-grade uptake, but prominent uptake may occur in the uncinate process. Within 4 h, all the administered activity is excreted, almost entirely by renal clearance [18,77–79].

[^{68}Ga]Ga-DOTA peptides have different affinity profiles for SSTR subtypes, which may lead to small differences in biodistribution. Whereas the affinity profile of [^{68}Ga]Ga-DOTATATE is limited to SSTR2, [^{68}Ga]Ga-DOTATOC and [^{68}Ga]Ga-DOTANOC have a wider receptor binding profile. [^{68}Ga]Ga-DOTATOC has high affinity for SSTR2 and SSTR5 and [^{68}Ga]Ga-DOTANOC for SSTR2, SSTR3, and SSTR5. Clinical choice of a particular [^{68}Ga]Ga-DOTA peptide is often driven by local availability because diagnostic performance appears to be comparable [77,80,81].

6.2. Indication

In particular, SSTR2 is highly expressed by neuroendocrine tumors such as gastroenteropancreatic neuroendocrine tumors, pheochromocytoma/paragangliomas [76], and most neuroblastomas (60–90%) [37,82–84]. High SSTR2 expression is mainly seen in more differentiated neuroblastoma [37]. [^{68}Ga]Ga-DOTA peptide imaging (and peptide receptor radionuclide therapy [PRRT]) is already well established in adult patients with SSTR-positive neuroendocrine tumors [77]. Despite increasing off-label use in mIBG non-avid neuroblastoma, there is still no established role for [^{68}Ga]Ga-DOTA peptide imaging in current guidelines.

6.3. Preparation

Somatostatin analog therapy may interfere with tracer distribution. Although evidence is lacking, it is recommended to avoid all short- and long-acting somatostatin agents. Acquisition is typically started 60 (range: 45–90) minutes after tracer administration [18].

6.4. Diagnostic Accuracy

The limited studies in patients with neuroblastoma suggest a higher sensitivity for lesion detection of [^{68}Ga]Ga-DOTA peptide imaging compared to [^{123}I]mIBG imaging.

Kroiss et al. (2011) compared [^{68}Ga]Ga-DOTATOC PET with [^{123}I]mIBG imaging (scintigraphy and SPECT) in four patients with neuroblastoma. [^{68}Ga]Ga-DOTATOC PET detected a total of 132 lesions, and [^{123}I]mIBG imaging detected 100 lesions. It is unknown whether [^{68}Ga]Ga-DOTATOC PET detected all lesions found on [^{123}I]mIBG imaging. Of the 107 lesions identified on CT/MRI, [^{68}Ga]Ga-DOTATOC PET detected 104 lesions (97.2%, $p < 0.0001$) and [^{123}I]mIBG SPECT detected 97 lesions (90.7%, $p < 0.09$) [85].

Kong et al. (2016) compared [^{68}Ga]Ga-DOTATATE PET-CT to mIBG imaging (pretreatment [^{123}I]mIBG scintigraphy and SPECT-CT or posttreatment [^{131}I]mIBG scintigraphy and SPECT) in eight patients with refractory neuroblastoma [86]. [^{68}Ga]Ga-DOTATATE uptake and immunohistological SSTR2 staining were positive in all patients and tumor samples, respectively. Even the smallest sub-centimeter lesions showed high tumor-to-background contrast and high SUV values. In three patients, [^{68}Ga]Ga-DOTATATE PET-CT identified additional disease compared to mIBG imaging. However, in two of these three patients, the time between paired scans was about 10 weeks. One patient underwent biopsy of a bone marrow lesion, which was histologically confirmed to be metastasis. Several tumor samples only showed mild SSTR2 staining but high uptake on [^{68}Ga]Ga-DOTATATE imaging. The authors postulated that the samples may have been collected from a tissue area with a lower expression and density of SSTR2.

Gains et al. (2020) compared [^{68}Ga]Ga-DOTATATE PET maximum intensity projection (MIP) images to [^{123}I]mIBG planar scintigraphy in 42 high-risk neuroblastoma patients. [^{68}Ga]Ga-DOTATATE was positive in all patients, whereas [^{123}I]mIBG was positive in 40 patients. [^{68}Ga]Ga-DOTATATE identified bone lesions in 97% (35/36) of the patients vs. 81% (29/36) for [^{123}I]mIBG and identified soft-tissue lesions in 100% (33/33) vs. 88% (29/33) of patients, respectively. Seven patients had [^{68}Ga]Ga-DOTATATE-positive bone lesions with negative [^{123}I]mIBG scans, whereas only one patient had [^{123}I]mIBG-positive bone lesions and a negative [^{68}Ga]Ga-DOTATATE PET. SIOPEN scores for [^{68}Ga]Ga-DOTATATE were significantly higher compared to [^{123}I]mIBG. [^{68}Ga]Ga-DOTATATE detected more (osteomedullary and soft tissue) lesions than [^{123}I]mIBG in 31–52% of patients, whereas [^{123}I]mIBG detected more lesions than [^{68}Ga]Ga-DOTATATE in 5% of patients [87].

With completely negative or weakly positive [^{123}I]mIBG imaging, extensive metastatic disease on [^{68}Ga]Ga-DOTA peptide imaging may be present (Figure 3). This has been described by several cases of neuroblastoma patients [79,88,89]. On the other hand, [^{68}Ga]Ga-DOTA peptide imaging may be negative in tumors with low SSTR expression, more likely seen in poorly differentiated tumors [90].

Physiological tracer distribution can potentially mask small-volume disease, for instance, when liver metastases show a similar degree of tracer accumulation to the normal liver. As SSTR uptake is not specific for tumoral pathologies, false-positive results can occur. Splenunculi or benign meningiomas may mimic focal metastatic disease. Uptake, usually low-grade, can be seen at sites of inflammation/infection, postradiotherapy changes, and osteoblastic activity (fractures, vertebral hemangioma, or epiphyseal growth plates) [78].

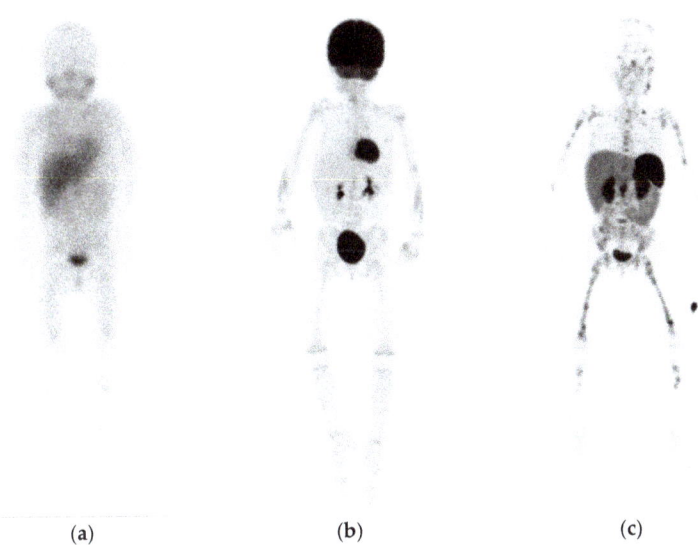

(a) (b) (c)

Figure 3. Example of a patient with neuroblastoma, showing diffuse pathological but faint osteomedullary uptake on planar [^{123}I]mIBG scintigraphy (**a**), without increased uptake on [^{18}F]FDG positron emission tomography (PET) maximum intensity projections (MIP) (**b**), but extensive pathological osteomedullary uptake on [^{68}Ga]Ga-DOTATATE PET MIP (**c**). Note the different physiological distribution between tracers.

6.5. Advantages and Limitations

First, [^{68}Ga]Ga-DOTA peptide imaging has shown to be safe and feasible in pediatric patients [18,79]. ^{68}Ga is derived from generators and, therefore, more easily available and practical for centers that do not have cyclotrons. Its short half-life (68 min) allows for 1-day imaging and results in a lower radiation exposure than [^{123}I]- and [^{18}F]-labeled tracers [18,91].

Second, [^{68}Ga]Ga-DOTA peptide uptake can have prognostic value. Low uptake has been shown to be an indicator of poor prognosis in adults with neuroendocrine tumors [92–94], but this has not been studied in neuroblastoma. Nevertheless, higher SSTR2 expression is correlated with higher [^{68}Ga]Ga-DOTATATE uptake [94]. Several studies found that higher SSTR2 expression is strongly associated with non-high-risk and differentiated neuroblastoma, and lack of SSTR expression has been found to correlate with advanced disease and decreased survival [82,90,95–97], while others did not find any prognostic relation [37].

Third, confirmation of [^{68}Ga]Ga-DOTA peptide uptake can be used to identify potential candidates for peptide receptor radionuclide therapy (PRRT) by replacing ^{68}Ga with lutetium-177 (^{177}Lu) [94]. The safety and feasibility of PRRT has been demonstrated in small groups of patients with refractory or relapsed neuroblastoma [86,98,99]. Gains et al. (2011) demonstrated that six out of eight patients with relapsed or refractory neuroblastoma showed sufficient [^{68}Ga]Ga-DOTATATE uptake (higher than the liver) to be treated with experimental [^{177}Lu]Lu-DOTATATE [98]. Recently, the same authors conducted a phase II trial, which was unfortunately terminated prematurely due to a lack of objective response and dose-limiting toxicity in one of the patients [100].

Last, along with the general advantages of PET imaging, [^{68}Ga]Ga-DOTA peptides have practical advantages such as simple patient preparation and few pharmacological interactions.

7. [^{18}F]F-DOPA

7.1. Uptake and Biodistribution

[^{18}F]Fluoro-L-DOPA ([^{18}F]F-DOPA) is L-DOPA (L-dihydroxyphenylalanine), the precursor of dopamine, norepinephrine, and epinephrine, labeled with PET radioisotope ^{18}F.

[^{18}F]F-DOPA is a metabolic compound that reflects locations of increased catecholamine metabolism. [^{18}F]F-DOPA is actively transported into cells via the large neutral amino acid transporter 1 (LAT1) system and subsequently converted by the enzyme L-amino acid decarboxylase (AADC) into [^{18}F]fluorodopamine [101]. In physiological situations, dopamine is stored intravesicularly and converted into norepinephrine and epinephrine [102]. Uptake and retention of [^{18}F]F-DOPA in neuroblastoma cells is dependent on increased intracellular transport and activity of AADC and less dependent on intravesicular storage [18,103].

Physiological activity is seen in the basal ganglia, pancreas, kidneys, adrenal glands, and epiphyseal growth plates in children [101,104]. Very intense activity is seen in the excretory tracts of the urinary system and biliary system [18]. Uptake in the pancreas and adrenal glands can occasionally be prominent, for instance, in the uncinate process of the pancreas. Mild diffuse uptake can be seen in the liver, myocardium, peripheral muscles, or gastrointestinal tract [77].

7.2. Indication

As a tumor-specific tracer, [^{18}F]F-DOPA can be used for the imaging of neuroendocrine tumors with increased catecholamine metabolism, mainly seen in tumors of the sympathetic nervous system. The main indication is as alternative to [^{68}Ga]Ga-DOTA peptide imaging [77].

[^{18}F]F-DOPA may be a promising PET alternative to [^{123}I]mIBG. Due to limited experience, [^{18}F]F-DOPA has no evident role in the current guidelines for the evaluation of neuroblastoma. In some clinics [^{18}F]F-DOPA is used as an off-label alternative tracer in mIBG-negative or weakly mIBG-positive neuroblastomas [18].

7.3. Preparation

Patients must fast for at least 4 h before tracer administration to avoid interaction with amino acids from food. Despite the lack of evidence, it is recommended to avoid AADC inhibitors such as carbidopa, catechol-O-methyl transferase inhibitors, and monoamine oxidase A inhibitors at least 48 h prior to tracer administration [18]. There is some evidence that carbidopa may actually reduce the physiological uptake of abdominal organs, but this effect is not fully elucidated [105]. Images are usually acquired 60–90 min postadministration [18].

7.4. Diagnostic Accuracy

The prospective pilot studies of Piccardo et al. (2012) and Lu et al. (2013) found that [^{18}F]F-DOPA PET-CT detected a significantly higher number of neuroblastoma lesions compared to [^{123}I]mIBG scintigraphy [103,106]. As SPECT-CT was not performed by all investigations, Piccardo et al. (2020) recently conducted another prospective study in 18 neuroblastoma patients comparing [^{18}F]F-DOPA PET-CT with [^{123}I]mIBG imaging (scintigraphy and SPECT-CT) using histological results or anatomical imaging (CT or MRI) as the reference standard [107]. [^{18}F]F-DOPA PET-CT was more sensitive than [^{123}I]mIBG SPECT-CT in detecting soft tissue lesions and small osteomedullary lesions, both at diagnosis and after chemotherapy. On a lesion-based analysis, the sensitivity at diagnosis for detecting soft tissue lesions was 86% for [^{18}F]F-DOPA vs. 41% for [^{123}I]mIBG, and for detecting osteomedullary lesions, 99% vs. 93%, respectively. After chemotherapy, the sensitivity for detecting soft tissue lesions was 77% [^{18}F]F-DOPA vs. 28% % for [^{123}I]mIBG, and for detecting osteomedullary lesions, 86% vs. 69%, respectively (all $p < 0.001$). It appears that even with a completely negative [^{123}I]mIBG or [^{18}F]FDG scan, [^{18}F]F-DOPA PET-CT can still reveal persistent disease [103,107].

In addition, false-positive findings as a result of atypical physiological uptake have been reported, for instance, in the case of asymmetrical intense uptake in one of the adrenal glands or the presence of biliary duct stasis [104].

7.5. Advantages and Limitations

[^{18}F]F-DOPA uptake seems to be of prognostic value. Piccardo and colleagues developed the [^{18}F]F-DOPA whole-body metabolic burden (WBMB) score, calculated as the sum of bone metabolic burden (SUV$_{mean}$ × SIOPEN score) of each bone-segment and the soft tissue metabolic burden (SUV$_{mean}$ × volume) of each soft tissue lesion [108]. A higher disease burden (WBMB > 7.5) after induction was independently and significantly associated with disease progression and mortality [107,108]. In contrast, Liu et al. (2017) found that lower [^{18}F]F-DOPA uptake (SUV$_{max}$ and metabolic active primary tumor volume) is related to a poor prognosis, and the authors contemplated this may be due to dedifferentiation on a molecular level [72]. There is a limited availability of this new tracer and lack of experience in pediatric applications.

8. Other

8.1. [^{11}C]mHED

Carbon-11 (^{11}C)-labeled *meta*-hydroxyephedrine ([^{11}C]mHED) is another norepinephrine analogue. The very hydrophilic [^{11}C]mHED shows rapid accumulation (within minutes) in sympathicomedullary tissue via NET and high retention in neural crest tumors [109]. Because of fast blood clearance by the liver and kidney, an optimal imaging time of 30 min after tracer administration was proposed [110]. The only two studies on [^{11}C]mHED imaging in neuroblastoma have demonstrated high diagnostic accuracy in the detection of neuroblastoma lesions. In six patients, Shulkin et al. (1996) showed that [^{11}C]mHED PET identified all lesions found on [^{123}I]mIBG scintigraphy, and SPECT and detected additional skull lesions in one patient [110]. After that Franzius et al. (2006) concluded that [^{11}C]mHED may be slightly less sensitive than [^{123}I]mIBG [111]. In one of six neuroblastoma patients [^{11}C]mHED PET-CT missed one large abdominal relapse that was visible on [^{123}I]mIBG imaging (scintigraphy and SPECT-CT). [^{11}C]mHED detected all other lesions detected by [^{123}I]mIBG imaging without detecting any additional lesions. Prominent physiological activity of [^{11}C]mHED is seen in the liver, kidneys, and urinary system, often exceeding tumor uptake, which may impede detection of small metastases in these regions [110,111]. The short half-life of ^{11}C (20 min) is a benefit because radiation exposure is considerably lower compared to [^{123}I]mIBG [110]. However, the short half-life is also the largest limitation because of the requirement of an onsite cyclotron, a complicated radiochemical labeling procedure, and a rigid time schedule [111].

8.2. Other Benzylguanidine Analogues

In recent years, many other benzylguanidine analogues have been developed [112]. ^{18}F-labeled fluoropropylbenzylguanidine (FPBG) PET-CT detected one extra (histologically confirmed) metastatic bone lesion compared to [^{123}I]mIBG scintigraphy in a case report of a neuroblastoma patient [113]. Other analogues that have only been studied in neuroblastoma cell lines are parafluorobenzylguanidine (PFBG) [114], LMI1195 (N-[3-bromo-4-(3-F-fluoro-propoxy)-benzyl]-guanidine) [115], FPOIBG (4-fluoropropoxy-3-iodobenzylguanidine) [116], and *meta*-bromobenzylguanidine (mBBG) [117].

8.3. Potential Theranostics

[^{123}I]/[^{131}I]mIBG and [^{68}Ga]/[^{177}Lu]Ga-DOTA peptides are examples of a theranostic approach, which involves the use of the same molecular target for diagnostic imaging and radionuclide therapy. These theranostics are still under investigation in clinical trials. New potential theranostics for neuroblastoma have been studied in preclinical studies, such as iodine-125 (^{125}I) labeled GPAID ((R)-(-)-5-[^{125}I]iodo-3'-O-[2-(ε-guanidinohexanoyl)-2-phenylacetyl]-2'-deoxyuridine), a norepinephrine analogue that co-targets DNA of proliferating cells [118]; an antagonist of CXC chemokine receptor 4 (CXCR4), frequently overexpressed in various tumor types in the form of ^{68}Ga-labeled pentixafor and ^{177}Lu-labeled pentixather [119]; and zirconium-89 (^{89}Zr)-labeled dinutuximab, a radiolabeled anti-GD2 immunotherapy [120].

9. Discussion

In this review, the use, characteristics, advantages and limitations of several new PET radiotracers for imaging of neuroblastoma are discussed (Table A1). At the moment, [^{123}I]mIBG scintigraphy (with SPECT-CT) is the best established and first-line nuclear imaging technique in neuroblastoma patients. However, there is an increasing use of PET imaging in neuroblastoma with multiple advantages over SPECT, such as superior resolution, full body tomographic range, accurate quantification of tracer uptake and the convenience of shorter acquisition times and often allowing for one-day imaging.

Regarding the diagnostic accuracy of PET imaging for lesion detection in neuroblastoma, preliminary reports in small patient cohorts have shown overall promising results. [^{124}I]mIBG, [^{18}F]mFBG, [^{68}Ga]Ga-DOTA peptides, and [^{18}F]F-DOPA appear to be sensitive and specific tracers, possibly even more sensitive than [^{123}I]mIBG imaging, especially for the detection of smaller lesions that are below the spatial resolution of SPECT. Only [^{18}F]FDG PET imaging seems less sensitive and specific than [^{123}I]mIBG imaging. Nevertheless, the difficulty of calculating sensitivity and specificity of PET imaging in neuroblastoma is that there is no real gold standard by which to measure its accuracy [78]. As histological confirmation of pathological uptake is often not feasible due to ethical and practical reasons, most studies use different surrogate reference standards, often a combination of imaging modalities and follow-up of lesions.

PET analogues of [^{123}I]mIBG, [^{18}F]mFBG, and [^{124}I]mIBG both visualize NET uptake in neuroblastoma. [^{124}I]mIBG is less appealing for diagnostic imaging because of its higher radiation exposure, 2-days imaging, and need for thyroid protection, but may have a purpose for dosimetry before [^{131}I]mIBG therapy. Given the potentially high diagnostic accuracy of [^{18}F]mFBG PET-CT, it is possible to further reduce radiation exposure [52]. [^{18}F]F-DOPA, [^{68}Ga]Ga-DOTA peptides, and [^{18}F]FDG use molecular targets other than NET and are increasingly used in mIBG non-avid neuroblastoma. Currently, [^{18}F]FDG is the only PET-tracer that has been recommended by the guidelines as alternative in the evaluation of mIBG-negative neuroblastoma or discrepancy between mIBG imaging and radiological/clinical findings [18]. The major limitation of [^{18}F]FDG is the physiological brain and variable bone marrow activity (f.e. reactive bone marrow activity after therapy) and, as a consequence, the impaired detection of skull and bone marrow lesions. In this case, [^{18}F]F-DOPA and [^{68}Ga]Ga-DOTA peptides may be more useful, especially when skull lesions are suspected. The advantages of [^{68}Ga]Ga-DOTA peptide imaging are high focal tumor-to-background contrast (high SUV values) even for small lesions, a lower radiation exposure, no requirement of a cyclotron, and the possibility of PRRT. However, [^{68}Ga]Ga-DOTA peptide uptake is not tumor-specific and can likewise be present in benign pathology. The prognostic value of quantified disease burden on PET has been demonstrated for [^{18}F]FDG and [^{18}F]F-DOPA. Measurements of tracer uptake in tumor lesions could identify patients who are more likely to relapse and are associated with poor outcome [74,107,108].

Other than the limited availability, the most important limitation that prevents the use of these new PET tracers is the limited experience and lack of knowledge, for example, on the normal distribution and radiation burden in young children. This may be overcome in the future if more centers install cyclotrons and/or generators and more studies are conducted. Currently, there are multiple ongoing prospective clinical trials comparing these PET tracers to [^{123}I]mIBG in patients with neuroblastoma, for instance, trial NL8152 and NCT02348749 on [^{18}F]mFBG and NCT02043899 on [^{124}I]mIBG. As suggested by Piccardo and colleagues, comparison of [^{18}F]F-DOPA or [^{68}Ga]Ga-DOTA peptides should be conducted with a PET analogue of [^{123}I]mIBG to eliminate any bias related to different imaging techniques [107].

The difficulty of introducing a more sensitive PET tracer is the uncertainty of the clinical relevance when more lesions are detected because this can have important implications on the overall management of patients. Improved imaging accuracy will likely lead to the upstaging of some patients. Nevertheless, a more accurate determination of disease extent could provide critical information and may lead to adequate intensification of treatment in children with inferior outcomes. Around 50–60% of patients deemed to be in complete remission on [^{123}I]mIBG imaging at end of treatment eventually relapse [8]. We hypothesize that persisting oligometastases only detectable by PET imaging, implying that these patients were not in complete remission, may be the cause of recurrent disease. In this case, these patients could benefit from maximum cytoreductive treatments, for instance, additional targeted radio(nuclide) therapy.

Before the current standard [^{123}I]mIBG imaging can be replaced by PET imaging, re-evaluation of diagnostic and treatment strategies is warranted. The prognostic value of current semiquantitative scoring systems is only validated for disease burden on mIBG scintigraphy. New scoring systems, ideally implementing quantification of tracer uptake, should be validated for these PET tracers.

It is unclear in which setting a patient may benefit most from imaging with a certain tracer. [^{18}F]DOPA could be useful in neuroblastoma with insufficient NET or SSTR expression, but this has not been studied yet. Variable tracer uptake on an interpatient, intrapatient and intratumoral level once again illustrates the heterogenous character of neuroblastoma and is a great challenge in the clinical practice. The exact reason for reduced NET or SSTR expression or a modified uptake mechanism is not fully understood but may partially be linked to tumor dedifferentiation. Heterogeneity of neuroblastoma indicate that that imaging with one molecular target may not fully depict disease extent. Therefore, expanding to imaging with a combination of radiotracers that use different molecular targets should be considered. [^{18}F]FDG PET-CT has already proven to complement [^{123}I]mIBG in selected patients with [^{123}I]mIBG-negative tumors. Despite extra radiation exposure and costs, routine implementation of [^{18}F]FDG PET-CT may have a role in high-risk patients to increase diagnostic accuracy while providing prognostic information. Furthermore, routine immunohistochemical identification of (molecular) target expression in all tumor samples may guide nuclear imaging and therapy. Molecular target heterogeneity needs to be studied in prospective studies and correlated to activity on PET imaging and clinical outcomes.

With ongoing developments of PET technologies, further improvement of image quality and reduction in radiation exposure can be expected. In the future, hybrid PET-MRI could eliminate the radiation exposure of CT and provide high soft tissue contrast images. In addition, improved tumor delineation may provide important information for radiotherapy planning. All in all, PET is expected to play an important role in the future of neuroblastoma imaging.

10. Conclusions

The advantages of PET imaging and the preliminary results on the diagnostic accuracy of new PET tracers for lesion detection in neuroblastoma, compared to current standard [^{123}I]mIBG imaging, are promising. PET imaging could have an important role in demonstrating full disease extent and guiding adequate therapy with the ultimate aim of improving outcome in patients at high risk for refractory and recurrent neuroblastoma. Heterogenous tracer uptake in tumor lesions can be a challenge in the management of neuroblastoma, with the risk of missing lesions. Therefore, it is important to investigate various tracers with different uptake mechanisms and possibly expand to multimodality nuclear imaging. Larger multicenter investigations are needed in order to establish the role of these new tracers in the management of neuroblastoma patients.

Author Contributions: Conceptualization, A.S., B.d.K. and G.A.M.T.; writing—original draft preparation, A.S., B.d.K. and G.A.M.T.; writing—review and editing, all authorsA.S., B.d.K., G.A.M.T., G.B., S.T.M.W., K.L.S.C., A.J.P., N.T., M.M.v.N., M.G.E.H.L.; visualization, A.S. and B.d.K; supervision, M.G.E.H.L. and M.M.v.N.; All authors have read and agreed to the published version of the manuscript.

Funding: This research received no external funding.

Institutional Review Board Statement: Not applicable.

Informed Consent Statement: Not applicable.

Conflicts of Interest: The authors declare no conflict of interest.

Appendix A

Table A1. characteristics of radiotracers for nuclear imaging of neuroblastoma.

Tracer	Molecular Target	Radioisotope (Half-Life)	Advantages	Limitations
[^{123}I]mIBG	norepinephrine transporter	iodine-123 (13 h)	- validated scoring systems - possible to select patients for [^{131}I]mIBG therapy	- two-day imaging - scintigraphy/SPECT imaging (limited spatial resolution, limited tomographic range, long acquisitions, as opposed to PET imaging) - need for thyroid protection - negative in 10% neuroblastomas
[^{124}I]mIBG	norepinephrine transporter	iodine-124 (100 h)	- PET imaging - possibility for [^{131}I]mIBG therapy dosimetry	- two-day imaging - high radiation exposure - poor image quality (only 23% positron abundance) - need for thyroid protection - limited experience & availability
[^{18}F]mFBG	norepinephrine transporter	fluorine-18 (110 min)	- PET imaging - one-day imaging	- limited experience & availability
[^{18}F]FDG	glucose metabolism	fluorine-18 (110 min)	- PET imaging - one-day imaging - widely available - often positive in mIBG non-avid neuroblastoma - prognostic value	- not tumor-specific - impaired detection of bone marrow and skull lesions - negative in neuroblastomas with low glucose metabolism - fasting - not possible to select patients for [^{131}I]mIBG therapy
[^{18}F]F-DOPA	catecholamine metabolism	fluorine-18 (110 min)	- PET imaging - one-day imaging - prognostic value	- fasting - not possible to select patients for [^{131}I]mIBG therapy - limited experience & availability
[^{68}Ga]Ga-DOTA peptides	somatostatin receptors	gallium-68 (68 min)	- PET imaging - one-day imaging - relatively low radiation exposure - gallium generator (often easier available than cyclotrons) - possible to select patients for peptide receptor radionuclide therapy	- not specific for tumors of sympathetic nervous system - negative in neuroblastomas with low SSTR expression - limited experience
[^{11}C]mHED	norepinephrine transporter	carbon-11 (20 min)	- PET imaging - one-day imaging - relatively low radiation exposure	- rigid time schedule - limited experience & availability

Abbreviations: *mIBG meta*-iodobenzylguanidine, *mFBG meta*-fluorobenzylguanidine, *FDG* fluorodeoxyglucose, *F-DOPA* fluoro-L-dihydroxyphenylalanine, *mHED meta*-hydroxyephedrine, *SPECT* single-photon emission computed tomography *PET* positron emission tomography.

References

1. Irwin, M.S.; Park, J.R. Neuroblastoma. *Pediatric Clin. N. Am.* **2015**, *62*, 225–256. [CrossRef]
2. Tas, M.L.; Reedijk, A.M.J.; Karim-Kos, H.E.; Kremer, L.C.M.; van de Ven, C.P.; Dierselhuis, M.P.; van Eijkelenburg, N.K.A.; van Grotel, M.; Kraal, K.C.J.M.; Peek, A.M.L.; et al. Neuroblastoma between 1990 and 2014 in the Netherlands: Increased incidence and improved survival of high-risk neuroblastoma. *Eur. J. Cancer* **2020**, *124*, 47–55. [CrossRef]
3. Morgenstern, D.A.; London, W.B.; Stephens, D.; Volchenboum, S.L.; Simon, T.; Nakagawara, A.; Shimada, H.; Schleiermacher, G.; Matthay, K.K.; Cohn, S.L.; et al. Prognostic significance of pattern and burden of metastatic disease in patients with stage 4 neuroblastoma: A study from the International Neuroblastoma Risk Group database. *Eur. J. Cancer* **2016**, *65*, 1–10. [CrossRef]
4. Monclair, T.; Brodeur, G.M.; Ambros, P.F.; Brisse, H.J.; Cecchetto, G.; Holmes, K.; Kaneko, M.; London, W.B.; Matthay, K.K.; Nuchtern, J.G.; et al. The International Neuroblastoma Risk Group (INRG) staging system: An INRG task force report. *J. Clin. Oncol.* **2009**, *27*, 298–303. [CrossRef] [PubMed]
5. Brodeur, G.M.; Pritchard, J.; Berthold, F.; Carlsen, N.L.T.; Castel, V.; Castleberry, R.P.; de Bernardi, B.; Evans, A.E.; Favrot, M.; Hedborg, F.; et al. Revisions of the international criteria for neuroblastoma diagnosis, staging, and response to treatment. *J. Clin. Oncol.* **1993**, *11*, 1466–1477. [CrossRef]
6. Cohn, S.L.; Pearson, A.D.J.; London, W.B.; Monclair, T.; Ambros, P.F.; Brodeur, G.M.; Faldum, A.; Hero, B.; Iehara, T.; Machin, D.; et al. The International Neuroblastoma Risk Group (INRG) classification system: An INRG task force report. *J. Clin. Oncol.* **2009**, *27*, 289–297. [CrossRef] [PubMed]
7. Simon, T.; Hero, B.; Benz-Bohm, G.; von Schweinitz, D.; Berthold, F. Review of image defined risk factors in localized neuroblastoma patients: Results of the GPOH NB97 trial. *Pediatric Blood Cancer* **2008**, *50*, 965–969. [CrossRef] [PubMed]
8. Maris, J.M. Recent advances in neuroblastoma. *N. Engl. J. Med.* **2010**, *362*, 2202–2211. [CrossRef] [PubMed]
9. Ladenstein, R.; Lambert, B.; Pötschger, U.; Castellani, M.R.; Lewington, V.; Bar-Sever, Z.; Oudoux, A.; Śliwińska, A.; Taborska, K.; Biassoni, L.; et al. Validation of the MIBG skeletal SIOPEN scoring method in two independent high-risk neuroblastoma populations: The SIOPEN/HR-NBL1 and COG-A3973 trials. *Eur. J. Nucl. Med. Mol. Imaging* **2018**, *45*, 292–305. [CrossRef]
10. Matthay, K.K.; Reynolds, C.P.; Seeger, R.C.; Shimada, H.; Adkins, E.S.; Haas-Kogan, D.; Gerbing, R.B.; London, W.B.; Villablanca, J.G. Long-term results for children with high-risk neuroblastoma treated on a randomized trial of myeloablative therapy followed by 13-cis-retinoic acid: A children's oncology group study. *J. Clin. Oncol.* **2009**, *27*, 1007–1013. [CrossRef] [PubMed]
11. London, W.B.; Castel, V.; Monclair, T.; Ambros, P.F.; Pearson, A.D.J.; Cohn, S.L.; Berthold, F.; Nakagawara, A.; Ladenstein, R.L.; Iehara, T.; et al. Clinical and biologic features predictive of survival after relapse of neuroblastoma: A report from the International Neuroblastoma Risk Group project. *J. Clin. Oncol.* **2011**, *29*, 3286–3292. [CrossRef] [PubMed]
12. Moreno, L.; Rubie, H.; Varo, A.; Le Deley, M.C.; Amoroso, L.; Chevance, A.; Garaventa, A.; Gambart, M.; Bautista, F.; Valteau-Couanet, D.; et al. Outcome of children with relapsed or refractory neuroblastoma: A meta-analysis of ITCC/SIOPEN European phase II clinical trials. *Pediatric Blood Cancer* **2017**, *64*, 25–31. [CrossRef] [PubMed]
13. Brisse, H.J.; McCarville, M.B.; Granata, C.; Krug, K.B.; Wootton-Gorges, S.L.; Kanegawa, K.; Giammarile, F.; Schmidt, M.; Shulkin, B.L.; Matthay, K.K.; et al. Guidelines for imaging and staging of neuroblastic tumors: Consensus report from the International Neuroblastoma Risk Group Project. *Radiology* **2011**, *261*, 243–257. [CrossRef] [PubMed]
14. Siegel, M.J.; Jaju, A. MR imaging of neuroblastic masses. *Magn. Reson. Imaging Clin. N. Am.* **2008**, *16*, 499–513. [CrossRef]
15. Rozovsky, K.; Koplewitz, B.Z.; Krausz, Y.; Revel-Vilk, S.; Weintraub, M.; Chisin, R.; Klein, M. Added value of SPECT/CT for correlation of MIBG scintigraphy and diagnostic CT in neuroblastoma and pheochromocytoma. *Am. J. Roentgenol.* **2008**, *190*, 1085–1090. [CrossRef] [PubMed]
16. Fukuoka, M.; Taki, J.; Mochizuki, T.; Kinuya, S. Comparison of diagnostic value of I-123 MIBG and high-dose I-131 MIBG scintigraphy including incremental value of SPECT/CT over planar image in patients with malignant pheochromocytoma/paraganglioma and neuroblastoma. *Clin. Nucl. Med.* **2011**, *36*, 1–7. [CrossRef] [PubMed]
17. Liu, B.; Servaes, S.; Zhuang, H. SPECT/CT MIBG imaging is crucial in the follow-up of the patients with high-risk neuroblastoma. *Clin. Nucl. Med.* **2018**, *43*, 232–238. [CrossRef]
18. Bar-Sever, Z.; Biassoni, L.; Shulkin, B.; Kong, G.; Hofman, M.S.; Lopci, E.; Manea, I.; Koziorowski, J.; Castellani, R.; Boubaker, A.; et al. Guidelines on nuclear medicine imaging in neuroblastoma. *Eur. J. Nucl. Med. Mol. Imaging* **2018**, *45*, 2009–2024. [CrossRef]
19. Biermann, M.; Schwarzlmüller, T.; Fasmer, K.E.; Reitan, B.C.; Johnsen, B.; Rosendahl, K. Is there a role for PET-CT and SPECT-CT in pediatric oncology? *Acta Radiol.* **2013**, *54*, 1037–1045. [CrossRef]
20. Sharp, S.E.; Trout, A.T.; Weiss, B.D.; Gelfand, M.J. MIBG in neuroblastoma diagnostic imaging and therapy. *Radiographics* **2016**, *36*, 258–278. [CrossRef]
21. Vallabhajosula, S.; Nikolopoulou, A. Radioiodinated metaiodobenzylguanidine (MIBG): Radiochemistry, biology, and pharmacology. *Semin. Nucl. Med.* **2011**, *41*, 324–333. [CrossRef] [PubMed]
22. Smets, L.A.; Loesberg, C.; Janssen, M.; Metwally, E.A.; Huiskamp, R. Active uptake and extravesicular storage of M-iodobenzylguanidine in human neuroblastoma SK-N-SH cells. *Cancer Res.* **1989**, *49*, 2941–2944. [PubMed]
23. Bombardieri, E.; Giammarile, F.; Aktolun, C.; Baum, R.P.; Bischof Delaloye, A.; Maffioli, L.; Moncayo, R.; Mortelmans, L.; Pepe, G.; Reske, S.N.; et al. 131I/123I-metaiodobenzylguanidine (MIBG) scintigraphy: Procedure guidelines for tumour imaging. *Eur. J. Nucl. Med. Mol. Imaging* **2010**, *37*, 2436–2446. [CrossRef] [PubMed]

24. Vik, T.A.; Pfluger, T.; Kadota, R.; Castel, V.; Tulchinsky, M.; Farto, J.C.A.; Heiba, S.; Serafini, A.; Tumeh, S.; Khutoryansky, N.; et al. (123)I-MIBG scintigraphy in patients with known or suspected neuroblastoma: Results from a prospective multicenter trial. *Pediatric Blood Cancer* **2009**, *52*, 784–790. [CrossRef] [PubMed]
25. Matthay, K.K.; Shulkin, B.; Ladenstein, R.; Michon, J.; Giammarile, F.; Lewington, V.; Pearson, A.D.J.; Cohn, S.L. Criteria for evaluation of disease extent by (123)I-metaiodobenzylguanidine scans in neuroblastoma: A report for the International Neuroblastoma Risk Group (INRG) task force. *Br. J. Cancer* **2010**, *102*, 1319–1326. [CrossRef]
26. Pfluger, T.; Schmied, C.; Porn, U.; Leinsinger, G.; Vollmar, C.; Dresel, S.; Schmid, I.; Hahn, K. Integrated imaging using MRI and 123I metaiodobenzylguanidine scintigraphy to improve sensitivity and specificity in the diagnosis of pediatric neuroblastoma. *AJR Am. J. Roentgenol.* **2003**, *181*, 1115–1124. [CrossRef]
27. Matthay, K.K.; Edeline, V.; Lumbroso, J.; Tanguy, M.L.; Asselain, B.; Zucker, J.M.; Valteau-Couanet, D.; Hartmann, O.; Michon, J. Correlation of early metastatic response by 123I- metaiodobenzylguanidine scintigraphy with overall response and event-free survival in stage IV neuroblastoma. *J. Clin. Oncol.* **2003**, *21*, 2486–2491. [CrossRef]
28. Lewington, V.; Lambert, B.; Poetschger, U.; Sever, Z.B.; Giammarile, F.; McEwan, A.J.B.; Castellani, R.; Lynch, T.; Shulkin, B.; Drobics, M.; et al. 123I-MIBG scintigraphy in neuroblastoma: Development of a SIOPEN semi-quantitative reporting, method by an international panel. *Eur. J. Nucl. Med. Mol. Imaging* **2017**, *44*, 234–241. [CrossRef]
29. Decarolis, B.; Schneider, C.; Hero, B.; Simon, T.; Volland, R.; Roels, F.; Dietlein, M.; Berthold, F.; Schmidt, M. Iodine-123 metaiodobenzylguanidine scintigraphy scoring allows prediction of outcome in patients with stage 4 neuroblastoma: Results of the cologne interscore comparison study. *J. Clin. Oncol.* **2013**, *31*, 944–951. [CrossRef]
30. Yanik, G.A.; Parisi, M.T.; Shulkin, B.L.; Naranjo, A.; Kreissman, S.G.; London, W.B.; Villablanca, J.G.; Maris, J.M.; Park, J.R.; Cohn, S.L.; et al. Semiquantitative MIBG scoring as a prognostic indicator in patients with stage 4 neuroblastoma: A report from the children's oncology group. *J. Nucl. Med.* **2013**, *54*, 541–548. [CrossRef]
31. Yanik, G.A.; Parisi, M.T.; Naranjo, A.; Nadel, H.; Gelfand, M.J.; Park, J.R.; Ladenstein, R.L.; Poetschger, U.; Boubaker, A.; Valteau-Couanet, D.; et al. Validation of postinduction curie scores in high-risk neuroblastoma: A children's oncology group and SIOPEN group report on SIOPEN/HR-NBL1. *J. Nucl. Med.* **2018**, *59*, 502–508. [CrossRef]
32. Bleeker, G.; Tytgat, G.A.M.; Adam, J.A.; Caron, H.N.; Kremer, L.C.M.; Hooft, L.; van Dalen, E.C. 123I-MIBG scintigraphy and 18F-FDG-PET imaging for diagnosing neuroblastoma. *Cochrane Database Syst. Rev.* **2015**, *2015*. [CrossRef] [PubMed]
33. Fendler, W.P.; Melzer, H.I.; Walz, C.; von Schweinitz, D.; Coppenrath, E.; Schmid, I.; Bartenstein, P.; Pfluger, T. High 123I-MIBG uptake in neuroblastic tumours indicates unfavourable histopathology. *Eur. J. Nucl. Med. Mol. Imaging* **2013**, *40*, 1701–1710. [CrossRef] [PubMed]
34. Biasotti, S.; Garaventa, A.; Villavecchia, G.P.; Cabria, M.; Nantron, M.; de Bernardi, B. False-negative metaiodobenzylguanidine scintigraphy at diagnosis of neuroblastoma. *Med. Pediatric Oncol.* **2000**, *35*, 153–155. [CrossRef]
35. DuBois, S.G.; Geier, E.; Batra, V.; Yee, S.W.; Neuhaus, J.; Segal, M.; Martinez, D.; Pawel, B.; Yanik, G.; Naranjo, A.; et al. Evaluation of norepinephrine transporter expression and metaiodobenzylguanidine avidity in neuroblastoma: A report from the children's oncology group. *Int. J. Mol. Imaging* **2012**, *2012*, 1–8. [CrossRef] [PubMed]
36. DuBois, S.G.; Mody, R.; Naranjo, A.; van Ryn, C.; Russ, D.; Oldridge, D.; Kreissman, S.; Baker, D.L.; Parisi, M.; Shulkin, B.L.; et al. MIBG avidity correlates with clinical features, tumor biology, and outcomes in neuroblastoma: A report from the children's oncology group. *Pediatric Blood Cancer* **2017**, *64*, 139–148. [CrossRef]
37. Gains, J.E.; Sebire, N.J.; Moroz, V.; Wheatley, K.; Gaze, M.N. Immunohistochemical evaluation of molecular radiotherapy target expression in neuroblastoma tissue. *Eur. J. Nucl. Med. Mol. Imaging* **2018**, *45*, 402–411. [CrossRef]
38. Colavolpe, C.; Guedj, E.; Cammilleri, S.; Taïeb, D.; Mundler, O.; Coze, C. Utility of FDG-PET:CT in the follow-up of neuroblastoma which became MIBG-negative. *Pediatric Blood Cancer* **2008**, *51*, 828–831. [CrossRef]
39. Mc Dowell, H.; Losty, P.; Barnes, N.; Kokai, G. Utility of FDG-PET/CT in the follow-up of neuroblastoma which became MIBG-negative. *Pediatric Blood Cancer* **2009**, *52*, 552. [CrossRef]
40. Schwarz, K.B.; Driver, I.; Lewis, I.J.; Taylor, R.E. Positive MIBG scanning at the time of relapse in neuroblastoma which was MIBG negative at diagnosis. *Br. J. Radiol.* **1997**, *70*, 90–92. [CrossRef]
41. Marachelian, A.; Shimada, H.; Sano, H.; Jackson, H.; Stein, J.; Sposto, R.; Matthay, K.K.; Baker, D.; Villablanca, J.G. The significance of serial histopathology in a residual mass for outcome of intermediate risk stage 3 neuroblastoma. *Pediatric Blood Cancer* **2012**, *58*, 675–681. [CrossRef]
42. Decarolis, B.; Simon, T.; Krug, B.; Leuschner, I.; Vokuhl, C.; Kaatsch, P.; von Schweinitz, D.; Klingebiel, T.; Mueller, I.; Schweigerer, L.; et al. Treatment and outcome of ganglioneuroma and ganglioneuroblastoma intermixed. *BMC Cancer* **2016**, *16*, 542. [CrossRef] [PubMed]
43. Rault, E.; Vandenberghe, S.; van Holen, R.; de Beenhouwer, J.; Staelens, S.; Lemahieu, I. Comparison of image quality of different iodine isotopes (I-123, I-124, and I-131). *Cancer Biother. Radiopharm.* **2007**, *22*, 423–430. [CrossRef]
44. Beijst, C.; de Keizer, B.; Lam, M.G.E.H.; Janssens, G.O.; Tytgat, G.A.M.; de Jong, H.W.A.M. A Phantom study: Should 124 I-MIBG PET/CT replace 123 I-MIBG SPECT/CT? *Med. Phys.* **2017**, *44*, 1624–1631. [CrossRef] [PubMed]
45. Cistaro, A.; Quartuccio, N.; Caobelli, F.; Piccardo, A.; Paratore, R.; Coppolino, P.; Sperandeo, A.; Arnone, G.; Ficola, U. 124I-MIBG: A new promising positron-emitting radiopharmaceutical for the evaluation of neuroblastoma. *Nucl. Med. Rev.* **2015**, *18*, 102–106. [CrossRef]

46. Huang, S.Y.; Bolch, W.E.; Lee, C.; van Brocklin, H.F.; Pampaloni, M.H.; Hawkins, R.A.; Sznewajs, A.; DuBois, S.G.; Matthay, K.K.; Seo, Y. Patient-specific dosimetry using pretherapy [124I]m-iodobenzylguanidine ([124I]MIBG) dynamic PET/CT imaging before [131I]MIBG targeted radionuclide therapy for neuroblastoma. *Mol. Imaging Biol.* **2015**, *17*, 284–294. [CrossRef] [PubMed]
47. Aboian, M.; Huang, S.; Pampaloni, M.H.; Hawkins, R.A.; Huh, Y.; Vo, K.; Gustafson, C.; Matthay, K.; Seo, Y. 124 I-MIBG PET-CT to monitor metastatic disease in children with relapsed neuroblastoma. *J. Nucl. Med.* **2020**, *62*, 43–47. [CrossRef] [PubMed]
48. Lee, C.-L.; Wahnishe, H.; Sayre, G.A.; Cho, H.-M.; Kim, H.-J.; Hernandez-Pampaloni, M.; Hawkins, R.A.; Dannoon, S.F.; VanBrocklin, H.F.; Itsara, M.; et al. Radiation dose estimation using preclinical imaging with 124I-metaiodobenzylguanidine (MIBG) PET. *Med. Phys.* **2010**, *37*, 4861–4867. [CrossRef]
49. Lassmann, M.; Treves, S.T. Paediatric radiopharmaceutical administration: Harmonization of the 2007 EANM paediatric dosage card (Version 1.5.2008) and the 2010 North American consensus guidelines. *Eur. J. Nucl. Med. Mol. Imaging* **2014**, *41*, 1036–1041. [CrossRef]
50. Seo, Y.; Gustafson, W.C.; Dannoon, S.F.; Nekritz, E.A.; Lee, C.L.; Murphy, S.T.; van Brocklin, H.F.; Hernandez-Pampaloni, M.; Haas-Kogan, D.A.; Weiss, W.A.; et al. Tumor dosimetry using [124I]miodobenzylguanidine micropet/CT for [131I]m-iodobenzylguanidine treatment of neuroblastoma in a murine xenograft model. *Mol. Imaging Biol.* **2012**, *14*, 735–742. [CrossRef]
51. Pentlow, K.S.; Graham, M.C.; Lambrecht, R.M.; Daghighian, F.; Bacharach, S.L.; Bendriem, B.; Finn, R.D.; Jordan, K.; Kalaigian, H.; Karp, J.S.; et al. Quantitative imaging of iodine-124 with PET. *J. Nucl. Med.* **1996**, *37*, 1557–1562.
52. Zhang, H.; Huang, R.; Cheung, N.K.V.; Guo, H.; Zanzonico, P.B.; Thaler, H.T.; Lewis, J.S.; Blasberg, R.G. Imaging the norepinephrine transporter in neuroblastoma: A comparison of [18F]-MFBG and 123I-MIBG. *Clin. Cancer Res.* **2014**, *20*, 2182–2191. [CrossRef]
53. Pandit-Taskar, N.; Zanzonico, P.; Staton, K.D.; Carrasquillo, J.A.; Reidy-Lagunes, D.; Lyashchenko, S.; Burnazi, E.; Zhang, H.; Lewis, J.S.; Blasberg, R.; et al. Biodistribution and dosimetry of 18 F-meta-fluorobenzylguanidine: A first-in-human PET/CT imaging study of patients with neuroendocrine malignancies. *J. Nucl. Med.* **2018**, *59*, 147–153. [CrossRef]
54. Pauwels, E.; Celen, S.; Vandamme, M.; Leysen, W.; Baete, K.; Bechter, O.; Bex, M.; Serdons, K.; van Laere, K.; Bormans, G.; et al. Improved resolution and sensitivity of [18F]MFBG PET compared with [123I]MIBG SPECT in a patient with a norepinephrine transporter–expressing tumour. *Eur. J. Nucl. Med. Mol. Imaging* **2020**. [CrossRef]
55. Plathow, C.; Weber, W.A. Tumor cell metabolism imaging. *J. Nucl. Med.* **2008**, *49*, 43S–63S. [CrossRef]
56. Shammas, A.; Lim, R.; Charron, M. Pediatric FDG PET/CT: Physiologic uptake, normal variants, and benign conditions. *Radiogr. Rev. Publ. Radiol. Soc. North Am. Inc* **2009**, *29*, 1467–1486. [CrossRef]
57. Sharp, S.E.; Shulkin, B.L.; Gelfand, M.J.; Salisbury, S.; Furman, W.L. 123I-MIBG scintigraphy and 18F-FDG PET in neuroblastoma. *J. Nucl. Med. Off. Publ. Soc. Nucl. Med.* **2009**, *50*, 1237–1243. [CrossRef]
58. Shulkin, B.L.; Sisson, C.; Castle, P.; Hutchinson, R.J.; Castle, V.P.; Yanik, G.A.; Shapiro, B.; Sisson, J.C. Neuroblastoma: Positron emission tomography with 2-[fluorine-18]-fluoro-2-deoxy-D-glucose compared with metaiodobenzylguanidine scintigraphy. *Radiology* **1996**, *199*, 743–750. [CrossRef]
59. Melzer, H.I.; Coppenrath, E.; Schmid, I.; Albert, M.H.; von Schweinitz, D.; Tudball, C.; Bartenstein, P.; Pfluger, T. 123I-MIBG scintigraphy/SPECT versus 18F-FDG PET in paediatric neuroblastoma. *Eur. J. Nucl. Med. Mol. Imaging* **2011**, *38*, 1648–1658. [CrossRef]
60. Papathanasiou, N.D.; Gaze, M.N.; Sullivan, K.; Aldridge, M.; Waddington, W.; Almuhaideb, A.; Bomanji, J.B. 18F-FDG PET/CT and 123I-metaiodobenzylguanidine imaging in high-risk neuroblastoma: Diagnostic comparison and survival analysis. *J. Nucl. Med.* **2011**, *52*, 519–525. [CrossRef] [PubMed]
61. Gil, T.Y.; Lee, D.K.; Lee, J.M.; Yoo, E.S.; Ryu, K.H. Clinical experience with 18F-fluorodeoxyglucose positron emission tomography and 123I-metaiodobenzylguanine scintigraphy in pediatric neuroblastoma: Complementary roles in follow-up of patients. *Korean J. Pediatrics* **2014**, *57*, 278–286. [CrossRef] [PubMed]
62. Kushner, B.H.; Yeung, H.W.D.; Larson, S.M.; Kramer, K.; Cheung, N.K.V. Extending positron emission tomography scan utility to high-risk neuroblastoma: Fluorine-18 fluorodeoxyglucose positron emission tomography as sole imaging modality in follow-up of patients. *J. Clin. Oncol.* **2001**, *19*, 3397–3405. [CrossRef] [PubMed]
63. Orr, K.E.; McHugh, K. The new international neuroblastoma response criteria. *Pediatric Radiol.* **2019**, *49*, 1433–1440. [CrossRef] [PubMed]
64. Park, J.R.; Bagatell, R.; Cohn, S.L.; Pearson, A.D.; Villablanca, J.G.; Berthold, F.; Burchill, S.; Boubaker, A.; McHugh, K.; Nuchtern, J.G.; et al. Revisions to the international neuroblastoma response criteria: A consensus statement from the National Cancer Institute clinical trials planning meeting. *J. Clin. Oncol.* **2017**, *35*, 2580–2587. [CrossRef]
65. Stauss, J.; Franzius, C.; Pfluger, T.; Juergens, K.U.; Biassoni, L.; Begent, J.; Kluge, R.; Amthauer, H.; Voelker, T.; Højgaard, L.; et al. Guidelines for 18F-FDG PET and PET-CT imaging in paediatric oncology. *Eur. J. Nucl. Med. Mol. Imaging* **2008**, *35*, 1581–1588. [CrossRef]
66. Taggart, D.R.; Han, M.M.; Quach, A.; Groshen, S.; Ye, W.; Villablanca, J.G.; Jackson, H.A.; Aparici, C.M.; Carlson, D.; Maris, J.; et al. Comparison of iodine-123 metaiodobenzylguanidine (MIBG) scan and [18F]fluorodeoxyglucose positron emission tomography to evaluate response after iodine-131 MIBG therapy for relapsed neuroblastoma. *J. Clin. Oncol.* **2009**, *27*, 5343–5349. [CrossRef]
67. Tolboom, N.; Servaes, S.E.; Zhuang, H. Neuroblastoma presenting as non-MIBG-avid widespread soft tissue metastases without bone involvement revealed by FDG PET/CT imaging. *Clin. Nucl. Med.* **2017**, *42*, 643–644. [CrossRef]

68. Wartski, M.; Jehanno, N.; Michon, J.; de Labriolle-Vaylet, C.; Montravers, F. Weak uptake of 123I-MIBG and 18F-FDOPA contrasting with high 18F-FDG uptake in stage i neuroblastoma. *Clin. Nucl. Med.* **2015**, *40*, 969–970. [CrossRef]
69. Codreanu, I.; Zhuang, H. Disparities in uptake pattern of (123)I-MIBG, (18)F-FDG, and (99m)Tc-MDP within the same primary neuroblastoma. *Clin. Nucl. Med.* **2014**, *39*, 184–186. [CrossRef]
70. Sato, Y.; Kurosawa, H.; Sakamoto, S.; Kuwashima, S.; Hashimoto, T.; Okamoto, K.; Tsuchioka, T.; Fukushima, K.; Arisaka, O.; Segura, M. Usefulness of 18F-fluorodeoxyglucose positron emission tomography for follow-up of 13-cis-retinoic acid treatment for residual neuroblastoma after myeloablative chemotherapy. *Medicine* **2015**, *94*, e1290. [CrossRef]
71. Garcia, J.R.; Bassa, P.; Soler, M.; Jaramillo, A.; Ortiz, S.; Riera, E. Benign differentiation of treated neuroblastoma as a cause of false positive by 123I-MIBG SPECT/CT. Usefulness of 18F-FDG PET/CT. *Rev. Española De Med. Nucl. E Imagen Mol. (Engl. Ed.)* **2019**, *38*, 389–390. [CrossRef]
72. Liu, C.-J.; Lu, M.-Y.; Liu, Y.-L.; Ko, C.-L.; Ko, K.-Y.; Tzen, K.-Y.; Chang, H.-H.; Yang, Y.-L.; Jou, S.-T.; Hsu, W.-M.; et al. Risk stratification of pediatric patients with neuroblastoma using volumetric parameters of 18F-FDG and 18F-DOPA PET/CT. *Clin. Nucl. Med.* **2017**, *42*, e142–e148. [CrossRef]
73. Kang, S.Y.; Rahim, M.K.; Kim, Y.-l.; Cheon, G.J.; Kang, H.J.; Shin, H.Y.; Kang, K.W.; Chung, J.K.; Kim, E.E.; Lee, D.S. Clinical significance of pretreatment FDG PET/CT in MIBG-avid pediatric neuroblastoma. *Nucl. Med. Mol. Imaging* **2017**, *51*, 154–160. [CrossRef]
74. Li, C.; Zhang, J.; Chen, S.; Huang, S.; Wu, S.; Zhang, L.; Zhang, F.; Wang, H. Prognostic value of metabolic indices and bone marrow uptake pattern on preoperative 18F–FDG PET/CT in pediatric patients with neuroblastoma. *Eur. J. Nucl. Med. Mol. Imaging* **2018**, *45*, 306–315. [CrossRef]
75. Lee, J.W.; Cho, A.; Yun, M.; Lee, J.D.; Lyu, C.J.; Kang, W.J. Prognostic value of pretreatment FDG PET in pediatric neuroblastoma. *Eur. J. Radiol.* **2015**, *84*, 2633–2639. [CrossRef]
76. Pauwels, E.; Cleeren, F.; Bormans, G.; Deroose, C.M. Somatostatin receptor PET ligands—The next generation for clinical practice. *Am. J. Nucl. Med. Mol. Imaging* **2018**, *8*, 311–331.
77. Bozkurt, M.F.; Virgolini, I.; Balogova, S.; Beheshti, M.; Rubello, D.; Decristoforo, C.; Ambrosini, V.; Kjaer, A.; Delgado-Bolton, R.; Kunikowska, J.; et al. Guideline for PET/CT imaging of neuroendocrine neoplasms with 68Ga-DOTA-conjugated somatostatin receptor targeting peptides and 18F-DOPA. *Eur. J. Nucl. Med. Mol. Imaging* **2017**, *44*, 1588–1601. [CrossRef]
78. Hofman, M.S.; Eddie Lau, W.F.; Hicks, R.J. Somatostatin receptor imaging With68Ga DOTATATE PET/CT: Clinical utility, normal patterns, pearls, and pitfalls in interpretation1. *Radiographics* **2015**, *35*, 500–516. [CrossRef]
79. Abongwa, C.; Mott, S.; Schafer, B.; McNeely, P.; Abusin, G.; O'Dorisio, T.; Zamba, G.; O'Dorisio, M.S.; Menda, Y. Safety and accuracy of 68Ga-DOTATOC PET/CT in children and young adults with solid tumors. *Am. J. Nucl. Med. Mol. Imaging* **2017**, *7*, 228–235. [PubMed]
80. Poeppel, T.D.; Binse, I.; Petersenn, S.; Lahner, H.; Schott, M.; Antoch, G.; Brandau, W.; Bockisch, A.; Boy, C. 68Ga-DOTATOC versus 68Ga-DOTATATE PET/CT in functional imaging of neuroendocrine tumors. *J. Nucl. Med. Off. Publ. Soc. Nucl. Med.* **2011**, *52*, 1864–1870. [CrossRef] [PubMed]
81. Kabasakal, L.; Demirci, E.; Ocak, M.; Decristoforo, C.; Araman, A.; Ozsoy, Y.; Uslu, I.; Kanmaz, B. Comparison of 68Ga-DOTATATE and 68Ga-DOTANOC PET/CT imaging in the same patient group with neuroendocrine tumours. *Eur. J. Nucl. Med. Mol. Imaging* **2012**, *39*, 1271–1277. [CrossRef] [PubMed]
82. O'Dorisio, M.S.; Chen, F.; O'Dorisio, T.M.; Wray, D.; Qualman, S.J. Characterization of somatostatin receptors on human neuroblastoma tumors. *Cell Growth Differ.* **1994**, *5*, 1–8. [PubMed]
83. Georgantzi, K.; Tsolakis, A.V.; Stridsberg, M.; Jakobson, A.; Christofferson, R.; Janson, E.T. Differentiated expression of somatostatin receptor subtypes in experimental models and clinical neuroblastoma. *Pediatric Blood Cancer* **2011**, *56*, 584–589. [CrossRef] [PubMed]
84. Albers, A.R.; O'Dorisio, M.S.; Balster, D.A.; Caprara, M.; Gosh, P.; Chen, F.; Hoeger, C.; Rivier, J.; Wenger, G.D.; O'Dorisio, T.M.; et al. Somatostatin receptor gene expression in neuroblastoma. *Regul. Pept.* **2000**, *88*, 61–73. [CrossRef]
85. Kroiss, A.; Putzer, D.; Uprimny, C.; Decristoforo, C.; Gabriel, M.; Santner, W.; Kranewitter, C.; Warwitz, B.; Waitz, D.; Kendler, D.; et al. Functional imaging in phaeochromocytoma and neuroblastoma with 68Ga-DOTA-Tyr3-octreotide positron emission tomography and 123I-metaiodobenzylguanidine. *Eur. J. Nucl. Med. Mol. Imaging* **2011**, *38*, 865–873. [CrossRef]
86. Kong, G.; Hofman, M.S.; Murray, W.K.; Wilson, S.; Wood, P.; Downie, P.; Super, L.; Hogg, A.; Eu, P.; Hicks, R.J. Initial experience with gallium-68 DOTA-octreotate PET/CT and peptide receptor radionuclide therapy for pediatric patients with refractory metastatic neuroblastoma. *J. Pediatric Hematol. Oncol.* **2016**, *38*, 87–96. [CrossRef]
87. Gains, J.E.; Aldridge, M.D.; Mattoli, M.V.; Bomanji, J.B.; Biassoni, L.; Shankar, A.; Gaze, M.N. 68Ga-DOTATATE and 123I-MIBG as imaging biomarkers of disease localisation in metastatic neuroblastoma: Implications for molecular radiotherapy. *Nucl. Med. Commun.* **2020**, *2*, 1169–1177. [CrossRef]
88. Telli, T.; Lay Ergün, E.; Volkan Salanci, B.; Özgen Kiratli, P. The complementary role of 68Ga-DOTATATE PET/CT in neuroblastoma. *Clin. Nucl. Med.* **2020**, *45*, 326–329. [CrossRef]
89. Torun, N. 68Ga-DOTA-TATE in neuroblastoma with marrow involvement. *Clin. Nucl. Med.* **2019**, *44*, 467–468. [CrossRef]
90. Alexander, N.; Marrano, P.; Thorner, P.; Naranjo, A.; van Ryn, C.; Martinez, D.; Batra, V.; Zhang, L.; Irwin, M.S.; Baruchel, S. Prevalence and clinical correlations of somatostatin receptor-2 (SSTR2) expression in neuroblastoma. *J. Pediatric Hematol. Oncol.* **2019**, *41*, 222–227. [CrossRef]

91. Machado, J.S.; Beykan, S.; Herrmann, K.; Lassmann, M. Recommended administered activities for 68Ga-labelled peptides in paediatric nuclear medicine. *Eur. J. Nucl. Med. Mol. Imaging* **2016**, *43*, 2036–2039. [CrossRef]
92. Campana, D.; Ambrosini, V.; Pezzilli, R.; Fanti, S.; Labate, A.M.M.; Santini, D.; Ceccarelli, C.; Nori, F.; Franchi, R.; Corinaldesi, R.; et al. Standardized uptake values Of68Ga-DOTANOC PET: A promising prognostic tool in neuroendocrine tumors. *J. Nucl. Med.* **2010**, *51*, 353–359. [CrossRef]
93. Kim, Y.-l.; Yoo, C.; Oh, S.J.; Lee, S.J.; Kang, J.; Hwang, H.S.; Hong, S.M.; Ryoo, B.Y.; Ryu, J.S. Tumour-to-liver ratio determined by [68Ga]Ga-DOTA-TOC PET/CT as a prognostic factor of lanreotide efficacy for patients with well-differentiated gastroenteropancreatic-neuroendocrine tumours. *Ejnmmi Res.* **2020**, *10*, 63. [CrossRef]
94. Zhang, L.; Vines, D.C.; Scollard, D.A.; McKee, T.; Komal, T.; Ganguly, M.; Do, T.; Wu, B.; Alexander, N.; Vali, R.; et al. Correlation of somatostatin receptor-2 expression with gallium-68-DOTA-TATE uptake in neuroblastoma xenograft models. *Contrast Media Mol. Imaging* **2017**, *2017*. [CrossRef] [PubMed]
95. Orlando, C.; Raggi, C.C.; Bagnoni, L.; Sestini, R.; Briganti, V.; La Cava, G.; Bernini, G.; Tonini, G.; Pazzagli, M.; Serio, M.; et al. Somatostatin receptor type 2 gene expression in neuroblastoma, measured by competitive RT-PCR, is related to patient survival and to somatostatin receptor imaging by indium -111-pentetreotide. *Med. Pediatric Oncol.* **2001**, *36*. [CrossRef]
96. Moertel, C.L.; Reubi, J.C.; Scheithauer, B.S.; Schaid, D.J.; Kvols, L.K. Expression of somatostatin receptors in childhood neuroblastoma. *Am. J. Clin. Pathol.* **1994**, *102*. [CrossRef] [PubMed]
97. Briganti, V.; Sestini, R.; Orlando, C.; Bernini, G.; La Cava, G.; Tamburini, A.; Raggi, C.C.; Serio, M.; Maggi, M. Imaging of somatostatin receptors by indium-111-pentetreotide correlates with quantitative determination of somatostatin receptor type 2 gene expression in neuroblastoma tumors. *Clin. Cancer Res.* **1997**, *3*, 2385–2391.
98. Gains, J.E.; Bomanji, J.B.; Fersht, N.L.; Sullivan, T.; D'Souza, D.; Sullivan, K.P.; Aldridge, M.; Waddington, W.; Gaze, M.N. 177Lu-DOTATATE molecular radiotherapy for childhood neuroblastoma. *J. Nucl. Med.* **2011**, *52*, 1041–1047. [CrossRef] [PubMed]
99. Menda, Y.; O'Dorisio, M.S.; Kao, S.; Khanna, G.; Michael, S.; Connolly, M.; Babich, J.; O'Dorisio, T.; Bushnell, D.; Madsen, M. Phase I trial of 90Y-DOTATOC therapy in children and young adults with refractory solid tumors that express somatostatin receptors. *J. Nucl. Med.* **2010**, *51*, 1524–1531. [CrossRef] [PubMed]
100. Gains, J.E.; Moroz, V.; Aldridge, M.D.; Wan, S.; Wheatley, K.; Laidler, J.; Peet, C.; Bomanji, J.B.; Gaze, M.N. A Phase IIa trial of molecular radiotherapy with 177-lutetium DOTATATE in children with primary refractory or relapsed high-risk neuroblastoma. *Eur. J. Nucl. Med. Mol. Imaging* **2020**, *47*, 2348–2357. [CrossRef] [PubMed]
101. Jager, P.L.; Chirakal, R.; Marriott, C.J.; Brouwers, A.H.; Koopmans, K.P.; Gulenchyn, K.Y. 6-L-18F-fluorodihydroxyphenylalanine PET in neuroendocrine tumors: Basic aspects and emerging clinical applications. *J. Nucl. Med.* **2008**, *49*, 573–586. [CrossRef]
102. Koopmans, K.P.; Neels, O.N.; Kema, I.P.; Elsinga, P.H.; Links, T.P.; de Vries, E.G.E.; Jager, P.L. Molecular imaging in neuroendocrine tumors: Molecular uptake mechanisms and clinical results. *Crit. Rev. Oncol. Hematol.* **2009**, *71*, 199–213. [CrossRef]
103. Lu, M.Y.; Liu, Y.L.; Chang, H.H.; Jou, S.T.; Yang, Y.L.; Lin, K.H.; Lin, D.T.; Lee, Y.L.; Lee, H.; Wu, P.Y.; et al. Characterization of neuroblastic tumors using 18F-FDOPA PET. *J. Nucl. Med.* **2013**, *54*, 42–49. [CrossRef] [PubMed]
104. Lopci, E.; Piccardo, A.; Nanni, C.; Altrinetti, V.; Garaventa, A.; Pession, A.; Cistaro, A.; Chiti, A.; Villavecchia, G.; Fanti, S. 18F-DOPA PET/CT in neuroblastoma: Comparison of conventional imaging with CT/MR. *Clin. Nucl. Med.* **2012**, *37*, e73–e78. [CrossRef]
105. Lopci, E.; D'Ambrosio, D.; Nanni, C.; Chiti, A.; Pession, A.; Marengo, M.; Fanti, S. Feasibility of carbidopa premedication in pediatric patients: A pilot study. *Cancer Biother. Radiopharm.* **2012**, *27*, 729–733. [CrossRef] [PubMed]
106. Piccardo, A.; Lopci, E.; Conte, M.; Garaventa, A.; Foppiani, L.; Altrinetti, V.; Nanni, C.; Bianchi, P.; Cistaro, A.; Sorrentino, S.; et al. Comparison of 18F-dopa PET/CT and 123I-MIBG scintigraphy in stage 3 and 4 neuroblastoma: A pilot study. *Eur. J. Nucl. Med. Mol. Imaging* **2012**, *39*, 57–71. [CrossRef]
107. Piccardo, A.; Morana, G.; Puntoni, M.; Campora, S.; Sorrentino, S.; Zucchetta, P.; Ugolini, M.; Conte, M.; Cistaro, A.; Ferrarazzo, G.; et al. Diagnosis, treatment response, and prognosis: The role of 18F-DOPA PET/CT in children affected by neuroblastoma in comparison with 123I-MIBG scan: The first prospective study. *J. Nucl. Med.* **2020**, *61*, 367–374. [CrossRef] [PubMed]
108. Piccardo, A.; Puntoni, M.; Lopci, E.; Conte, M.; Foppiani, L.; Sorrentino, S.; Morana, G.; Naseri, M.; Cistaro, A.; Villavecchia, G.; et al. Prognostic value of 18F-DOPA PET/CT at the time of recurrence in patients affected by neuroblastoma. *Eur. J. Nucl. Med. Mol. Imaging* **2014**, *41*, 1046–1056. [CrossRef]
109. Rischpler, C.; Fukushima, K.; Isoda, T.; Javadi, M.S.; Dannals, R.F.; Abraham, R.; Wahl, R.; Bengel, F.M.; Higuchi, T. Discrepant uptake of the radiolabeled norepinephrine analogues hydroxyephedrine (HED) and metaiodobenzylguanidine (MIBG) in rat hearts. *Eur. J. Nucl. Med. Mol. Imaging* **2013**, *40*, 1077–1083. [CrossRef] [PubMed]
110. Shulkin, B.L.; Wieland, D.M.; Baro, M.E.; Ungar, D.R.; Mitchell, D.S.; Dole, M.G.; Rawwas, J.B.; Castle, V.P.; Sisson, J.C.; Hutchinson, R.J. PET hydroxyephedrine imaging of neuroblastoma. *J. Nucl. Med.* **1996**, *37*, 16–21.
111. Franzius, C.; Hermann, K.; Weckesser, M.; Kopka, K.; Juergens, K.U.; Vormoor, J.; Schober, O. Whole-body PET/CT with 11C-meta-hydroxyephedrine in tumors of the sympathetic nervous system: Feasibility study and comparison with 123I-MIBG SPECT/CT. *J. Nucl. Med.* **2006**, *47*, 1635–1642. [PubMed]
112. Chen, X.; Kudo, T.; Lapa, C.; Buck, A.; Higuchi, T. Recent advances in radiotracers targeting norepinephrine transporter: Structural development and radiolabeling improvements. *J. Neural Transm.* **2020**, *127*, 851–873. [CrossRef] [PubMed]

113. Suh, M.; Park, H.J.; Choi, H.S.; So, Y.; Lee, B.C.; Lee, W.W. Case report of PET/CT imaging of a patient with neuroblastoma using18f-FPBG. *Pediatrics* **2014**, *134*, e1731–e1734. [CrossRef] [PubMed]
114. Zhang, H.; Huang, R.; Pillarsetty, N.V.K.; Thorek, D.L.J.; Vaidyanathan, G.; Serganova, I.; Blasberg, R.G.; Lewis, J.S. Synthesis and evaluation of 18F-labeled benzylguanidine analogs for targeting the human norepinephrine transporter. *Eur. J. Nucl. Med. Mol. Imaging* **2014**, *41*, 322–332. [CrossRef]
115. Yu, M.; Bozek, J.; Lamoy, M.; Guaraldi, M.; Silva, P.; Kagan, M.; Yalamanchili, P.; Onthank, D.; Mistry, M.; Lazewatsky, J.; et al. Evaluation of LMI1195, a novel 18F-labeled cardiac neuronal PET imaging agent, in cells and animal models. *Circ. Cardiovasc. Imaging* **2011**, *4*, 435–443. [CrossRef]
116. Vaidyanathan, G.; McDougald, D.; Koumarianou, E.; Choi, J.; Hens, M.; Zalutsky, M.R. Synthesis and evaluation of 4-[18F]fluoropropoxy-3-iodobenzylguanidine ([18F]FPOIBG): A novel 18F-labeled analogue of MIBG. *Nucl. Med. Biol.* **2015**, *42*, 673–684. [CrossRef]
117. Hampel, T.; Bruns, M.; Bayer, M.; Handgretinger, R.; Bruchelt, G.; Brückner, R. Synthesis and biological effects of new hybrid compounds composed of benzylguanidines and the alkylating group of busulfan on neuroblastoma cells. *Bioorganic Med. Chem. Lett.* **2014**, *24*, 2728–2733. [CrossRef]
118. Kortylewicz, Z.P.; Coulter, D.W.; Han, G.; Baranowska-Kortylewicz, J. Radiolabeled (R)-(–)-5-Iodo-3′-O-[2-(ε-guanidinohexanoyl)-2-phenylacetyl]-2′-deoxyuridine: A new theranostic for neuroblastoma. *J. Label. Compd. Radiopharm.* **2020**, *63*, 312–324. [CrossRef]
119. Liu, D.; Li, M.; Bellizzi, A.; Menda, Y.; Lee, D.; Nourmahnad, K.; Ghobrial, S.; Schultz, M.; O'Dorisio, M.S. Preclinical evaluation of CXCR4 as novel radio-theranostic target for high grade neuroendocrine and neuroblastoma tumors. *J. Nucl. Med.* **2018**, *59*, 1313.
120. Butch, E.; Mishra, J.; Amador-Diaz, V.; Vavere, A.; Snyder, S. Selective detection of GD2-positive pediatric solid tumors using 89Zr-dinutuximab PET to facilitate anti-GD2 immunotherapy. *J. Nucl. Med.* **2018**, *59*, 170.

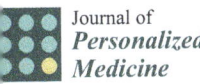

Journal of Personalized Medicine

Review

A Review on the Value of Imaging in Differentiating between Large Vessel Vasculitis and Atherosclerosis

Pieter H. Nienhuis [1,*], Gijs D. van Praagh [1], Andor W. J. M. Glaudemans [1], Elisabeth Brouwer [2] and Riemer H. J. A. Slart [1,3]

1. Department of Nuclear Medicine and Molecular Imaging, Medical Imaging Center, University of Groningen, University Medical Center Groningen, 9700 RB Groningen, The Netherlands; g.d.van.praagh@umcg.nl (G.D.v.P.); a.w.m.j.glaudemans@umcg.nl (A.W.J.M.G.); r.h.j.a.slart@umcg.nl (R.H.J.A.S.)
2. Department of Rheumatology and Clinical Immunology, University of Groningen, University Medical Center Groningen, 9700 RB Groningen, The Netherlands; e.brouwer@umcg.nl
3. Department of Biomedical Photonic Imaging, Faculty of Science and Technology, University of Twente, 7500 AE Enschede, The Netherlands
* Correspondence: p.h.nienhuis@umcg.nl

Abstract: Imaging is becoming increasingly important for the diagnosis of large vessel vasculitis (LVV). Atherosclerosis may be difficult to distinguish from LVV on imaging as both are inflammatory conditions of the arterial wall. Differentiating atherosclerosis from LVV is important to enable optimal diagnosis, risk assessment, and tailored treatment at a patient level. This paper reviews the current evidence of ultrasound (US), 2-deoxy-2-[18F]fluoro-D-glucose positron emission tomography (FDG-PET), computed tomography (CT), and magnetic resonance imaging (MRI) to distinguish LVV from atherosclerosis. In this review, we identified a total of eight studies comparing LVV patients to atherosclerosis patients using imaging—four US studies, two FDG-PET studies, and two CT studies. The included studies mostly applied different methodologies and outcome parameters to investigate vessel wall inflammation. This review reports the currently available evidence and provides recommendations on further methodological standardization methods and future directions for research.

Keywords: large vessel vasculitis; atherosclerosis; imaging; FDG-PET; radiological imaging

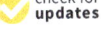

Citation: Nienhuis, P.H.; van Praagh, G.D.; Glaudemans, A.W.J.M.; Brouwer, E.; Slart, R.H.J.A. A Review on the Value of Imaging in Differentiating between Large Vessel Vasculitis and Atherosclerosis. *J. Pers. Med.* **2021**, *11*, 236. https://doi.org/10.3390/jpm11030236

Academic Editor: Pim A. de Jong

Received: 22 January 2021
Accepted: 15 March 2021
Published: 23 March 2021

Publisher's Note: MDPI stays neutral with regard to jurisdictional claims in published maps and institutional affiliations.

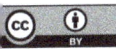

Copyright: © 2021 by the authors. Licensee MDPI, Basel, Switzerland. This article is an open access article distributed under the terms and conditions of the Creative Commons Attribution (CC BY) license (https://creativecommons.org/licenses/by/4.0/).

1. Introduction

Large vessel vasculitis (LVV) is an inflammatory condition of the blood vessel wall affecting large- and medium-sized arteries. This may cause obstruction, ischemia, or aneurysm formation, resulting in vascular events, such as vision loss, cerebrovascular accidents, or aortic rupture [1].

The two major variants of LVV are giant cell arteritis (GCA) and Takayasu arteritis (TA). GCA and TA differ mainly in age of onset—older than 50 years and younger than 40 years, respectively—and the affected arteries. The aorta and its major branches are often affected in both variants. In GCA however, third-order branches of the aorta in the head and neck region, such as the temporal artery, are also commonly involved [2].

An early and accurate diagnosis is vital to prevent complications in patients with LVV. However, the diagnosis is difficult as there are no disease-specific signs, symptoms, or laboratory tests that can definitively prove or reject the presence of GCA or TA [3,4]. The "gold standard" for diagnosing GCA, a temporal artery biopsy, has a high specificity but lower sensitivity, depending on the included patients [5,6].

Consequently, to improve diagnosis, the role of imaging in LVV has been emerging over the past decade. Current recommendations include imaging early upon clinical suspicion of LVV [7]. Imaging techniques used to investigate LVV include ultrasound

(US), magnetic resonance imaging (MRI), computed tomography (CT), and 2-deoxy-2-[18F]fluoro-D-glucose positron emission tomography (FDG-PET).

Similar to LVV, atherosclerosis is an inflammatory condition of the blood vessel wall characterized by an accumulation of activated immune cells, such as macrophages. Changes in vessel wall morphology also develop, mostly on the intimal side. Atherosclerotic lesions are patchy and result in plaque formation and calcification. Therefore, when imaging LVV patients, it may be difficult to distinguish between vasculitis and atherosclerosis. Distinguishing atherosclerosis from vasculitis is vital because both diseases require different treatment methods, and a personalized medicine approach [8].

The most commonly used imaging modalities in LVV are US and FDG-PET/CT. Several studies using these modalities reported atherosclerosis as a potential mimic for LVV. For US, the mainstay of recognizing LVV is based on the presence of a "halo sign"—a hypoechoic ring around the vessel wall [9]. However, there is evidence that the halo sign is also present in other vasculopathies, such as atherosclerosis [10]. Differentiating may be further complicated by the fact that the accuracy of US in LVV highly depends on the skills of the examiner and the US system used [5]. FDG-PET/CT displays glycolytic activity in tissues such as inflammatory lesions. Therefore, it is widely used to assess inflammation of the middle and large systemic arteries. Elevated FDG uptake can also be noticed in atheromatous plaques, making atherosclerosis a known confounder in the diagnosis of LVV with FDG-PET [11,12]. Currently, there is no clear consensus on how to distinguish FDG uptake by a vasculitic lesion from an atheromatous plaque [13].

MRI is mainly used in the smaller arteries of the head and neck for investigation of inflammation by LVV [9]. Typical vasculitic lesions show concentric wall thickening and contrast uptake around the inflamed artery [14], according to expert opinion. Atherosclerosis does not show any contrast enhancement and has a visible eccentric appearance. However, to the best of our knowledge, there is still much unknown about differentiating these lesions on MRI and recommendations for vasculitis do not mention how to differentiate. CT (angiography) visualizes vessel wall thickening and luminal changes in inflamed arteries [15]. Calcified plaques can be detected well on CT due to their high attenuating structures. Quantification of calcifications for risk assessment is done frequently, e.g., with the Agatston score [16]. Imaging noncalcified or high-risk atheromatous plaques with CT is, however, more challenging and may thus be difficult to distinguish from vasculitis [17].

Optimal diagnosis, risk assessment, and tailored treatment on patient-level is necessary, and this starts with the ability to discriminate LVV and atherosclerosis.

This review aims to evaluate the current evidence of imaging techniques to distinguish LVV from atherosclerosis.

2. Materials and Methods

2.1. Research Questions

The main research question of this review is: Can imaging findings of US, FDG-PET, CT, and MRI differentiate between large vessel vasculitis and atherosclerosis?

2.2. Search Strategy

The inclusion of appropriate studies was based on a literature search performed in the MEDLINE, EMBASE, and Web of Science electronic databases. The search strings used for each database is shown in the Appendix A.

Article title, authors, year of publication, and abstract were exported from the electronic databases and subsequently imported into Mendeley reference manager. Duplicates were removed based on suggestions in Mendeley and manually verified.

Reviewers independently screened all abstracts in Rayyan based on inclusion criteria. In case of disagreement about the eligibility of abstracts, consensus was reached through discussion. The resulting eligible articles were reviewed in full-text. These articles were cross-checked for important references. When these cited studies met our inclusion criteria, they were also included.

2.3. Inclusion Criteria

The resulting criteria for article inclusion were as follows: (1) studies including LVV patients, defined as GCA or TA; (2) studies including atherosclerosis patients; (3) studies in which US, MRI, CT, FDG-PET, or a combination of those were performed; (4) studies using parameters of vascular inflammation; (5) original research articles; (6) studies written in English.

2.4. Exclusion Criteria

Exclusion criteria were: (1) studies including patients with other types of vasculitis, such as Kawasaki or Behçet disease; (2) case reports, conference papers, animal studies, or (systematic) reviews.

2.5. Extraction of Study Characteristics

Several data were extracted from the included full-text papers. Study characteristics regarding the main study, including year of publication, type of study (prospective or retrospective), primary aim, methods used, and primary outcome of the study, were collected.

The outcome parameters regarding vascular inflammation (including—but not limited to—vessel wall thickness, tissue enhancement, FDG uptake, or the presence of a halo sign) were collected for the LVV patient group and the atherosclerosis patient group.

3. Results

An overview of the results of the literature search is shown in Figure 1. In total, eight original research articles met the inclusion criteria—a comparison of LVV patients and atherosclerosis patients imaged with US, CT, MRI, or FDG-PET—and, therefore, were included in this review.

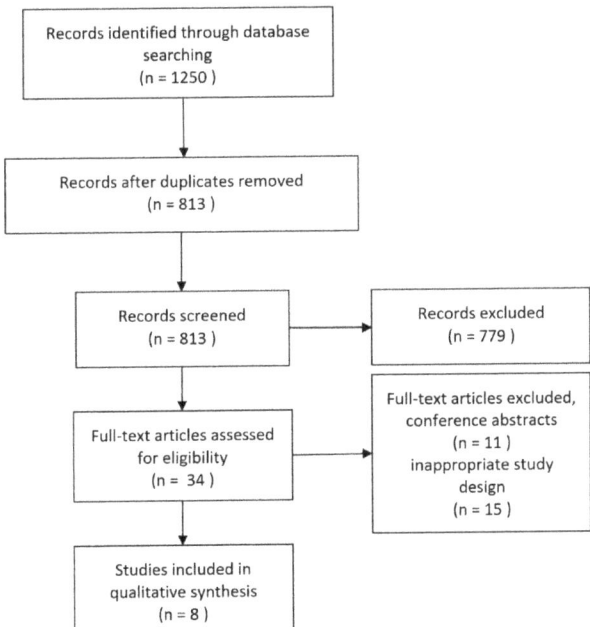

Figure 1. Flowchart of the literature review article selection process. Inappropriate study design refers to studies that did not include a well-defined LVV or atherosclerosis group or did not perform a comparative analysis between both.

Table 1 reveals the main characteristics of the included studies. Four studies were performed with US, two with FDG-PET, and two with CT. No studies with MRI were found.

Table 1. Overview of the included studies and their aims and primary outcomes.

First Author	Year	Imaging Modality	Primary Aim	Primary Outcome
Sharma	1995	CT	Assess vessel wall changes in TA	TA patients show distinct changes in vessel wall morphology
Murgatroyd	2003	US	Evaluate the diagnostic accuracy of US in GCA	US shows a sensitivity 86% and a specificity of 68%
Tsai	2005	US	Identify the main cause of carotid artery occlusion	Atherosclerosis and TA are the two most common causes of carotid artery occlusion
Karahaliou	2006	US	Evaluate the diagnostic accuracy of US in GCA	US shows high sensitivity when bilateral halo sign is present
Chowdhary	2013	CT	Identify CT angiographic findings in aortitis	Idiopathic aortitis causes larger dilatation than noninflammatory aneurysms
Stellingwerff	2015	FDG-PET	To define optimal scoring methods for GCA	Visual scoring of vascular uptake compared to liver demonstrated the highest accuracy
Grayson	2018	FDG-PET	Assessing the role of FDG-PET as a biomarker in GCA	Higher FDG-PET scores resulted in a higher chance of relapse
Fernàndez-Fernàndez	2020	US	Frequency of US halo sign in non-GCA patients	There are other conditions than GCA that reveal the halo sign

CT = computed tomography; US = ultrasound; FDG-PET = 2-deoxy-2-[18F]fluoro-D-glucose positron emission tomography; TA = Takayasu Arteritis; GCA = Giant Cell Arteritis.

In four studies, the primary objective was to assess the diagnostic accuracy of the imaging modality. Two studies included only TA patients, four studies included only GCA patients, and two studies included both. The included studies were heterogeneous in their study methods and did not use the same outcome parameters. Therefore, a direct comparison of the study results could not be performed, and only descriptive data are noted.

3.1. Ultrasound

Four studies contained data on US imaging in both LVV and atherosclerosis patients, see Table 2. Three studies considered a hypoechoic ring, or halo sign, as an outcome parameter to diagnose LVV. All three studies found that the presence of a halo sign was highly sensitive for GCA. However, two studies found that the halo sign can also be present in atherosclerosis. The study by Murgatroyd et al. found histologic evidence of moderate to severe atherosclerosis in patients with false-positive halo sign [18]. In a recent study, Fernàndez-Fernàndez et al. found that in a group of 305 patients with GCA-positive US examinations, 14 (4.6%) of patients were initially not diagnosed with GCA. Three out of these fourteen false-positive cases turned out to be atherosclerosis patients [19].

No other parameter of vascular inflammation was measured in the US studies. Karahaliou et al. demonstrated that blood flow abnormalities, mainly due to all degrees of stenosis, were present in both LVV and atherosclerosis and therefore not useful to differentiate between the diseases [20].

Table 2. Overview Outcome Parameters Ultrasound Studies.

First Author	Year	Study Design	Type of Vasculitis (GCA; TA)	Vasculitis Patients			Atherosclerosis Patients			Presence of Hypoechoic Ring (Halo Sign) Temporal Artery (%)		Blood Flow Abnormality (%)		Homogenous Echogenicity Carotid Artery (%)	
				Reference Diagnosis	Number of Patients	Mean Age	Reference Diagnosis	Number of Patients	Mean Age	Vasculitis Patients	Atherosclerosis Patients	Vasculitis Patients	Atherosclerosis Patients	Vasculitis Patients	Atherosclerosis Patients
Murgatroyd	2003	Prospective	GCA	Positive Temporal Artery Biopsy	7	-	Histology	8	-	6 (86)	6 (75)	-	-	-	-
Tsai	2005	Prospective	TA	Ishikawa Criteria	11	36	Clinical Diagnosis	17	70	-	-	-	-	0 (0)	11 (100)
Karahaliou	2006	Prospective	GCA	Clinical Diagnosis	22	70	Clinical Diagnosis of DM Type II or Stroke	15	73	18 (82)	0 (0)	9 (41)	6 (40)	-	-
Fernández-Fernández	2020	Retrospective	GCA	Clinical Diagnosis	291	-	3	-	-	291 * (100)	3 * (100)	-	-	-	-

* Patients included in this study were selected based on an US positive for GCA and, therefore, 100% of patients show the halo sign. GCA = Giant Cell Arteritis; TA = Takayasu Arteritis.

Tsai et al. compared carotid artery occlusion between atherosclerosis and TA patients. Homogeneous intima media thickening was considered a specific finding in TA patients, as opposed to heterogeneous thickening in atherosclerosis patients [21]. Moreover, they concluded that TA lesions were often more concentric (circumferential) compared with the eccentric ("off-center") lesions in atherosclerosis. They also indicated the involvement of different locations of the diseases. Atherosclerosis had a predilection for occlusion of the carotid bifurcation, with 88% involvement in atherosclerosis patients compared with 27% in TA patients. Conversely, all included TA patients had some degree of stenosis of the subclavian artery compared with only 18% of atherosclerosis patients.

3.2. FDG-PET

Both studies on FDG-PET/CT imaging that were included used visual assessment methods as outcome parameters (Table 3). Grayson et al. included FDG-PET/CT assessment based on expert opinion ("gestalt"). Of all clinically active LVV (GCA and TA) patients, 85% was considered positive [22]. Using this method, 17% of patients in the hyperlipidemia group were falsely positive assigned as LVV on FDG-PET/CT.

A more standardized approach was taken in the study by Stellingwerff et al. by visually scoring FDG uptake in the vessels compared to the liver [23]. In grade 1, the vessel uptake was lower than the liver, in grade 2 equal to the liver, and in grade 3 higher than the liver. Considering grade 2 and 3 as positive for LVV, resulted in 100% sensitivity, considering only grade 3 as positive resulted in a 92% sensitivity. Importantly, sensitivity decreased for patients who were on treatment with glucocorticoids. Using the first threshold (similar to or higher than liver) resulted in diagnosing 63% of atherosclerosis patients as GCA. The latter threshold (higher than liver) was more specific for GCA with 21% of atherosclerosis cases being falsely positive for GCA.

Apart from uptake intensity, FDG uptake pattern can also be scored. A diffuse (homogeneous) FDG uptake pattern was present in all GCA patients, but only in 21% of atherosclerosis patients. When combining uptake intensity (uptake compared to liver) and a diffuse uptake pattern, GCA can be well differentiated from atherosclerosis with a 95% specificity. However, sensitivity for GCA decreased to 83%.

A semiquantitative approach to visual scoring was used in both studies. By counting the number of arteries and the intensity uptake grade, it is possible to better distinguish between LVV and (atherosclerotic) controls. Such a composite score, like the PETVAS score devised by Grayson et al., is likely to be higher in LVV compared to atherosclerosis, because of more intense FDG uptake in a higher number of arteries [22].

In the study by Stellingwerff et al., the maximal standardized uptake value (SUVmax) was also measured. This uptake parameter was, on average, higher in GCA patients compared to atherosclerosis patients but also showed overlap [23].

3.3. CT(A)

Two studies gathered data in vasculitis and atherosclerosis patients using CT Angiography, see Table 4. Both studies investigated the aorta. In 1995, Sharma et al. described vessel wall abnormalities in both abdominal and thoracic aorta, such as stenosis, dilatation, and wall thickening in patients with TA [24]. None of these vessel wall abnormalities was noticed in atherosclerosis patients. Calcification was present in all atherosclerosis patients and in 54% of TA patients.

Table 3. Overview Outcome Parameters FDG-PET studies.

First Author	Year	Study Design	Vasculitis Patients			Atherosclerosis Patients			Number of Patients with Visual Uptake Similar to Liver (%); Higher than Liver (%)		Number of Patients with Diffuse Visual Uptake		Mean Number of Arteries with Increased Visual FDG Uptake (range)		Mean SUVmax in the Aorta (SD)		Number of Scans ** with Positive Visual 'Gestalt' LVV Assessment	
			Type of Vasculitis (GCA; TA)	Reference Diagnosis	Number of Patients	Mean Age	Reference Diagnosis	Number of Patients	Mean Age	Vasculitis Patients	Atherosclerosis Patients	Vasculitis Patients	Atherosclerosis Patients	Vasculitis Patients	Atherosclerosis Patients	Vasculitis Patients	Atherosclerosis Patients	Vasculitis Patients	Atherosclerosis Patients
Stellingwerff	2015	Retrospective	GCA	ACR Criteria; Positive TAB; Established Clinical Diagnosis	12	70	CT Calcified Plaque Score > 2	19	69	12 (100); 11 (92)	12 (63); 4 (21)	12 (100)	4 (21)	35 (19-40)	13 (5-27)	3.81 (1.10)	2.82 (0.76)	-	-
Grayson	2018	Prospective	GCA; TA *	ACR Criteria; Clinically Active Disease	25, 15 *	67; 44 *	Hyperlipidemia (>55 years and statin use)	35	64	-	-	-	-	22 (·); 19 * (·)***	14***	-	-	34 (85)	6 (17)

* Data for the second patient group in this study. ** The study using this parameter used data for the number of scans, not numbers. *** The parameter in this study included two fewer arteries than the other study. LVV = Large vessel vasculitis; GCA = Giant Cell Arteritis; TA = Takayasu Arteritis.

Table 4. Overview Outcome Parameters CT(A) studies.

First Author	Year	Study Design	Vasculitis Patients			Atherosclerosis Patients			Patients with Aortic Stenosis or occlusion (%)		Patients with Aortic Dilative Lesions (%)		Patients with Aortic Wall Thickening (%)		Patients with Aortic Calcification (%)		Diameter Ascending Aorta mm (SD)		Diameter Aortic Arch mm (SD)		Diameter Descending Aorta mm (SD)	
			Type of Vasculitis (GCA; TA)	Reference Diagnosis	Number of Patients	Mean Age	Reference Diagnosis	Number of Patients	Mean Age	Vasculitis Patients	Atherosclerosis Patients	Vasculitis Patients	Atherosclerosis Patients	Vasculitis Patients	Atherosclerosis Patients	Vasculitis Patients	Atherosclerosis Patients	Vasculitis Patients	Atherosclerosis Patients	Vasculitis Patients	Atherosclerosis Patients	Vasculitis Patients	Atherosclerosis Patients
Sharma	1996	Prospective	TA	-	24	70	-	12	63	10 (42)	0 (0)	9 (38)	0 (0)	20 (83)	0 (0)	13 (54)	12 (100)	-	-	-	-	-	-
Chowdhary	2013	Retrospective	GCA ****	Clinical Diagnosis of Secondary Aortitis	16	36	Patients with noninflammatory aneurysms	18	70	-	-	-	-	1 (6)	4 (22)	1 (6)	10 (56)	53 (10)	49 (12)	35 (6)	31 (4)	36 (7)	33 (13)

**** This patient group included 10 GCA, 2 TA, 2 with bicuspid aortic valve, 1 seronegative arthritis, and 1 lupus patient. GCA = Giant cell arteritis; TA = Takayasu Arteritis.

Chowdhary et al. investigated patients with thoracic aortic aneurysms [25]. Patients with noninflammatory aneurysms more frequently had hyperlipidemia. These atherosclerotic patients showed increased aortic calcification compared to TA patients. This study also found aortic wall thickening of more than 3 mm in four atherosclerosis patients and in one LVV patient.

Additionally, the same study measured aortic diameters in the thoracic aorta. Aortic diameters differed in the aortic arch, where LVV patients had a slightly higher mean diameter than atherosclerosis patients.

4. Discussion

This review aimed to gather the currently available evidence for distinguishing LVV and atherosclerosis on imaging. Eight imaging studies were included based on their inclusion of separate groups of LVV and atherosclerosis patients. Several studies indicated that the most used diagnostic signs of LVV in US and FDG-PET, respectively, the halo sign and visual FDG uptake, may also be present in atherosclerosis patients. When visually scoring FDG uptake intensity and pattern, FDG-PET/CT attained 95% specificity for diagnosing LVV against an atherosclerotic control group. The two included CTA studies indicated calcification was more often seen in atherosclerosis patients. No MRI studies comparing LVV and atherosclerosis were found.

Three US studies indicated the presence of the halo sign in atherosclerosis patients. One study showed histologic evidence of atherosclerosis on temporal artery biopsy in patients with a positive halo sign [18]. However, these patients were clinically suspected of having GCA, and the temporal artery biopsy may have been a false negative. Two of these three articles were published 14 and 17 years ago. In more recent studies, the requirements for the halo sign were more standardized [26]. The included study from 2020 did show the presence of a halo sign using these standardized measures [19].

Another recent US study in atherosclerosis patients showed that thickening of the carotid artery walls correlated with thickening of the temporal artery walls, mimicking the halo sign [10]. As US is increasingly being used to diagnose LVV, there is a growing need to identify diseases that may mimic LVV diagnosis on US.

FDG-PET is already a proven method for measuring vascular inflammation in atherosclerotic plaques as well as in LVV [13,27]. However, only two studies identified in this review directly compared FDG-PET in atherosclerosis and LVV [22,23]. The presence of FDG uptake in atherosclerosis patients decreased the specificity of FDG-PET when diagnosing LVV. When used in conjunction with CT, an overlap of calcification and FDG uptake may be used to identify atherosclerosis [11]. However, FDG uptake is most prominent in the early stages of atherosclerosis and decreases when the plaque is calcified (stabilized nonvulnerable) [27,28]. Distinguishing between noncalcified atherosclerotic plaques and LVV may, thus, be extra challenging.

One way to discriminate between atherosclerosis and LVV is by objectivating the pattern of FDG uptake. One study included in this review showed that using a diffuse uptake pattern as a diagnostic criterium decreases the number of false positives, especially the number of false-positive atherosclerosis patients [23]. Atherosclerosis typically has more focal or "patchy" FDG uptake. Diffuse uptake as a diagnostic criterion has also been used in previous research [12], and recommended in the analysis of LVV [13,29]. In addition to uptake pattern, FDG uptake intensity is thought to be higher in LVV than in atherosclerosis [30]. This is reflected in the studies included in this review, where using a threshold for uptake higher than liver resulted in fewer false-positive atherosclerosis patients. Also, semiquantitative measurements such as SUVmax were higher in LVV patients. Careful interpretation of LVV patients with moderate FDG uptake is, therefore, important.

The location of the vessels may also differentiate between LVV and atherosclerosis, with atherosclerosis being more common in the abdominal aorta and iliofemoral arteries [30]. Cumulative FDG uptake scores—using the sum of uptake scores of multiple arteries—can help differentiate between LVV and atherosclerosis patients. However, such a cumulative score does not discriminate on the level of a single artery and, therefore, does not aid identifying atherosclerotic disease in LVV affected arteries.

A recent recommendation paper on FDG-PET/CT in LVV proposes further standardization of interpretation criteria and acknowledges the possible difficulties distinguishing atherosclerosis and LVV [13]. These include visually scoring uptake intensity compared to liver and noting its uptake pattern, with patchy uptake being more suggestive of atherosclerosis. The authors also recommended the use of a cumulative vascular FDG uptake score. Worldwide adoption of these standardized interpretation criteria will enable better comparison of LVV and atherosclerosis with FDG-PET/CT, expanding the current limited evidence on this subject.

The use of more semiquantitative measurements when interpreting FDG-PET/CT is mentioned by recommendation/position papers for both LVV and atherosclerosis [13,31]. Both papers mention the highest reproducibility when calculating the ratio of the standardized uptake values (SUV) of the vessel wall compared to SUV in a background organ. The use target-to-background ratio (TBR) may further increase standardization of FDG-PET/CT interpretation as well as provide an opportunity for monitoring vessel wall inflammation.

Two studies included in this review investigated CTA in TA patients. Apart from increased calcification in atherosclerosis patients, the results from these studies are less clear. One of the studies was published 25 years ago and only stated an absence of vessel wall abnormalities in atherosclerosis [24]. Additionally, the reference standard for the atherosclerosis group was not defined. The other CTA study compared aneurysm patients and found increased aortic vessel wall thickness in atherosclerosis and LVV patients. Importantly, this study also included 5 patients without LVV in the group of 17. Nonetheless, the study was included in this review because all patients in this group had aortitis.

Whereas calcified plaques are easily discernable on CT, detecting noncalcified, fatty plaques is more difficult [32]. Consequently, determining whether the cause of stenosis is atherosclerotic or vasculitic may also be challenging, especially in arteries that are commonly affected in both atherosclerosis and LVV, such as the carotid arteries. Distinguishing here may be especially important as severe complications such as transient ischemic attack and cerebrovascular accident can result from both atherosclerosis and LVV when the head/neck arteries are affected. CTA can be used to diagnose LVV based on morphological vessel wall abnormalities, showing concentric thickening stretching a long segment of an artery [33]. Atherosclerotic non-calcified plaques and vulnerability can also be assessed using CTA, showing eccentric and focal thickening of the arterial wall [34]. Although there is little evidence on the combined use of FDG-PET and CTA in LVV, its combined use may reliably diagnose LVV while also showing morphological changes to the vessel wall. This way, atherosclerosis may be distinguished reliably from LVV, also at the level of an individual artery.

No MRI studies met the inclusion criteria of this review. MRI is not commonly used in atherosclerosis imaging nor is it a first-line imaging technique in LVV [7]. Several MRI studies on intracranial vasculopathies did include vasculitis patients, although not identified as GCA or TA [14,35,36]. Schwarz et al. concluded MRI could be used well in differentiating between vasculitis and atherosclerosis, but the distinction in this study was mainly based on expert opinion. Vasculitis shows perivascular contrast enhancement and wall thickening can be characterized as concentric and in a long vessel segment. Conversely, atherosclerosis does not show any contrast enhancement, and wall thickening is eccentric and focal. The exact value of MRI in this matter should be further investigated.

The most frequently used imaging techniques in LVV, US and FDG-PET, may cause false-positive diagnoses in atherosclerosis patients. Discriminating atherosclerosis from vasculitis in LVV patients is vital to prevent unnecessary GC treatment in atherosclerotic patients. Moreover, there is evidence of accelerated atherosclerosis in LVV patients, in particular in TA [37]. GCA affects patients in the same age range where atherosclerosis is common, meaning they often overlap. Future studies will need to elucidate the extent to which atherosclerosis can mimic LVV and study the degree of atherosclerosis in LVV patients. Including atherosclerotic comparator groups in future LVV imaging studies is pivotal to addressing this question.

Additionally, studies using modern imaging systems are needed. High-resolution US, digital PET imaging, combined PET/MR, and previously mentioned combined PET/CTA may detect (noncalcified) underlying atheromatous plaques in LVV patients by visualizing the arterial wall in more detail [31]. Importantly, future imaging studies will need to include more quantified and standardized parameters with which these types of vascular inflammation can be differentiated. These parameters will subsequently allow us to recognize atherosclerotic plaques within LVV patients beyond using vascular calcification. Lastly, new identified parameters may allow the study of the interaction between the atherosclerotic and vasculitic process.

The reference standards used in the studies were also heterogeneous and 3 out of 8 studies were of retrospective design. Some studies defined those with an increased cardiovascular risk profile as atherosclerosis patients, based on clinical diagnosis or by hyperlipidemia. Other studies used histology or a plaque score. As there are no set criteria for diagnosing patients with atherosclerosis, multiple reference standards are possible. However, well defined and standardized methods are important to ensure reproducibility. Standardized cardiovascular risk profile scores and calcification scores may therefore be best suitable to define an atherosclerosis group. The latter may be achieved by using (low dose) CT scans to quantify the level of calcification, similar to the Agatston score [16]. Visual methods to assess the degree of calcification measurements may also be used, provided that CT is available [38]. Furthermore, artificial intelligence could be a valuable tool in differentiating between the (mixed) diseases. For example, neural networks have been proven to be strong in segmentation tasks and as classifiers [39]. One of the outcomes of the included studies of the current paper was that atherosclerotic uptake was more focal, while vasculitic uptake was more diffuse. Textural analysis of these neural networks and/or radiomics has the potential to prove this in more detail, including the location of the disease, as LVV is mainly in the adventitia and media of the arterial wall, and atherosclerosis at the intima, including the use of high resolution (digital) scanners to distinguish the vascular wall layers. In addition, it could vastly reduce analysis time of all vessels and potentially improve quantification of the diseases.

In general, there is a lack of common study methods and outcome parameters in the included studies, which prohibited us to perform a meta-analysis. However, this is, to the best of our knowledge, the first review to assess the studies in which atherosclerosis and LVV are compared on imaging. Hence, the little available evidence this review presents is important as a starting point for future research.

5. Conclusions

In conclusion, the evidence available in literature suggests that atherosclerosis can mimic imaging findings of LVV on US and FDG-PET. Hence, it may be difficult in some cases to differentiate between LVV and atherosclerosis, which lowers the diagnostic accuracy of these frequently used imaging methods. High intensity and diffuse uptake pattern on FDG-PET/CT showed the highest specificity distinguishing LVV from atherosclerosis. However, only few imaging studies directly compared atherosclerosis and LVV, and there is little standardization of study methods. Future, randomized, prospective study set-ups comparing atherosclerosis and LVV should be performed with standardized inclusion criteria and assessment methods.

Author Contributions: Conceptualization, R.H.J.A.S. and P.H.N.; methodology, G.D.v.P. and P.H.N.; software, P.H.N.; validation, G.D.v.P., P.H.N. and R.H.J.A.S.; formal analysis, G.D.v.P. and P.H.N.; investigation, P.H.N.; resources, P.H.N.; data curation, P.H.N.; writing—original draft preparation, P.H.N.; writing—review and editing, G.D.v.P., P.H.N., R.H.J.A.S., A.W.J.M.G., and E.B.; visualization, P.H.N. and G.D.v.P.; supervision, R.H.J.A.S.; project administration, P.H.N.; funding acquisition, N/A. All authors have read and agreed to the published version of the manuscript.

Funding: This research received no external funding.

Institutional Review Board Statement: Not applicable.

Informed Consent Statement: Not applicable.

Data Availability Statement: Not applicable.

Conflicts of Interest: Pieter H. Nienhuis, Riemer H.J.A. Slart, Elisabeth Brouwer, and Andor W.J. Glaudemans declare no conflicts of interest. Gijs D. van Praagh was supported in part by an unconditional grant from PUSH: a collaboration between Siemens Healthineers and the University Medical Center Groningen. The sponsor had no role in the conceptualization, interpretation of findings, writing or publication of the article.

Appendix A

Search string MEDLINE (search date: 01-12-2020, 424 results)

("Diagnostic Imaging"[Mesh] OR Diagnostic Ima*[tiab] OR Ultraso*[tiab] OR US[tiab] OR magnetic resonance [tiab] OR MRI[tiab] OR MRA[tiab] OR angiography[tiab] OR computed tomography[tiab] OR CT[tiab] OR CTA[tiab] OR positron emission tomography[tiab] OR PET[tiab])

AND

("Giant Cell Arteritis"[Mesh] OR Vasculi*[tiab] OR LVV[tiab] OR large vessel vasculitis[tiab] OR giant cell arteritis[tiab] OR GCA[tiab] OR "Takayasu Arteritis"[Mesh] OR takayasu arteritis[tiab] OR TAK[tiab])

AND

("Atherosclerosis"[Mesh] OR "Arteriosclerosis"[Mesh] OR athero*[tiab] OR vascular calcification[tiab])

NOT "Case Reports" [Publication Type]

Search string EMBASE (search date: 01-12-2020, 519 results)

(('Diagnostic Ima*' OR Ultraso* OR US OR 'magnetic resonance' OR MRI OR MRA OR angiography OR 'computed tomography' OR CT OR CTA OR 'positron emission tomography' OR PET):ab,ti)

AND

((Vasculi* OR LVV OR 'large vessel vasculitis' OR 'giant cell arteritis' OR GCA OR 'takayasu arteritis' OR TAK):ab,ti)

AND

((athero* OR 'vascular calcification'):ab,ti)

NOT 'case report'/exp

Search string Web of Science, Core Collection (search date: 01-12-2020, 104 results)

TS = ("Diagnostic Imaging" OR "Diagnostic Ima*" OR "Ultraso*" OR "US" OR "magnetic resonance" OR "MRI" OR "MRA" OR "angiography" OR "computed tomography" OR

"CT" OR "CTA" OR "positron emission tomography" OR "PET")

AND

TI = ("Giant Cell Arteritis" OR "Vasculi*" OR "LVV" OR "large vessel vasculitis" OR "giant cell arteritis" OR "GCA" OR "Takayasu Arteritis" OR "TAK")

AND

TS = ("Atherosclerosis" OR "Arteriosclerosis" OR "athero*" OR "vascular calcification")

References

1. Jennette, J. Overview of the 2012 revised International Chapel Hill Consensus Conference nomenclature of vasculitides. *Clin. Exp. Nephrol.* **2013**, *17*, 603–606. [CrossRef] [PubMed]
2. Watanabe, R.; Berry, G.J.; Liang, D.H.; Goronzy, J.J.; Weyand, C.M. Pathogenesis of Giant Cell Arteritis and Takayasu Arteritis—Similarities and Differences. *Curr. Rheumatol. Rep.* **2020**, *22*, 68. [CrossRef] [PubMed]
3. Van Der Geest, K.S.M.; Sandovici, M.; Brouwer, E.; Mackie, S.L. Diagnostic Accuracy of Symptoms, Physical Signs, and Laboratory Tests for Giant Cell Arteritis: A Systematic Review and Meta-analysis. *JAMA Intern. Med.* **2020**, *180*, 1295–1304. [CrossRef] [PubMed]
4. Kim, E.S.H.; Beckman, J. Takayasu arteritis: Challenges in diagnosis and management. *Heart* **2018**, *104*, 558–565. [CrossRef]
5. Luqmani, R.; Lee, E.; Singh, S.; Gillett, M.; Schmidt, W.A.; Bradburn, M.; Dasgupta, B.; Diamantopoulos, A.P.; Forrester-Barker, W.; Hamilton, W.; et al. The role of ultrasound compared to biopsy of temporal arteries in the diagnosis and treatment of giant cell arteritis (TABUL): A diagnostic accuracy and cost-effectiveness study. *Health Technol Assess* **2016**, *20*, 313. [CrossRef]
6. MacKie, S.L.; Brouwer, E. What can negative temporal artery biopsies tell us? *Rheumatology* **2020**, *59*, 925–927. [CrossRef]
7. Dejaco, C.; Ramiro, S.; Duftner, C.; Besson, F.L.; Bley, T.A.; Blockmans, D.; Brouwer, E.; Cimmino, M.A.; Clark, E.; Dasgupta, B.; et al. EULAR recommendations for the use of imaging in large vessel vasculitis in clinical practice. *Ann. Rheum. Dis.* **2018**, *77*, 636–643. [CrossRef] [PubMed]
8. Larivière, D.; Sacre, K.; Klein, I.; Hyafil, F.; Choudat, L.; Chauveheid, M.P.; Papo, T. Extra- and intracranial cerebral vasculitis in giant cell arteritis: An observational study. *Medicine* **2014**, *93*, e265. [CrossRef] [PubMed]
9. Duftner, C.; Dejaco, C.; Sepriano, A.; Falzon, L.; Schmidt, W.A.; Ramiro, S. Imaging in diagnosis, outcome prediction and monitoring of large vessel vasculitis: A systematic literature review and meta-Analysis informing the EULAR recommendations. *RMD Open* **2018**, *4*. [CrossRef]
10. De Miguel, E.; Beltran, L.M.; Monjo, I.; Deodati, F.; Schmidt, W.A.; Garcia-Puig, J. Atherosclerosis as a potential pitfall in the diagnosis of giant cell arteritis. *Rheumatology* **2018**, *57*, 318–321. [CrossRef] [PubMed]
11. Ben-Haim, S.; Kupzov, E.; Tamir, A.; Israel, O. Evaluation of 18F-FDG uptake and arterial wall calcifications using 18F-FDG PET/CT. *J. Nucl. Med.* **2004**, *45*, 1816–1821. [PubMed]
12. Lensen, K.D.F.; Comans, E.F.I.; Voskuyl, A.E.; Van Der Laken, C.J.; Brouwer, E.; Zwijnenburg, A.T.; Pereira Arias-Bouda, L.M.; Glaudemans, A.W.J.M.; Slart, R.H.J.A.; Smulders, Y.M. Large-vessel vasculitis: Interobserver agreement and diagnostic accuracy of ^{18}F-FDG-PET/CT. *Biomed Res. Int.* **2015**, *2015*. [CrossRef] [PubMed]
13. Slart, R.H.J.A.; Glaudemans, A.W.J.M.; Chareonthaitawee, P.; Treglia, G.; Besson, F.L.; Bley, T.A.; Blockmans, D.; Boellaard, R.; Bucerius, J.; Carril, J.M.; et al. FDG-PET/CT(A) imaging in large vessel vasculitis and polymyalgia rheumatica: Joint procedural recommendation of the EANM, SNMMI, and the PET Interest Group (PIG), and endorsed by the ASNC. *Eur. J. Nucl. Med. Mol. Imaging* **2018**, *45*, 1250–1269. [CrossRef] [PubMed]
14. Schwarz, F.; Strobl, F.F.; Cyran, C.C.; Helck, A.D.; Hartmann, M.; Schindler, A.; Nikolaou, K.; Reiser, M.F.; Saam, T. Reproducibility and differentiation of cervical arteriopathies using in vivo high-resolution black-blood MRI at 3 T. *Neuroradiology* **2016**, *58*, 569–576. [CrossRef] [PubMed]
15. Broncano, J.; Vargas, D.; Bhalla, S.; Cummings, K.W.; Raptis, C.A.; Luna, A. CT and MR imaging of cardiothoracic vasculitis. *Radiographics* **2018**, *38*, 997–1021. [CrossRef] [PubMed]
16. Agatston, A.S.; Janowitz, W.R.; Hildner, F.J.; Zusmer, N.R.; Viamonte, M.; Detrano, R. Quantification of coronary artery calcium using ultrafast computed tomography. *J. Am. Coll. Cardiol.* **1990**, *15*, 827–832. [CrossRef]
17. Das, M.; Braunschweig, T.; Mühlenbruch, G.; Mahnken, A.H.; Krings, T.; Langer, S.; Koeppel, T.; Jacobs, M.; Günther, R.W.; Mommertz, G. Carotid Plaque Analysis: Comparison of Dual-Source Computed Tomography (CT) Findings and Histopathological Correlation. *Eur. J. Vasc. Endovasc. Surg.* **2009**, *38*, 14–19. [CrossRef] [PubMed]
18. Murgatroyd, H.; Nimmo, M.; Evans, A.; MacEwen, C. The use of ultrasound as an aid in the diagnosis of giant cell arteritis: A pilot study comparing histological features with ultrasound findings. *EYE* **2003**, *17*, 415–419. [CrossRef] [PubMed]
19. Fernández-Fernández, E.; Monjo-Henry, I.; Bonilla, G.; Plasencia, C.; Miranda-Carús, M.-E.; Balsa, A.; De Miguel, E. False positives in the ultrasound diagnosis of giant cell arteritis: Some diseases can also show the halo sign. *Rheumatology* **2020**. [CrossRef]

20. Karahaliou, M.; Vaiopoulos, G.; Papaspyrou, S.; Kanakis, M.A.; Revenas, K.; Sfikakis, P.P. Colour duplex sonography of temporal arteries before decision for biopsy: A prospective study in 55 patients with suspected giant cell arteritis. *Arthritis Res. Ther.* **2006**, *8*, R116. [CrossRef]
21. Tsai, C.-F.; Jeng, J.-S.; Lu, C.-J.; Yip, P.-K. Clinical and ultrasonographic manifestations in major causes of common carotid artery occlusion. *J. Neuroimaging* **2005**, *15*, 50–56. [CrossRef] [PubMed]
22. Grayson, P.C.; Alehashemi, S.; Bagheri, A.A.; Civelek, A.C.; Cupps, T.R.; Kaplan, M.J.; Malayeri, A.A.; Merkel, P.A.; Novakovich, E.; Bluemke, D.A.; et al. 18F-Fluorodeoxyglucose–Positron Emission Tomography As an Imaging Biomarker in a Prospective, Longitudinal Cohort of Patients With Large Vessel Vasculitis. *Arthritis Rheumatol.* **2018**, *70*, 439–449. [CrossRef] [PubMed]
23. Stellingwerff, M.D.; Brouwer, E.; Lensen, K.J.D.F.; Rutgers, A.; Arends, S.; Van Der Geest, K.S.M.; Glaudemans, A.W.J.M.; Slart, R.H.J.A. Different scoring methods of FDG PET/CT in Giant cell arteritis need for standardization. *Medicine* **2015**, *94*, 1–9. [CrossRef] [PubMed]
24. Sharma, S.; Sharma, S.; Taneja, K.; Gupta, A.K.; Rajani, M. Morphologic mural changes in the aorta revealed by CT in patients with nonspecific aortoarteritis (Takayasu's arteritis). *Am. J. Roentgenol.* **1996**, *167*, 1321–1325. [CrossRef] [PubMed]
25. Chowdhary, V.R.; Crowson, C.S.; Bhagra, A.S.; Warrington, K.J.; Vrtiska, T.J. CT angiographic imaging characteristics of thoracic idiopathic aortitis. *J. Cardiovasc. Comput. Tomogr.* **2013**, *7*, 297–302. [CrossRef] [PubMed]
26. Chrysidis, S.; Duftner, C.; Dejaco, C.; Schaefer, V.S.; Ramiro, S.; Carrara, G.; Scire, C.A.; Hocevar, A.; Diamantopoulos, A.P.; Iagnocco, A.; et al. Definitions and reliability assessment of elementary ultrasound lesions in giant cell arteritis: A study from the OMERACT Large Vessel Vasculitis Ultrasound Working Group. *RMD Open* **2018**, *4*. [CrossRef]
27. Tarkin, J.M.; Joshi, F.R.; Rudd, J.H.F. PET imaging of inflammation in atherosclerosis. *Nat. Rev. Cardiol.* **2014**, *11*, 443–457. [CrossRef]
28. Meirelles, G.S.P.; Gonen, M.; Strauss, H.W. 18F-FDG uptake and calcifications in the thoracic aorta on positron emission tomography/computed tomography examinations: Frequency and stability on serial scans. *J. Thorac. Imaging* **2011**, *26*, 54–62. [CrossRef]
29. Slart, R.H.; Glaudemans, A.W.; Gheysens, O.; Lubberink, M.; Kero, T.; Dweck, M.R.; Habib, G.; Gaemperli, O.; Saraste, A.; Gimelli, A.; et al. Procedural recommendations of cardiac PET/CT imaging: Standardization in inflammatory-, infective-, infiltrative-, and innervation (4Is)-related cardiovascular diseases: A joint collaboration of the EACVI and the EANM. *Eur. J. Nucl. Med. Mol. Imaging* **2020**. [CrossRef]
30. Belhocine, T.; Blockmans, D.; Hustinx, R.; Vandevivere, J.; Mortelmans, L. Imaging of large vessel vasculitis with 18FDG PET: Illusion or reality? A critical review of the literature data. *Eur. J. Nucl. Med. Mol. Imaging* **2003**, *30*, 1305–1313. [CrossRef]
31. Bucerius, J.; Hyafil, F.; Verberne, H.J.; Slart, R.H.J.A.; Lindner, O.; Sciagra, R.; Agostini, D.; Übleis, C.; Gimelli, A.; Hacker, M. Position paper of the Cardiovascular Committee of the European Association of Nuclear Medicine (EANM) on PET imaging of atherosclerosis. *Eur. J. Nucl. Med. Mol. Imaging* **2016**, *43*, 780–792. [CrossRef]
32. Schlett, C.L.; Ferencik, M.; Celeng, C.; Maurovich-Horvat, P.; Scheffel, H.; Stolzmann, P.; Do, S.; Kauczor, H.U.; Alkadhi, H.; Bamberg, F.; et al. How to assess non-calcified plaque in CT angiography: Delineation methods affect diagnostic accuracy of low-attenuation plaque by CT for lipid-core plaque in histology. *Eur. Heart J. Cardiovasc. Imaging* **2013**, *14*, 1099–1105. [CrossRef] [PubMed]
33. Prieto-González, S.; Arguis, P.; García-Martínez, A.; Espígol-Frigolé, G.; Tavera-Bahillo, I.; Butjosa, M.; Sánchez, M.; Hernández-Rodríguez, J.; Grau, J.M.; Cid, M.C. Large vessel involvement in biopsy-proven giant cell arteritis: Prospective study in 40 newly diagnosed patients using CT angiography. *Ann. Rheum. Dis.* **2012**, *71*, 1170–1176. [CrossRef] [PubMed]
34. Menezes, L.J.; Kotze, C.W.; Agu, O.; Richards, T.; Brookes, J.; Goh, V.J.; Rodriguez-Justo, M.; Endozo, R.; Harvey, R.; Yusuf, S.W.; et al. Investigating vulnerable atheroma using combined 18F-FDG PET/CT angiography of carotid plaque with immunohistochemical validation. *J. Nucl. Med.* **2011**, *52*, 1698–1703. [CrossRef] [PubMed]
35. Perren, F.; Vargas, M.I.; Kargiotis, O. Etiology of Intracranial Arterial Stenosis: Are Transcranial Color-Coded Duplex Ultrasound and 3T Black Blood MR Imaging Complementary? *J. Neuroimaging* **2016**, *26*, 426–430. [CrossRef]
36. Park, J.E.; Jung, S.C.; Lee, S.H.; Jeon, J.Y.; Lee, J.Y.; Kim, H.S.; Choi, C.-G.; Kim, S.-O.S.J.; Lee, D.H.; Kim, S.-O.S.J.; et al. Comparison of 3D magnetic resonance imaging and digital subtraction angiography for intracranial artery stenosis. *Eur. Radiol.* **2017**, *27*, 4737–4746. [CrossRef] [PubMed]
37. Hong, J.; Maron, D.J.; Shirai, T.; Weyand, C.M. Accelerated atherosclerosis in patients with chronic inflammatory rheumatologic conditions. *Int. J. Clin. Rheumtol.* **2015**, *10*, 365–381. [CrossRef] [PubMed]
38. Rominger, A.; Saam, T.; Wolpers, S.; Cyran, C.C.; Schmidt, M.; Foerster, S.; Nikolaou, K.; Reiser, M.F.; Bartenstein, P.; Hacker, M. 18F-FDG PET/CT identifies patients at risk for future vascular events in an otherwise asymptomatic cohort with neoplastic disease. *J. Nucl. Med.* **2009**, *50*, 1611–1620. [CrossRef] [PubMed]
39. Al'Aref, S.J.; Anchouche, K.; Singh, G.; Slomka, P.J.; Kolli, K.K.; Kumar, A.; Pandey, M.; Maliakal, G.; Van Rosendael, A.R.; Beecy, A.N.; et al. Clinical applications of machine learning in cardiovascular disease and its relevance to cardiac imaging. *Eur. Heart J.* **2019**, *40*, 1975–1986. [CrossRef]

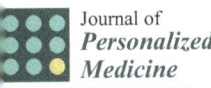

Article

Analysis of Morphological-Hemodynamic Risk Factors for Aneurysm Rupture Including a Newly Introduced Total Volume Ratio

Ui Yun Lee [1] and Hyo Sung Kwak [2,*]

[1] Division of Mechanical Design Engineering, College of Engineering, Jeonbuk National University, Jeon-ju 54896, Korea; euiyun93@naver.com
[2] Department of Radiology and Research Institute of Clinical Medicine of Jeonbuk National University, Biomedical Research Institute of Jeonbuk National University Hospital, Jeon-ju 54907, Korea
* Correspondence: kwak8140@jbnu.ac.kr; Tel.: +82-63-250-2582

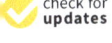

Citation: Lee, U.Y.; Kwak, H.S. Analysis of Morphological-Hemodynamic Risk Factors for Aneurysm Rupture Including a Newly Introduced Total Volume Ratio. *J. Pers. Med.* 2021, 11, 744. https://doi.org/10.3390/jpm11080744

Academic Editors: Pim A. de Jong, Nelleke Tolboom and Wouter Foppen

Received: 5 July 2021
Accepted: 27 July 2021
Published: 29 July 2021

Publisher's Note: MDPI stays neutral with regard to jurisdictional claims in published maps and institutional affiliations.

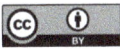

Copyright: © 2021 by the authors. Licensee MDPI, Basel, Switzerland. This article is an open access article distributed under the terms and conditions of the Creative Commons Attribution (CC BY) license (https://creativecommons.org/licenses/by/4.0/).

Abstract: The purpose of this study was to evaluate morphological and hemodynamic factors, including the newly developed total volume ratio (TVR), in evaluating rupture risk of cerebral aneurysms using ≥7 mm sized aneurysms. Twenty-three aneurysms (11 unruptured and 12 ruptured) ≥ 7 mm were analyzed from 3-dimensional rotational cerebral angiography and computational fluid dynamics (CFD). Ten morphological and eleven hemodynamic factors of the aneurysms were qualitatively and quantitatively compared. Correlation analysis between morphological and hemodynamic factors was performed, and the relationship among the hemodynamic factors was analyzed. Morphological factors (ostium diameter, ostium area, aspect ratio, and bottleneck ratio) and hemodynamic factors (TVR, minimal wall shear stress of aneurysms, time-averaged wall shear stress of aneurysms, oscillatory shear index, relative residence time, low wall shear stress area, and ratio of low wall stress area) were statistically different between ruptured and unruptured aneurysms ($p < 0.05$). By simple regression analysis, the morphological factor aspect ratio and the hemodynamic factor TVR were significantly correlated ($r^2 = 0.602$, $p = 0.001$). Ruptured aneurysms had complex and unstable flow. In ≥7 mm ruptured aneurysms, high aspect ratio, bottleneck ratio, complex flow, unstable flow, low TVR, wall shear stress at aneurysm, high oscillatory shear index, relative resistance time, low wall shear stress area, and ratio of low wall stress area were significant in determining the risk of aneurysm rupture.

Keywords: cerebral aneurysm; computational fluid dynamics; hemodynamic; morphological; rupture

1. Introduction

The size of cerebral aneurysms is correlated with the risk of rupture and is the most widely used determinant of treatment; aneurysms ≥7 mm are at increased risk of rupture [1,2]. However, according to the guidelines of the American Heart Association and American Stroke Association, morphological and hemodynamic factors, in addition to size, should be considered when estimating the risk of rupture [3]. Comparison of the features of ruptured aneurysms with those of unruptured aneurysms can help in identifying the risk factors for rupture and in the clinical management of the aneurysms [4,5].

Morphological factors, such as aspect ratio (AR) and flow angle of aneurysms are associated with rupture [6], and hemodynamic factors, identified with computational fluid dynamics (CFD) simulations, play a role in the pathogenesis, growth, and rupture of aneurysms. Among the hemodynamic factors are wall shear stress (WSS), oscillatory shear index (OSI), and relative residence time (RRT) [7,8]. These hemodynamic factors are used in the risk assessment and decision-making of aneurysm management [2,9], and potential additional factors should be considered.

The aim of the present study was to evaluate indicators to be used in determining the rupture risk of an aneurysm by validating the morphological and hemodynamic factors already used as well as a newly developed hemodynamic factor, total volume ratio (TVR), in unruptured and ruptured aneurysms ≥7 mm [10]. We quantitatively and qualitatively analyzed the morphological and hemodynamic factors and the correlations among the factors.

2. Materials and Methods

2.1. Patient Data

Patients with a cerebral aneurysm diagnosed during October 2015 and December 2018 at Jeonbuk National University Hospital were reviewed. The collection of patient data and the study design were approved by the hospital's institutional review board (The Ethics Committee of Jeonbuk National University Hospital; JUH 2019-10-040). The acquisition time point of brain imaging of patients with ruptured aneurysms was as soon as the patients visited the emergency room. Inclusion criteria were as follows: (1) a source image performed with 3-dimensional rotational cerebral angiography; (2) saccular aneurysm shape; (3) aneurysm location (posterior communicating artery, distal internal carotid artery, cavernous, paraclinoid, and ophthalmic); (4) and aneurysm size ≥7 mm. Most patient data were excluded because of aneurysm size (mostly < 7 mm), aneurysm location, insufficient image quality to be used for CFD modeling, and the presence of fusiform or partially thrombosed aneurysms. Thus, 11 unruptured aneurysms and 12 ruptured aneurysms constituted the study population (posterior communicating artery, 17; distal internal carotid artery, 1; cavernous, 1; paraclinoid, 3; ophthalmic, 1). The age range of patients with unruptured aneurysms was between 40 and 80 years (62.81 ± 13.71 years), and those with ruptured aneurysms were between 41 and 86 years (62.16 ± 14.94 years).

2.2. Image Data Acquisition and Geometry Reconstruction

All image data were acquired with 3-dimensional rotational cerebral angiography (Axiom Artis dBA; Siemens Medical Solutions, Erlangen, Germany) with 1.5-degree rotation, 8-second-rotational image acquisition and 29 frames per second. Digital Imaging and Communications in Medicine(DICOM) format of the source image for each patient was obtained and imported into Materialise Mimics software (version 20.0; Materialise NV, Leuven, Belgium) for geometry reconstruction. Based on our previous work [11], we used threshold segmentation to obtain 3-dimensional geometry and a cropping method to designate the desired region of vessels. Images of small and unnecessary branches were removed and truncated for CFD analysis, and a smoothing method was used for rough and sharp surfaces of the reconstructed 3-dimensional geometry. The regenerated model was saved in a Standard Triangle Language format file for CFD simulation.

2.3. Measurement and Calculation of Morphological Variables

To quantitatively compare morphological variables between unruptured and ruptured aneurysms, height, width, size, ostium diameter (neck of aneurysm), ostium area, the surface area of the aneurysm, and volume of the aneurysm were measured. The largest distance between the tip of aneurysm domes and necks was defined as height, and the maximum diameter orthogonal to the height was defined as width. The size of aneurysms was defined as the longest diameter between height and width [12]. The maximum distance of the neck plane was defined as the ostium diameter [13]. The known morphological risk factors of aneurysm rupture, such as AR, bottleneck ratio (BR), and nonsphericity index (NSI), were calculated based on the measured morphological variables. AR was the ratio between the height of the aneurysm dome and the neck of the aneurysm dome, and BR was the ratio between the width of the aneurysm dome and the neck of the aneurysm dome [14]. NSI was calculated from the volume and surface area of the aneurysm dome [15]. The detailed equations are listed in Table 1 [6,15].

Table 1. List of equations used for evaluation of morphologic and hemodynamic variables.

	Equations
Morphological variables	
AR	$\frac{\text{height of aneurysm dome}}{\text{neck of aneurysm dome}}$
BR	$\frac{\text{width of aneurysm dome}}{\text{neck of aneurysm dome}}$
NSI	$1 - (18\pi)^{1/3} \frac{\text{volume of aneurysm dome}^{2/3}}{\text{surface area of aneurysm dome}}$
Hemodynamic variables	
Time-averaged WSS	$\frac{1}{T}\int_0^T |WSS_i| dt$
OSI	$\frac{1}{2}\left\{1 - \frac{\left|\int_0^T WSS dt\right|}{\int_0^T |WSS| dt}\right\}$
RRT	$\frac{1}{(1-2\times OSI)\times TAWSS}$
Ratio of LSA	$\frac{LSA}{\text{surface area of aneurysm dome}} \times 100$

Morphological variables: AR: aspect ratio; BR: bottleneck ratio; NSI: nonsphericity index. Hemodynamic variables: WSS: wall shear stress; TAWSS: time-averaged wall shear stress; OSI: oscillatory shear index; RRT: relative residence time; LSA: low wall shear stress area (area of low WSS below 10% of wall shear stress at parent artery).

2.4. CFD Modeling

COMSOL Multiphysics Modeling software (version 5.2a; COMSOL Inc., Burlington, MA, USA) was used to generate mesh and solve the incompressible Navier–Stokes equation for computation of blood flow [16]. The following parameters of mesh element size were adjusted to find the optimal condition of mesh: maximum element growth rate, minimum element size, maximum element size, resolution of narrow regions, and curvature factor. The optimal condition of mesh was observed when no more changes in velocity and pressure were found. The mesh independence was confirmed. Tetrahedral meshes with approximately 500,000 elements were formed. Blood vessel walls were assumed to be rigid and to have a no-slip condition due to a lack of patient-specific information [17]. Assumptions of laminar flow, Newtonian fluid with a viscosity of 0.0035 Pa·s and density of 1066 kg/m^3 were applied to the simulation [1,18]. The published flow rate (2.6 mL/s) and inlet area of each patient were used to calculate the patient-specific velocity profiles. The utilized flow rate for inlet boundary condition is shown in Figure 1 [8,17,18]. All simulations were computed during four cardiac cycles, and the second cardiac cycle was taken for quantitative and qualitative analysis [4].

2.5. Hemodynamic Data Analysis

After CFD simulation, the following hemodynamic variables were calculated for comparison of unruptured and ruptured aneurysms. (1) Time-averaged WSS (TAWSS) of the aneurysm was calculated by integration of the magnitude of the WSS during one cardiac cycle. The minimum and maximum WSS were also evaluated over the entire wall of the aneurysm dome. The time-averaged WSS of the parent artery was recorded for comparison with the aneurysm dome to the parent artery [4]. (2) OSI was defined as the fluctuation of WSS over one cardiac cycle. OSI is a non-dimensional parameter and ranges from 0 (no change) to 0.5 (oscillating flow) [19]. (3) RRT was calculated from WSS and OSI and defined as the residence time of blood near the aneurysm wall [6]. (4) Low wall shear stress area (LSA) was defined as the wall area of the aneurysm dome, indicating less than 10% WSS of the parent artery. The percentage ratio of LSA was calculated by dividing the LSA by the surface area of the aneurysm [20]. The detailed equations for TAWSS, OSI, RRT, and the ratio of LSA are listed in Table 1. (5) Flow complexity and stability: Flow complexity was classified as simple flow and complex flow. Simple flow had one recirculation zone, and complex flow had two or more recirculation zones. Stable flow and unstable flow were included in flow stability. Stable flow had no flow change during one cardiac cycle, whereas unstable flow had flow separation, change, and movement during one cardiac cycle [21].

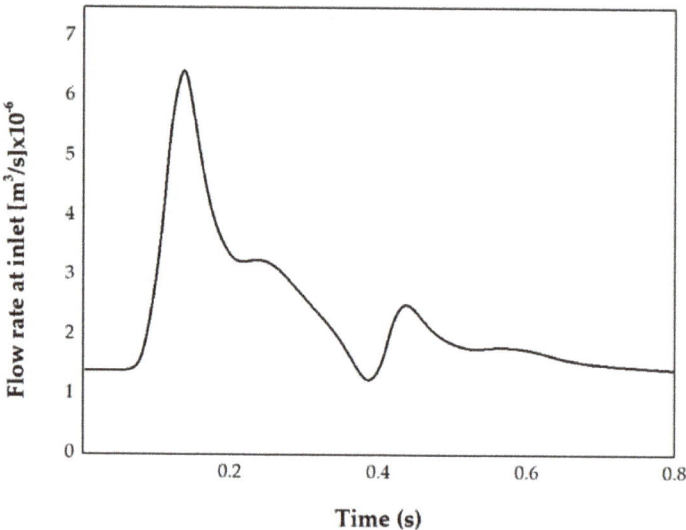

Figure 1. One cardiac cycle of flow rate according to time [18]. Using the flow rate and patient-specific inlet area, the velocity profiles for each patient were calculated for inlet boundary conditions.

2.6. Total Volume Ratio (TVR)

TVR is a recently developed quantitative hemodynamic factor that might analyze the rupture risk of an aneurysm. It is the ratio of blood volume through the aneurysm neck per one cardiac cycle to aneurysm volume.

$$\text{TVR} = \frac{\int_{T_i}^{T_e} Q_{AN} dt}{AV} = \frac{\text{blood volume through aneurysm neck per one cardiac cycle}}{\text{aneurysm volume}} \quad (1)$$

The volume flow rate of the blood through the aneurysm neck during one cardiac cycle is integrated and then divided by aneurysm volume for each patient. In Equation (1), T_i and T_e denote the initial time of the cardiac cycle and end time of the cardiac cycle, respectively. Q_{AN} denotes blood volume through the aneurysm neck per one cardiac cycle, and AV denotes aneurysm volume.

Simply expressed, high TVR means that blood flows well into the aneurysm and flows out well, whereas low TVR means that blood in the aneurysm is not fully circulating. For example, we assumed that aneurysm models A and B have the same aneurysm volume (250 mm^3), and integrated blood volume flow rates of models A and B are 500 and 2500 mm^3 per one cardiac cycle, respectively. Under these assumptions, the TVR of model A is $\frac{500 \text{ mm}^3}{250 \text{ mm}^3} = 2$, and the TVR of model B is $\frac{2500 \text{ mm}^3}{250 \text{ mm}^3} = 10$ (Figure 2). The low TVR in model A means that the ratio of the amount of circulating blood in the aneurysm to the aneurysm volume is five times lower than in model B. The cause of the low TVR is unstable and complex blood flow within the aneurysm, with blood stagnation. Low TVR is the comprehensive outcome of unstable, complex flow, low WSS, high OSI, and high RRT in the aneurysm. Thus, low TVR can be the combined results of morphological and hemodynamic variables.

2.7. Statistical Analyses

The measured and calculated morphological and hemodynamic variables were expressed as mean ± standard deviation. To compare values of unruptured and ruptured aneurysms, we used the Mann–Whitney test for non-normally distributed parameters and the independent sample t-test for normally distributed parameters. To analyze the relationships between morphological and hemodynamic factors, we used Pearson correlation analysis and simple linear regression. A *p*-value less than 0.05 was considered statistically significant.

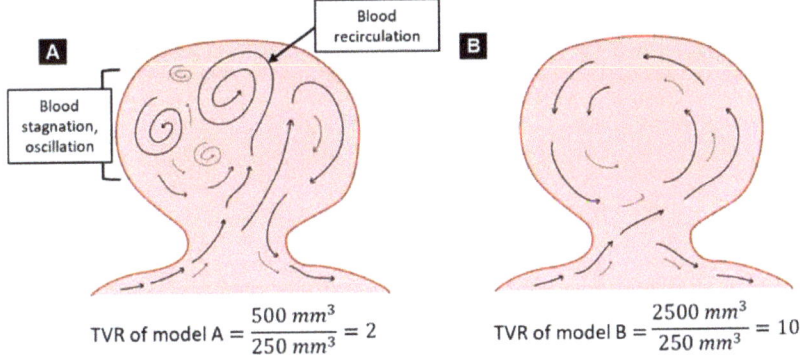

Figure 2. Two examples of a newly developed hemodynamic risk factor, total volume ratio (TVR). (**A**) TVR of model A shows lower TVR compared to model B due to blood recirculation, blood stagnation, and oscillation. (**B**) TVR of model B shows higher TVR compared to model A.

3. Results

3.1. Morphological Analysis of Unruptured and Ruptured Aneurysms

Comparison of measured and calculated morphological variables of unruptured and ruptured aneurysms are presented in Table 2. Ostium diameters of ruptured aneurysms were significantly less than those of unruptured aneurysms (6.08 ± 1.58 mm vs. 7.49 ± 1.40 mm; $p = 0.035$), as was ostium area (20.99 ± 11.51 vs. 33.92 ± 11.17; $p = 0.013$). The AR was significantly higher for ruptured aneurysms (1.32 ± 0.27) than for unruptured aneurysms (0.87 ± 0.26; $p = 0.001$). Similarly, BR was significantly more in ruptured aneurysms (1.62 ± 0.50) than in unruptured aneurysms ((1.18 ± 0.22), $p = 0.009$). Height, width, size, surface area, and volume of ruptured aneurysms and unruptured aneurysms were not significantly different. The NSI of unruptured aneurysms (0.29 ± 0.08) and ruptured aneurysms (0.30 ± 0.03) was very similar, and no significant difference was observed ($p = 0.695$).

Table 2. Quantification of morphological variables.

Variables (Unit)	Unruptured Aneurysm (n = 11)	Ruptured Aneurysm (n = 12)	p Value *
Patients			
Age (yr)	62.81 ± 13.71	62.16 ± 14.94	0.915
Measured morphological variables			
Height of aneurysm (mm)	6.45 ± 1.81	7.98 ± 2.54	0.115
Width of aneurysm (mm)	8.84 ± 2.01	9.54 ± 3.00	0.608
Size of aneurysm (mm)	9.10 ± 1.73	9.78 ± 2.93	0.512
Ostium diameter (mm)	7.49 ± 1.40	6.08 ± 1.58	0.035 *
Calculated morphological variables			
AR	0.87 ± 0.26	1.32 ± 0.27	0.001 *
BR	1.18 ± 0.22	1.62 ± 0.50	0.009 *
Ostium area (mm^2)	33.92 ± 11.17	20.99 ± 11.51	0.013 *
Surface area of aneurysm (mm^2)	183.57 ± 87.83	243.90 ± 175.91	0.260
Volume of aneurysm (mm^3)	212.23 ± 175.70	361.32 ± 480.94	0.190
NSI	0.29 ± 0.08	0.30 ± 0.03	0.695

Values given are mean ± standard deviation, and * indicates $p < 0.05$. AR: aspect ratio, BR: bottleneck ratio, NSI: nonsphericity index

3.2. Quantitative Analysis of Hemodynamic Variables

The nine calculated hemodynamic factors of the two aneurysm groups are presented in Table 3. Values of the new hemodynamic factor, TVR, were significantly lower in ruptured aneurysms (5.02 ± 3.20) than in unruptured aneurysms ((10.62 ± 5.27), p = 0.005), and TVR had the lowest p-value among the calculated hemodynamic factors, which might allow for the most significant and representative results. TVR of unruptured aneurysms was two times larger than that of ruptured aneurysms. With respect to WSS, ruptured aneurysms had lower minimal WSS at the aneurysm, TAWSS at the aneurysm, and maximal WSS at the aneurysm than did unruptured aneurysms as shown in Table 3. Minimal WSS at aneurysms (p = 0.032) and TAWSS at aneurysms (p = 0.037) were significantly different between the two groups. TAWSS at the parent artery was higher than TAWSS at the aneurysm, and no statistically significant difference between TAWSS of the parent artery in unruptured and ruptured groups was found. Moreover, maximal WSS at the aneurysm was not significantly different between ruptured and unruptured aneurysms. Ruptured aneurysms had significantly higher OSI and RRT values compared to unruptured aneurysms (p = 0.031 and p = 0.006 for OSI and RRT, respectively). Similar to OSI and RRT, LSA and the ratio of LSA were significantly higher in ruptured aneurysms (55.92 ± 55.07 and 21.73 ± 9.79 for LSA and the ratio of LSA, respectively) compared with unruptured aneurysm (22.72 ± 21.95 and 12.71 ± 13.97 for LSA and ratio of LSA, respectively).

Table 3. Quantification of hemodynamic variables.

Variables (Unit)	Unruptured Aneurysm (n = 11)	Ruptured Aneurysm (n = 12)	p Value *
TVR	10.62 ± 5.27	5.02 ± 3.20	0.005 *
Minimal WSS at aneurysm (Pa)	0.69 ± 0.37	0.42 ± 0.24	0.032 *
Time-averaged WSS at aneurysm (Pa)	1.17 ± 0.62	0.73 ± 0.42	0.037 *
Maximal WSS at aneurysm (Pa)	3.40 ± 2.17	2.14 ± 1.47	0.051
Time-averaged WSS at parent artery (Pa)	2.76 ± 1.08	3.30 ± 2.34	0.695
OSI	0.28 ± 0.11	0.37 ± 0.07	0.031 *
RRT	3.19 ± 2.00	11.56 ± 10.69	0.006 *
LSA (mm^2)	22.72 ± 21.95	55.92 ± 55.07	0.037 *
Ratio of LSA (%)	12.71 ± 13.97	21.73 ± 9.79	0.023 *

Values given are mean ± standard deviation, and * indicates p < 0.05. TVR: total volume ratio, WSS: wall shear stress, OSI: oscillatory shear index, RRT: relative residence time, LSA: low wall shear stress area.

3.3. Qualitative Analysis of Hemodynamic Variables

Figure 3 shows the simulated flow streamlines of unruptured aneurysms at end-diastole. The streamline showed that all ruptured aneurysms had complex flow, whereas 72% of unruptured aneurysms had simple flow. Among the unruptured aneurysms, UR 6, 10, and 11 had complex flow; the remaining unruptured aneurysms had a single recirculation zone. In Figure 4, simulated flow streamlines of ruptured aneurysms are presented. All ruptured aneurysms had complex flow at end-diastole; the recirculation zones are indicated with black arrows. For example, RU 3 and 4 had two recirculation zones. RU 2 and 9 had one recirculation zone at the aneurysm tip. RU 1, 6, and 12 had multiple recirculation zones. The difference in flow complexity between the two aneurysm groups was statistically significant (p = 0.002) (Table 4).

Representative cases of unruptured aneurysms for flow stability and WSS are shown in Figure 5. UR 4 and 7 had no flow change during the cardiac cycle, and a small area of low WSS at the aneurysm domes was present. For comparison with ruptured aneurysms, scale bars of blood flow and WSS were the same (0 to 0.6 m/s for blood flow and 0 to 2 Pa for WSS). As presented in Figure 6, changes and movement of flow during the cardiac cycle were present in RU 1 and 3. Compared with RU 1 at peak-systole, blood flow at end-diastole became more complex. Similar to RU 1, RU 3 had unstable flow during the cardiac cycle. The changes in flow are marked with black arrows. Ruptured aneurysms had larger areas of low WSS at aneurysm domes compared to unruptured aneurysms. Unlike the WSS in unruptured aneurysms, because the region of low WSS area was large in ruptured aneurysms, a definite difference in WSS between the parent artery and the aneurysm dome was observed.

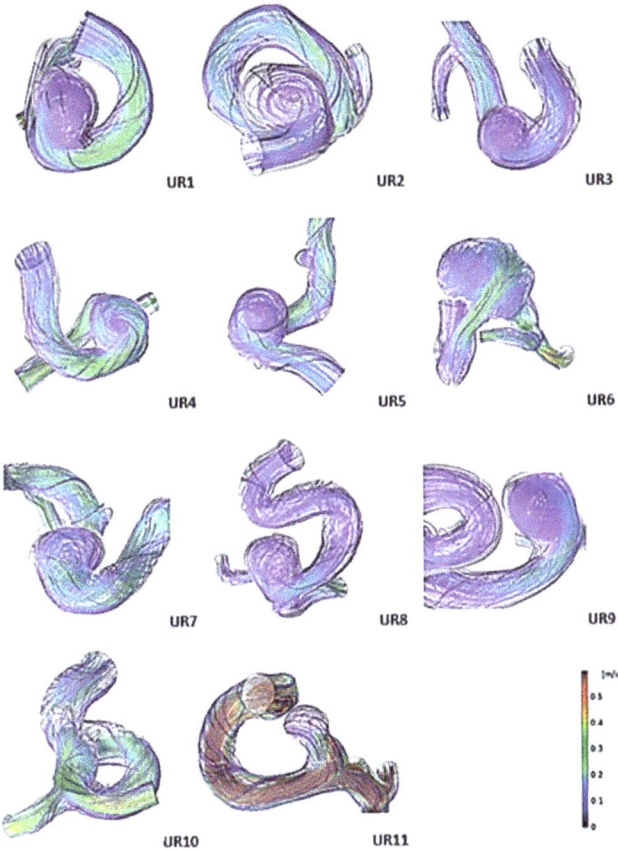

Figure 3. Simulated flow streamlines of unruptured aneurysms showing flow complexity at end-diastole. UR: unruptured aneurysm.

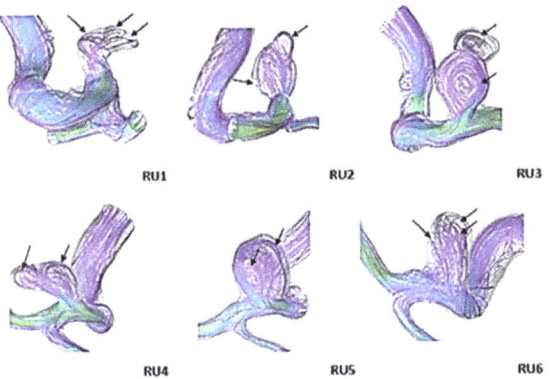

Figure 4. *Cont.*

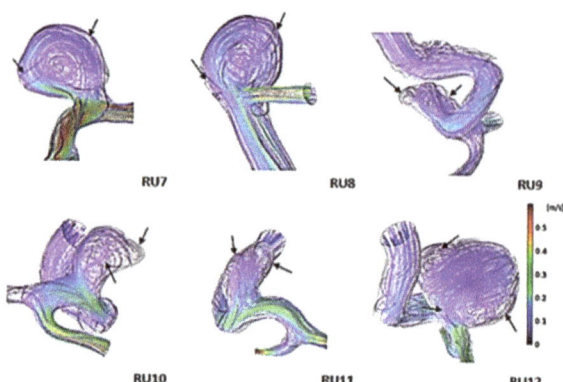

Figure 4. Simulated flow streamlines of ruptured aneurysms showing flow complexity at end-diastole. The black arrow indicates the recirculation region of the aneurysm. RU: ruptured aneurysm.

Table 4. Quantification of hemodynamic variables.

Complexity	Unruptured Aneurysm (n = 11)	Ruptured Aneurysm (n = 12)	p Value *
Simple	8	0	0.002 *
Complex	3	12	

* indicates $p < 0.05$.

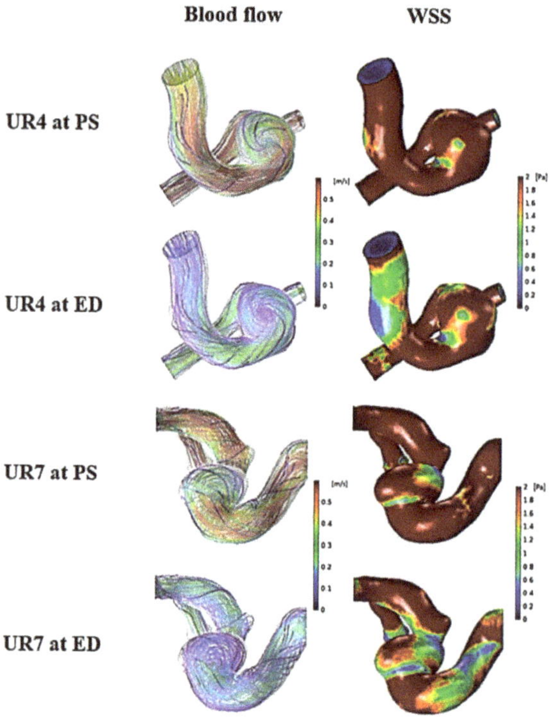

Figure 5. Two representative cases (UR4 and UR7) for unruptured aneurysms at peak-systole and end-diastole. The streamlines showing flow stability of the unruptured aneurysms (blood flow column). The distribution of wall shear stress on the aneurysm, showing low wall shear stress area (WSS column). PS: peak-systole; ED: end-diastole; UR: unruptured aneurysm; WSS: wall shear stress.

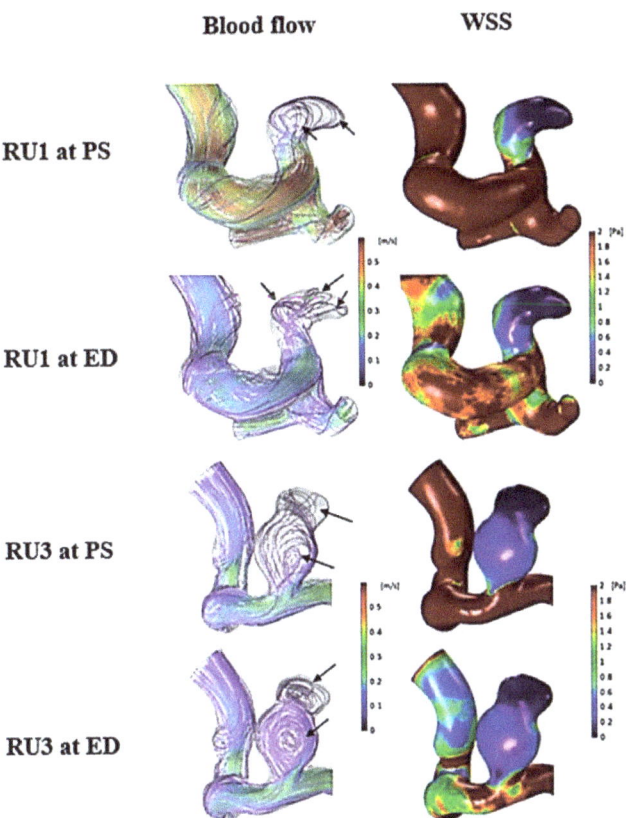

Figure 6. Two representative cases (RU1 and RU3) of ruptured aneurysms at peak-systole and end-diastole. The streamlines showing the flow stability of the ruptured aneurysm (blood flow column). The black arrow indicates the recirculation region of the aneurysm. The distribution of wall shear stress on the aneurysms showing low wall-shear stress area (WSS column). PS: peak-systole; ED: end-diastole; RU: ruptured aneurysm; WSS: wall shear stress.

4. Discussion

Many studies have focused on finding risk factors of rupture of cerebral aneurysms by comparing morphological and hemodynamic factors between unruptured and ruptured aneurysms [2,4,8]. In this study, we analyzed 10 widely used morphological factors and 11 hemodynamic factors, including the new factor, TVR, for correlation with the rupture of aneurysms.

4.1. Morphological Variables

Ruptured aneurysms tended to have larger values of all factors except for neck diameter and area. The difference between unruptured and ruptured aneurysms was statistically significant only in neck diameter, neck area, AR, and BR (Table 2). Because the neck diameter of ruptured aneurysms was smaller than unruptured aneurysms, the values of AR and BR were increased. Moreover, ruptured aneurysms are known to have higher AR and BR, according to other studies [13,22].

AR is the most useful morphological factor in determining aneurysm rupture risk, so many researchers have conducted studies to set thresholds of AR [23]. For example, Ujiie et al. [24] studied 78 unruptured and 129 ruptured aneurysms and found that 90% of unruptured aneurysms had lower AR (less than 1.6), and 80% of ruptured aneurysms had greater AR (more than 1.6). However, Jing et al. [4] reviewed 86 unruptured and 69 ruptured aneurysms and found that AR of more than 1.064 was related to aneurysm rupture. Backes et al. [2] reported that, regardless of aneurysm size and location, AR more than 1.3 was associated with the risk of aneurysm rupture. In this study, we compared the average AR of unruptured and ruptured aneurysms and found that the AR of ruptured aneurysms was consistent with that reported by Backes et al. [2]. The average value of AR in ruptured aneurysms was 1.32, and the difference between the two aneurysms was statistically significant (Table 2). Although AR is a well-known morphological risk factor, reported threshold values vary among studies. In this study, the tendency of aspect ratio showed similar or different results compared to other literature. The results might be affected due to differences in the number of the study population, aneurysm location, and aneurysm size. Thus, validation of AR in large populations is needed.

4.2. Hemodynamic Variables

In previous studies, there has been a consensus between in vivo measurement and CFD analysis, and hemodynamic factors can discriminate between unruptured and ruptured aneurysms. Thus, we calculated quantitative and qualitative hemodynamic factors using CFD simulation [8,25]. Complex flow, which increases infiltration of inflammatory cells from aneurysm walls, is associated with aneurysm rupture [4]. Cebral et al. [7] studied 210 patients with intracranial aneurysms and found that simple and stable flow were often present in unruptured aneurysms, whereas complex and unstable flow were correlated with aneurysm rupture. Similarly, in this study, most unruptured aneurysms had simple and stable flow, whereas ruptured aneurysms had complex and unstable flow significantly more often.

Xiang et al. [8]. performed a quantitative hemodynamic analysis with 81 unruptured and 38 ruptured aneurysms. Xiang et al. found the difference between unruptured aneurysms and ruptured aneurysms. Ruptured aneurysms had lower WSS (0.68 Pa, unruptured vs. 0.33 Pa, ruptured), higher OSI (0.0035, unruptured vs. 0.016, ruptured), and higher RRT (2.70, unruptured vs. 7.52, ruptured) compared to unruptured aneurysms. In this study, we found that the ruptured group had lower WSS (1.17 Pa, unruptured vs. 0.73 Pa, ruptured), higher OSI (0.28, unruptured vs. 0.37, ruptured), and higher RRT (3.19, unruptured vs. 11.56, ruptured) compared to the unruptured group. The tendency of Xiang et al.'s study and this study was similar, but the values of hemodynamic factors were different due to the size variations. According to Xiang et al., the sizes of unruptured and ruptured aneurysms were 4.01 mm and 5.15 mm, respectively. However, we included only aneurysms larger than 7 mm in this study.

Chung et al. [1] compared unruptured and ruptured aneurysms with various hemodynamic factors. Lower minimal WSS (0.8 Pa, unruptured vs. 0.4 Pa, ruptured), higher LSA (45.8 mm^2, unruptured vs. 51.6 mm^2, ruptured), and higher OSI (0.25, unruptured vs. 0.31, ruptured) were found in ruptured aneurysms compared to unruptured aneurysms. We observed similar tendencies and values of hemodynamic factors compared to the Chung et al. study due to the similar aspect ratio of the aneurysm (0.879, unruptured vs. 1.304, ruptured in Chung et al.; 0.87, unruptured vs. 1.32, ruptured in this study). Jou et al. [26] conducted a comparison study between unruptured and ruptured aneurysms. The sizes of the unruptured aneurysms and ruptured aneurysms were 6.9 mm and 11 mm, respectively. The ratio of LSA was 11 for unruptured aneurysms and 27 for ruptured aneurysms. In this study, the ratio of LSA was 12.71 in the unruptured group and 21.73 in the ruptured group. Since this study included aneurysms larger than 7 mm, the tendencies and values of the ratio of LSA were similar to Jou et al.'s study. Minimal and time-averaged WSS at aneurysms were statistically significantly different between ruptured and unruptured aneurysms. However, maximal WSS at aneurysms and time-averaged WSS of parent arteries were not different. We only compared unruptured with ruptured aneurysms, but WSS was higher in parent arteries than in aneurysm domes because of the tortuosity of the vessels. A sudden change in morphology of blood vessels induces oscillating blood and high OSI in the aneurysm dome [27]. High OSI and low WSS promote damage to endothelial cells and degradation of the aneurysm wall, leading to aneurysm rupture [19]. Other studies have found that high OSI and low WSS are related to aneurysm rupture [28], and our results are consistent with those observations. Prolonged RRT and high OSI are associated with atherosclerotic changes in cerebral aneurysms [29].

Based on our observations on hemodynamic factors, the characteristics of ruptured aneurysms can help analyze the risk of rupture. Complex and unstable flow have multiple recirculation and oscillating zones. This feature causes decreased WSS and increased OSI. Due to the stagnation of blood flow, the region of low WSS is widened, and the residence time of blood flow near the aneurysm wall is longer. Thus, the LSA and RRT are increased.

4.3. TVR

The newly introduced hemodynamic factor, TVR, is defined as the ratio of the integrated blood volume through the aneurysm neck per one cardiac cycle to aneurysm volume. We examined the correlation of TVR with morphological factor AR and hemodynamic factor TAWSS of aneurysms in Figures 2a and 2b, respectively. In this study, ruptured aneurysms had complex, unstable flow, multiple recirculation zones, and stagnation of blood flow, which resulted in lower TVR of ruptured aneurysms compared to unruptured aneurysms. Low TVR denotes that circulating blood flow to aneurysm volume is relatively low, which means that recirculation zone and stagnation of blood are present in the aneurysm. Prolonged stay of blood flow promotes thrombus formation, and as thrombi get closer to the wall of the aneurysm, it promotes inflammation in the wall. The inflammatory reaction can lead to aneurysm rupture as various destructive enzymes are released [7].

As to the correlation between TVR and AR, due to the low TVR of ruptured aneurysms, low blood flow and stagnant flow in aneurysm domes are correlated with atherosclerosis and inflammatory reaction, resulting in the growth of aneurysms, and the growth might lead to an increase of AR [4]. In this study, TVR and AR were highly correlated (coefficient of determination: $r^2 = 0.602$, $p = 0.001$). Thus, TVR might be a useful hemodynamic factor related to aneurysm rupture. For clinical use of TVR, calculation of TVR in more patient groups and various locations of aneurysms, such as the middle cerebral artery and anterior communicating artery, will be needed.

4.4. Limitations of the Present Study

First of all, due to the small number of patients, there were several limitations as follows: (1) Small sample size limits the feasibility of statistical analysis (i.e., regression analysis); (2) This study focused on comparing unruptured and ruptured aneurysm groups rather than predicting rupture risk of the aneurysm due to the small number of patients; (3) The average values of the morphological factor (i.e., AR) and hemodynamic factor (i.e., TAWSS) could not be considered as a cutoff point due to the low number of cases. Studies in larger populations and multiple centers are needed to assess the validity of our results. Second, we conducted analysis on aneurysms larger than 7 mm. The results might limit the application of TVR in aneurysms smaller than 7 mm. Third, there might be errors in regenerating the geometry for each patient using the threshold segmentation method. However, since the images were acquired with 3-dimensional rotational cerebral angiography with high resolution, this might not be a significant limitation. Fourth, we assumed the vessels to have rigid walls and did not consider the real conditions of elasticity and thickness. Lastly, for CFD simulation, blood was assumed to be a Newtonian fluid since we did not have viscosity data to allow comparison of patients' blood viscosity. The real physical property of blood is non-Newtonian, and blood flow becomes slower in aneurysm domes [30]. Ideally, we would have considered the non-Newtonian properties of blood, but the serious condition of patients with ruptured aneurysms was prohibitive.

5. Conclusions

A detailed comparison of morphological and hemodynamic factors of modeled unruptured and ruptured aneurysms was conducted. In morphological analysis, large AR and BR were independently associated with rupture of aneurysms. In hemodynamic analysis, unstable flow, complex flow, low WSS, high OSI, RRT, LSA, and ratio of LSA were good indicators of rupture risk. A new hemodynamic factor, TVR, was significantly different between unruptured and ruptured aneurysms. These findings should be tested in multi-center, large population studies.

Author Contributions: U.Y.L. was involved in formal analysis, writing, visualization. H.S.K. was involved in supervision, validation, and funding acquisition. All authors have read and agreed to the published version of the manuscript.

Funding: This research was supported by the Basic Science Research Program (NRF-2019R1I1A3A 01060695, NRF-2019R1I1A3A01059720, NRF-2020R1A2C1008089, and NRF-2020R1A4A2002817) by the National Research Foundation of Korea (NRF) funded by the Ministry of Education.

Institutional Review Board Statement: The present research was approved by our institutional review board and was conducted in accordance with the Declaration of Helsinki (The Ethics Committee of Jeonbuk National University Hospital; JUH 2019-10-040).

Informed Consent Statement: Informed consent was obtained from all subjects involved in the study.

Data Availability Statement: The data presented in this study are available on request from the corresponding author. The data are not publicly available due to privacy restrictions.

Conflicts of Interest: The authors declare no conflict of interest.

References

1. Chung, B.; Mut, F.; Putman, C.; Hamzei-Sichani, F.; Brinjikji, W.; Kallmes, D.; Jimenez, C.; Cebral, J. Identification of hostile hemodynamics and geometries of cerebral aneurysms: A case-control study. *Am. J. Neuroradiol.* **2018**, *39*, 1860–1866. [CrossRef] [PubMed]
2. Backes, D.; Vergouwen, M.D.; Velthuis, B.K.; van der Schaaf, I.C.; Bor, A.S.E.; Algra, A.; Rinkel, G.J. Difference in aneurysm characteristics between ruptured and unruptured aneurysms in patients with multiple intracranial aneurysms. *Stroke* **2014**, *45*, 1299–1303. [CrossRef]
3. Connolly Jr, E.S.; Rabinstein, A.A.; Carhuapoma, J.R.; Derdeyn, C.P.; Dion, J.; Higashida, R.T.; Hoh, B.L.; Kirkness, C.J.; Naidech, A.M.; Ogilvy, C.S. Guidelines for the management of aneurysmal subarachnoid hemorrhage: A guideline for healthcare professionals from the American Heart Association/American Stroke Association. *Stroke* **2012**, *43*, 1711–1737. [CrossRef] [PubMed]
4. Jing, L.; Fan, J.; Wang, Y.; Li, H.; Wang, S.; Yang, X.; Zhang, Y. Morphologic and hemodynamic analysis in the patients with multiple intracranial aneurysms: Ruptured versus unruptured. *PLoS ONE* **2015**, *10*, e0132494. [CrossRef] [PubMed]
5. Ramachandran, M.; Retarekar, R.; Raghavan, M.L.; Berkowitz, B.; Dickerhoff, B.; Correa, T.; Lin, S.; Johnson, K.; Hasan, D.; Ogilvy, C. Assessment of image-derived risk factors for natural course of unruptured cerebral aneurysms. *J. Neurosurg.* **2016**, *124*, 288–295. [CrossRef] [PubMed]
6. Amigo, N.; Valencia, Á. Determining Significant Morphological and Hemodynamic Parameters to Assess the Rupture Risk of Cerebral Aneurysms. *J. Med Biol. Eng.* **2018**, *39*, 329–335. [CrossRef]
7. Cebral, J.R.; Mut, F.; Weir, J.; Putman, C.M. Association of hemodynamic characteristics and cerebral aneurysm rupture. *Am. J. Neuroradiol.* **2011**, *32*, 264–270. [CrossRef] [PubMed]
8. Xiang, J.; Natarajan, S.K.; Tremmel, M.; Ma, D.; Mocco, J.; Hopkins, L.N.; Siddiqui, A.H.; Levy, E.I.; Meng, H. Hemodynamic–morphologic discriminants for intracranial aneurysm rupture. *Stroke* **2011**, *42*, 144–152. [CrossRef] [PubMed]
9. Jansen, I.; Schneiders, J.; Potters, W.; van Ooij, P.; van den Berg, R.; van Bavel, E.; Marquering, H.; Majoie, C. Generalized versus patient-specific inflow boundary conditions in computational fluid dynamics simulations of cerebral aneurysmal hemodynamics. *Am. J. Neuroradiol.* **2014**, *35*, 1543–1548. [CrossRef]
10. Lee, U.Y. Analysis of Morphological and Hemodynamic Risk Factors for Cerebral Aneurysm Rupture Using Patient-Specific Computational Fluid Dynamics Modeling. Ph. D. Thesis, Jeonbuk National University, Jeonbuk, Korea, 2019.
11. Lee, U.Y.; Jung, J.; Kwak, H.S.; Lee, D.H.; Chung, G.H.; Park, J.S.; Koh, E.J. Wall Shear Stress and Flow Patterns in Unruptured and Ruptured Anterior Communicating Artery Aneurysms Using Computational Fluid Dynamics. *J. Korean Neurosurg. Soc.* **2018**, *61*, 689. [CrossRef]

12. Lauric, A.; Baharoglu, M.I.; Malek, A.M. Ruptured status discrimination performance of aspect ratio, height/width, and bottleneck factor is highly dependent on aneurysm sizing methodology. *Neurosurgery* **2012**, *71*, 38–46. [CrossRef]
13. Skodvin, T.Ø.; Johnsen, L.-H.; Gjertsen, Ø.; Isaksen, J.G.; Sorteberg, A. Cerebral aneurysm morphology before and after rupture: Nationwide case series of 29 aneurysms. *Stroke* **2017**, *48*, 880–886. [CrossRef]
14. Ryu, C.-W.; Kwon, O.-K.; Koh, J.S.; Kim, E.J. Analysis of aneurysm rupture in relation to the geometric indices: Aspect ratio, volume, and volume-to-neck ratio. *Neuroradiology* **2011**, *53*, 883–889. [CrossRef]
15. Chien, A.; Sayre, J. Morphologic and hemodynamic risk factors in ruptured aneurysms imaged before and after rupture. *Am. J. Neuroradiol.* **2014**, *35*, 2130–2135. [CrossRef]
16. Varble, N.; Rajabzadeh-Oghaz, H.; Wang, J.; Siddiqui, A.; Meng, H.; Mowla, A. Differences in morphologic and hemodynamic characteristics for "PHASES-based" intracranial aneurysm locations. *Am. J. Neuroradiol.* **2017**, *38*, 2105–2110. [CrossRef] [PubMed]
17. Takao, H.; Murayama, Y.; Otsuka, S.; Qian, Y.; Mohamed, A.; Masuda, S.; Yamamoto, M.; Abe, T. Hemodynamic differences between unruptured and ruptured intracranial aneurysms during observation. *Stroke* **2012**, *43*, 1436–1439. [CrossRef]
18. Morales, H.G.; Larrabide, I.; Geers, A.J.; Aguilar, M.L.; Frangi, A.F. Newtonian and non-Newtonian blood flow in coiled cerebral aneurysms. *J. Biomech.* **2013**, *46*, 2158–2164. [CrossRef]
19. Russell, J.H.; Kelson, N.; Barry, M.; Pearcy, M.; Fletcher, D.F.; Winter, C.D. Computational fluid dynamic analysis of intracranial aneurysmal bleb formation. *Neurosurgery* **2013**, *73*, 1061–1069. [CrossRef]
20. Farnoush, A.; Avolio, A.; Qian, Y. Effect of bifurcation angle configuration and ratio of daughter diameters on hemodynamics of bifurcation aneurysms. *Am. J. Neuroradiol.* **2013**, *34*, 391–396. [CrossRef] [PubMed]
21. Byrne, G.; Mut, F.; Cebral, J. Quantifying the large-scale hemodynamics of intracranial aneurysms. *Am. J. Neuroradiol.* **2014**, *35*, 333–338. [CrossRef] [PubMed]
22. Zeng, Z.; Kallmes, D.F.; Durka, M.; Ding, Y.; Lewis, D.; Kadirvel, R.; Robertson, A.M. Hemodynamics and anatomy of elastase-induced rabbit aneurysm models: Similarity to human cerebral aneurysms? *Am. J. Neuroradiol.* **2011**, *32*, 595–601. [CrossRef]
23. Lall, R.R.; Eddleman, C.S.; Bendok, B.R.; Batjer, H.H. Unruptured intracranial aneurysms and the assessment of rupture risk based on anatomical and morphological factors: Sifting through the sands of data. *Neurosurg. Focus* **2009**, *26*, E2. [CrossRef]
24. Ujiie, H.; Tamano, Y.; Sasaki, K.; Hori, T. Is the aspect ratio a reliable index for predicting the rupture of a saccular aneurysm? *Neurosurgery* **2001**, *48*, 495–503. [CrossRef] [PubMed]
25. Karmonik, C.; Yen, C.; Diaz, O.; Klucznik, R.; Grossman, R.G.; Benndorf, G. Temporal variations of wall shear stress parameters in intracranial aneurysms—importance of patient-specific inflow waveforms for CFD calculations. *Acta Neurochir.* **2010**, *152*, 1391–1398. [CrossRef] [PubMed]
26. Jou, L.-D.; Lee, D.; Morsi, H.; Mawad, M. Wall shear stress on ruptured and unruptured intracranial aneurysms at the internal carotid artery. *Am. J. Neuroradiol.* **2008**, *29*, 1761–1767. [CrossRef] [PubMed]
27. Xiao, W.; Qi, T.; He, S.; Li, Z.; Ou, S.; Zhang, G.; Liu, X.; Huang, Z.; Liang, F. Low Wall Shear Stress Is Associated with Local Aneurysm Wall Enhancement on High-Resolution MR Vessel Wall Imaging. *Am. J. Neuroradiol.* **2018**, *39*, 2082–2087. [CrossRef]
28. Shojima, M.; Oshima, M.; Takagi, K.; Torii, R.; Hayakawa, M.; Katada, K.; Morita, A.; Kirino, T. Magnitude and role of wall shear stress on cerebral aneurysm: Computational fluid dynamic study of 20 middle cerebral artery aneurysms. *Stroke* **2004**, *35*, 2500–2505. [CrossRef]
29. Furukawa, K.; Ishida, F.; Tsuji, M.; Miura, Y.; Kishimoto, T.; Shiba, M.; Tanemura, H.; Umeda, Y.; Sano, T.; Yasuda, R. Hemodynamic characteristics of hyperplastic remodeling lesions in cerebral aneurysms. *PLoS ONE* **2018**, *13*, e0191287. [CrossRef]
30. Ohta, M.; Wetzel, S.G.; Dantan, P.; Bachelet, C.; Lovblad, K.O.; Yilmaz, H.; Flaud, P.; Rüfenacht, D.A. Rheological changes after stenting of a cerebral aneurysm: A finite element modeling approach. *Cardiovasc. Interv. Radiol.* **2005**, *28*, 768–772. [CrossRef]

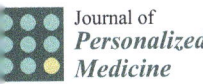

Article

Different Lower Extremity Arterial Calcification Patterns in Patients with Chronic Limb-Threatening Ischemia Compared with Asymptomatic Controls

Louise C. D. Konijn [1,*], Richard A. P. Takx [2], Willem P. Th. M. Mali [2], Hugo T. C. Veger [3] and Hendrik van Overhagen [1]

1. Department of Diagnostic and Interventional Radiology, Haga Teaching Hospital, Els Borst-Eilersplein 275, 2545 AA The Hague, The Netherlands; h.voverhagen@hagaziekenhuis.nl
2. Department of Diagnostic and Interventional Radiology, University Medical Center Utrecht and Utrecht University, Heidelberglaan 100, 3584 CX Utrecht, The Netherlands; r.a.p.takx@umcutrecht.nl (R.A.P.T.); w.mali@umcutrecht.nl (W.P.T.M.M.)
3. Department of Vascular Surgery, Haga Teaching Hospital, 2545 AA The Hague, The Netherlands; h.veger@hagaziekenhuis.nl
* Correspondence: l.konijn@hagaziekenhuis.nl; Tel.: +31-(0)-70-210-5046

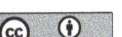

Abstract: *Objectives:* The most severe type of peripheral arterial disease (PAD) is critical limb-threatening ischemia (CLI). In CLI, calcification of the vessel wall plays an important role in symptoms, amputation rate, and mortality. However, calcified arteries are also found in asymptomatic persons (non-PAD patients). We investigated whether the calcification pattern in CLI patients and non- PAD patients are different and could possibly explain the symptoms in CLI patients. *Materials and Methods:* 130 CLI and 204 non-PAD patients underwent a CT of the lower extremities. This resulted in 118 CLI patients (mean age 72 ± 12, 70.3% male) that were age-matched with 118 non-PAD patients (mean age 71 ± 11, 51.7% male). The characteristics severity, annularity, thickness, and continuity were assessed in the femoral and crural arteries and analyzed by binary multiple logistic regression. *Results:* Nearly all CLI patients have calcifications and these are equally frequent in the femoropopliteal (98.3%) and crural arteries (97.5%), while the non-PAD patients had in just 67% any calcifications with more calcifications in the femoropopliteal (70.3%) than in the crural arteries (55.9%, $p < 0.005$). The crural arteries of CLI patients had significantly more complete annular calcifications (OR 2.92, $p = 0.001$), while in non-PAD patients dot-like calcifications dominated. In CLI patients, the femoropopliteal arteries had more severe, irregular/patchy, and thick calcifications (OR 2.40, 3.27, 1.81, $p \leq 0.05$, respectively) while in non-PAD patients, thin continuous calcifications prevailed. *Conclusions:* Compared with non-PAD patients, arteries of the lower extremities of CLI patients are more frequently and extensively calcified. Annular calcifications were found in the crural arteries of CLI patients while dot-like calcifications were mostly present in non-PAD patients. These different patterns of calcifications in CLI point at different etiology and can have prognostic and eventually therapeutic consequences.

Keywords: chronic limb-threatening ischemia; peripheral arterial disease; calcification pattern

1. Introduction

Recent studies have shown that calcification across the vascular wall of patients with peripheral arterial disease (PAD) and chronic limb-threatening ischemia (CLI) play an important role [1–3]. These calcifications are of clinical importance since they are associated with symptoms, treatment outcome, and mortality [4–6]. These studies have also shown that in PAD and CLI, two different types of calcifications can be found: (1) calcifications based on calcified atherosclerotic plaques located in the intimal layer of the vessel wall and (2) calcification of the tunica media and internal elastic lamina of the vessel wall as a separate metabolic disease, causing stiffness and limit remodeling [7].

Medial calcifications are not only present in the arteries of the lower extremities but also for example in the carotid siphon and in the arteries of the breast [8–10]. However medial calcifications are almost absent in the coronary arteries. Although the differentiation between intimal and medial calcification on a CT scan is not completely reliable, annular calcifications most likely represent medial calcifications.

Medial wall calcification is an active metabolic process with bone progression proteins, instead of solely deposition of bisphosphonates in the arterial walls [7,11]. Medial calcifications can be reversible over time as showed in the arteries of the breast, for example, after kidney transplantation, but not all patients have a clear cause for regression of these calcifications [8,12]. Thus, regression of calcifications can presumably occur partially Indeed, a histological study of the arteries of the lower limbs found osteoclasts, however scarce [13]. Extensive regression of calcifications therefore does not seem plausible.

It has been shown that medial calcifications can be halted by bisphosphonate etidronate in patients with pseudoxanthoma elasticum [14,15], a rare monogenetic disease resulting in medial calcifications of the arteries. Since we know that CLI patients with complete annular calcifications, most likely medial arterial calcifications, have worse survival than patients without these calcifications, treatment of these patients with etidronate could therefore be a therapeutic option.

Since it is known that vascular calcifications also occur in asymptomatic people [16], we wanted to compare CLI patients with these asymptomatic patients and investigate whether the calcification pattern perhaps could be associated with the symptomatology in CLI patients.

Therefore, the primary aim of this present study was to examine differences in presence, severity, and characteristics of arterial calcifications in the lower extremities between CLI patients and patients without known PAD using CT.

2. Materials and Methods

2.1. CLI Patients

This study consisted of data from two trials with CLI patients. The PADI trial (Percutaneous transluminal Angioplasty and Drug-eluting stents for infrapopliteal lesions in critical limb ischemia), and the PADI Imaging Trial.

From the PADI trial extensive study details and mid- to long-term results have been published elsewhere [17–20]. Briefly, the PADI Trial was an investigator-initiated prospective, multicenter RCT in CLI patients due to infrapopliteal pathology to assess the value of drug eluting stents (DES) compared to the current reference treatment with bare-metal stents (BMS). Included in the PADI trial were 137 patients. DES provided better 6-month patency rates and less amputations after 6 and 12 months. From these 137 patients 87 patients underwent a CT angiography of the lower extremity and were included in the present study. Patients were scanned on a 256-slice CT scanner (Siemens Definition Flash Scanner, Siemens Healthineers, Forchheim, Germany). Slice thickness was set between 0.625 and 1 mm.

The subsequent PADI Imaging Trial was an investigator-initiated prospective study developed to investigate atherosclerosis and arteriosclerosis in the whole body in patients with CLI. Patients with CLI were recruited in the outpatient clinic of the department of vascular surgery in a large teaching hospital in The Hague, the Netherlands. Patients were excluded from the study if they were unable to give consent, if they were younger than 18 years, if patients were allergic for intravenous contrast. All included patients gave written consent. Extensive clinical assessment, routine cardiovascular laboratory tests, and a whole-body spectral CT were done including a CT angiography of the lower extremities, which was used for this current study. Patients were scanned on a 256-slice CT scanner (Siemens Definition Flash Scanner, Siemens Healthineers, Forchheim, Germany). Slice thickness was set between 0.625 and 1 mm. All 43 participants in the PADI Imaging Trial enrolled to date were included in the current study.

A total of 130 CLI patients from the PADI Trial and PADI Imaging Trial were analyzed in this study.

2.2. Non-PAD Patients

As control group we used patients from a different study without known vascular disease as stated in their electronic patient file. Patient details have been published elsewhere [21]. In short, patients with an indication for a full-body PET-CT because of melanoma, infection, unknown fever, or lymphadenopathy were selected. These scans were matched to medical record data for cardiovascular risk factors and symptomatic PAD status. A total of 204 patients without known PAD were included in this study.

2.3. Study Approval

The medical ethical board of the participating centers approved the prospective PADI Imaging Trial (Unique identifier number: NL64059.098.17) and to re-use data from the PADI trial (ClinicalTrials.gov trial register Unique identifier number: NCT00471289) as a post hoc analysis.

Regarding the patients without PAD, the medical ethical board of the University Medical Center Utrecht (UMCU) waived review because of its non-invasive, retrospective character (study number: 17-897/C). This study was also approved by the ethical board of the Haga Teaching Hospital (study number: T18-003).

2.4. Baseline Measurements and Definitions

The following variables were included for analysis: age, gender, diabetes mellitus (DM), weight, current smoking status, systolic blood pressure, diastolic blood pressure, and renal function (eGFR). Obesity was defined as a body mass index (BMI) ≥ 30 kg/m^2. Hypertension was defined as a systolic blood pressure at admission >140 mmHg or diastolic blood pressure of >90 mmHg. Chronic kidney disease (CKD) was defined as an eGFR < 60 mL/min/1.73 m^2, mildly decreased kidney function to renal failure (G3a-G5) [22]. We also showed severely decreased kidney function (G4-G5) with a cut-off value of <30 mL/min/1.73 m^2, since this is the best prognostic factor in patients with CLI [23].

2.5. Calcification Assessment

All patients underwent a CT scan of the lower extremities and were evaluated on 3 mm slice thickness reconstructions. For evaluation of arterial calcifications, bone settings were used for all CT exams (Window Settings: Window = 300 Hounsfield Units; Width = 1600 Hounsfield Units). This made it possible to distinguish between calcium and other densities on both CT angiographies and non-contrast CT. Both the femoropopliteal and crural arteries were scored. Vascular calcification patterns were examined in a semi-quantitative way; severity (absent, mild, moderate, severe), annularity (absent, dot(s), <90°, 90–270°, 270–360°), thickness (absent, ≥ 1.5 mm, <1.5 mm), and continuity (indistinguishable, irregular/patchy, or continuous). In case more patterns were present, the most dominant characteristic was chosen to score. Figures 1 and 2 provide different types of calcifications and illustrative examples of the CT scoring system. Extensive details on the calcification measurements are described elsewhere [21] and is based on the recently developed and CT-histologically validated score for the carotid siphon by Kockelkoren et al. with a proven reproducible scoring system (inter-observer kappa 0.54–0.99) [24,25]. All measurements were performed by a radiology resident with more than 4 years of experience with the scoring system (LCDK) who was blinded to the patients' clinical data. In one of our other studies with a similar set of CLI patients with Fontaine 3 and 4, test–retest reliability was calculated based on second reader measurements scored by a senior radiologist (WPThM) with over 40 years of radiological experience. Cohen's weighted Kappa tests (Kw) showed good agreement of interreader test–retest reproducibility. Kw values were for severity 0.72 (95% CI 0.55–0.90, $p < 0.001$), annularity 0.77 (95% CI 00.58–0.95, $p < 0.001$), thickness 0.65 (95% CI 0.29–1.01, $p < 0.001$), and continuity 0.62 (95% CI 0.31–0.94, $p < 0.001$).

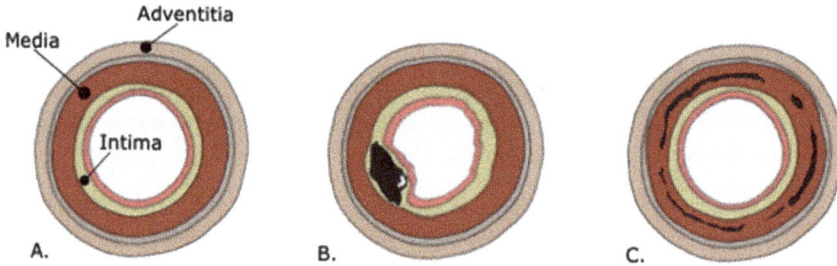

Figure 1. (**A**) Wall layers in a normal artery from inside to outside: endothelium, tunica intima (internal elastic membrane and fibrocollagenous tissue), tunica media (smooth muscle), tunica adventitia (external elastic lamina and fibrocollagenous tissue). (**B**) Calcifications in the intimal wall: thick and non-annular. (**C**) calcifications in the medial wall and in the internal elastic lamina: thin and annular.

2.6. Statistical Considerations

2.6.1. Case Matching

Due to an age difference of approximately 9 years in the CLI (cases) and non-PAD patients (controls), age matching was performed. The intention was to construct patient groups with a comparable age, as the occurrence of arterial calcification is age-dependent. The match tolerance (fuzz) factor was set on 5 years. There were 118 matches, 98 patients were excluded of further analysis. This resulted in a final sample of 236 patients, whereof 118 patients with CLI and 118 patients without clinical known PAD. Matching was performed blinded to outcomes.

2.6.2. Statistical Analysis

Descriptive data are presented as mean ± standard deviation (SD) for normally distributed continuous variables, for non-normally distributed continuous variables as median (interquartile range (IQR)). Regarding categorical variables, characteristics were presented as number (percentages). Groups were compared using the Chi-squared test for categorical variables and the Student's t test for continuous variables.

The prevalence of different calcifications characteristics (severity, annularity, thickness, and continuity) in the femoropopliteal and crural arteries was plotted graphically for both absolute numbers and percentages.

Regarding evaluation of similarities and differences between these CT calcification characteristics for both the femoropopliteal and crural arteries, patients without calcifications were excluded from this analysis (4 CLI patients and 57 non-PAD patients). Of the remaining 114 CLI patients and 61 non-PAD patients with any calcifications, type, and pattern analysis were performed.

Binary multiple logistic regression was performed to evaluate these different CT calcification characteristics. To adjust for confounding, correction for gender was performed. A p-value of less than 0.05 was considered to be significant. Data analysis was carried out using SPSS version 27.0 (IBM Corporation, New York, NY, USA).

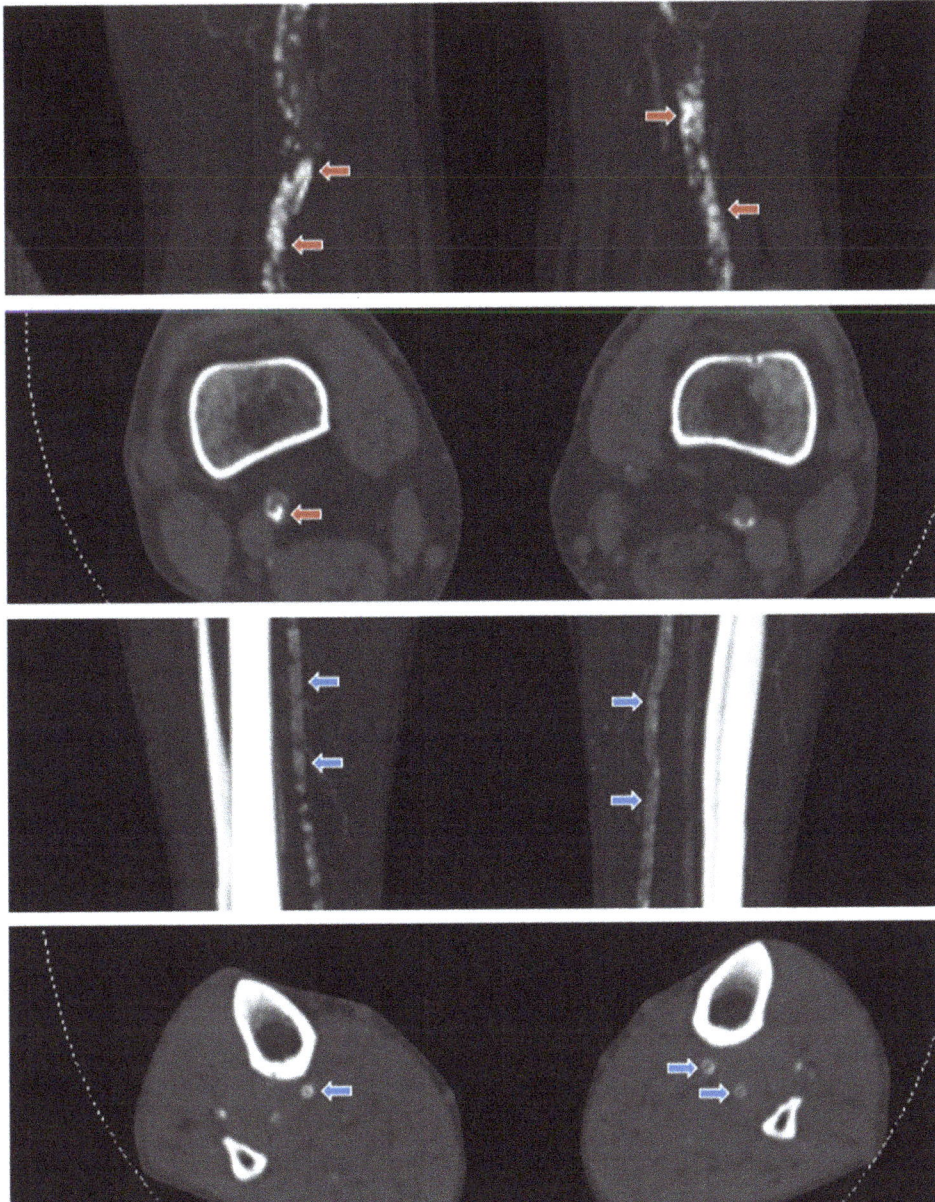

Figure 2. Examples of different calcification patterns in patients with CLI. Shown are coronal MIP and axial 3 mm CT angiography images of the lower extremities. A. Top two figures: the red arrows in femoropopliteal arteries showing irregular/patchy, thick, and non-annular calcifications corresponding to a dominant intimal calcification pattern. B. Bottom two figures: the blue arrows in the crural arteries showing continuous, thin, and annular calcifications corresponding to a dominant medial calcification pattern.

3. Results

3.1. Baseline Characteristics

Mean age was 74 years (range 40–95; SD 11). There were 61% (n = 236) male patients Patients with CLI were significantly more likely to be male, had a higher prevalence of diabetes mellitus, smokers, hypertension and lower eGFR. Baseline characteristics and comorbidities of both CLI and non-PAD are shown in Table 1.

Table 1. Baseline variables of the age-matched CLI patients and the control non-PAD patients.

	Non-PAD (n = 118)	CLI (n = 118)	p-Value
Age (years)	71 ± 11	72 ± 12	0.461
Sex (male)	61 (51.7%)	83 (70.3%)	0.003 *
BMI	27.9 (6.0%)	25.2 (3.9%)	0.053
Diabetes mellitus	11 (9.6%)	68 (57.6%)	<0.001 *
History of PAD	0 (0%)	71 (60.7%)	
Stroke	0 (0%)	12 (10.3%)	
CAD	0 (0%)	45 (38.1%)	
Smoking	32 (30.2%)	63 (54.3%)	<0.001 *
eGFR	67 (93)	61 (142)	0.069
Chronic kidney disease (eGFR < 60)	30 (37.5%)	50 (62.5%)	<0.006 *
Severely decreased kidney function (eGFR < 30)	10 (43.5%)	13 (56.5%)	<0.510
Systolic blood pressure	137 ± 20	153 ± 26	<0.001 *
Diastolic blood pressure	78 ± 13	83 ± 12	<0.001 *
Hypertension	54 (45.8%)	64 (69.6%)	<0.001 *
Any Calcification			
Crural	66/118 (55.9%)	115/118 (97.5%)	<0.001 *
Femoropopliteal	83/118 (70.3%)	116/118 (98.3%)	<0.001 *

Values are mean ± SD, median (IQR) or n (%) as appropriate. Abbreviations: BMI = body mass index; PAD = peripheral arterial disease; CAD = coronary artery disease; eGFR = estimated glomerular filtration rate (mL/min/1.73 m^2). * = statistically significant p-value.

3.2. Prevalence of Lower Extremity Arterial Calcifications

The prevalence of any calcification in the crural arteries was 97.5% (115/118) in CLI patients and 55.9% (66/118) in non-PAD patients, $p < 0.005$. In the femoropopliteal arteries, the prevalence of calcifications was 98.3% (116/118) in CLI patients and in non-PAD patients 70.3% (83/118), $p < 0.005$.

3.3. Differences in Lower Extremity Arterial Calcification Patterns between CLI and Non-PAD Patients

Patients without calcifications were excluded for further analysis. This resulted in the CLI patient group in the loss of only three (2.5%) patients without crural arterial calcifications and only two patients (1.7%) without femoropopliteal arterial calcifications. In the non-PAD group, 52 (44.1%) patients without crural arterial calcifications were excluded from analysis and 35 (29.7%) non-PAD patients without femoropopliteal arterial calcifications. Baseline characteristics of these subpopulations were not markedly different on any of the variables compared to the primary case-match cohort of 236 patients. These baseline characteristics are shown in Table S1. A further subdivision in baseline characteristics between patients with calcifications and without calcifications in non-PAD patients, showed that patients with calcifications in this group were older, more likely to be male, smoker, and had more often hypertension. See Tables S2 and S3.

Comparing all patients with lower extremity arterial calcifications in the crural arteries, most calcifications were severe (CLI vs. non-PAD: 71.3% (82/115) vs. 60.0% (39/65) without a significant difference between these two patient groups. The majority of femoropopliteal arteries were also severely calcified with 78.4% (91/116) in CLI patients compared to 60.2% (50/83) in non-PAD patients, here, a significant OR was found (OR 2.40, 95% CI 1.29–4.48, $p = 0.006$). See Figure 3A,B for stacked graphs and Tables 2 and 3 for corresponding logistic regression analysis. See Tables S4 and S5 for the severity of calcifications by decade.

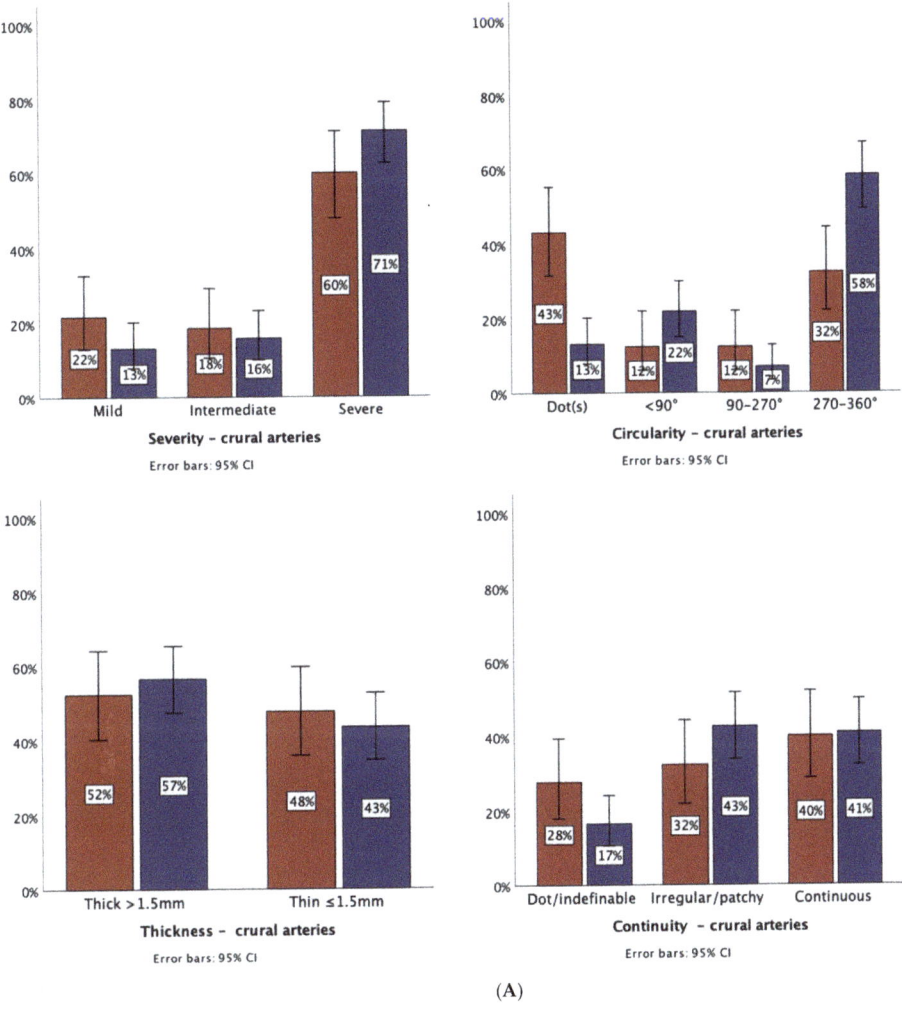

(A)

Figure 3. Cont.

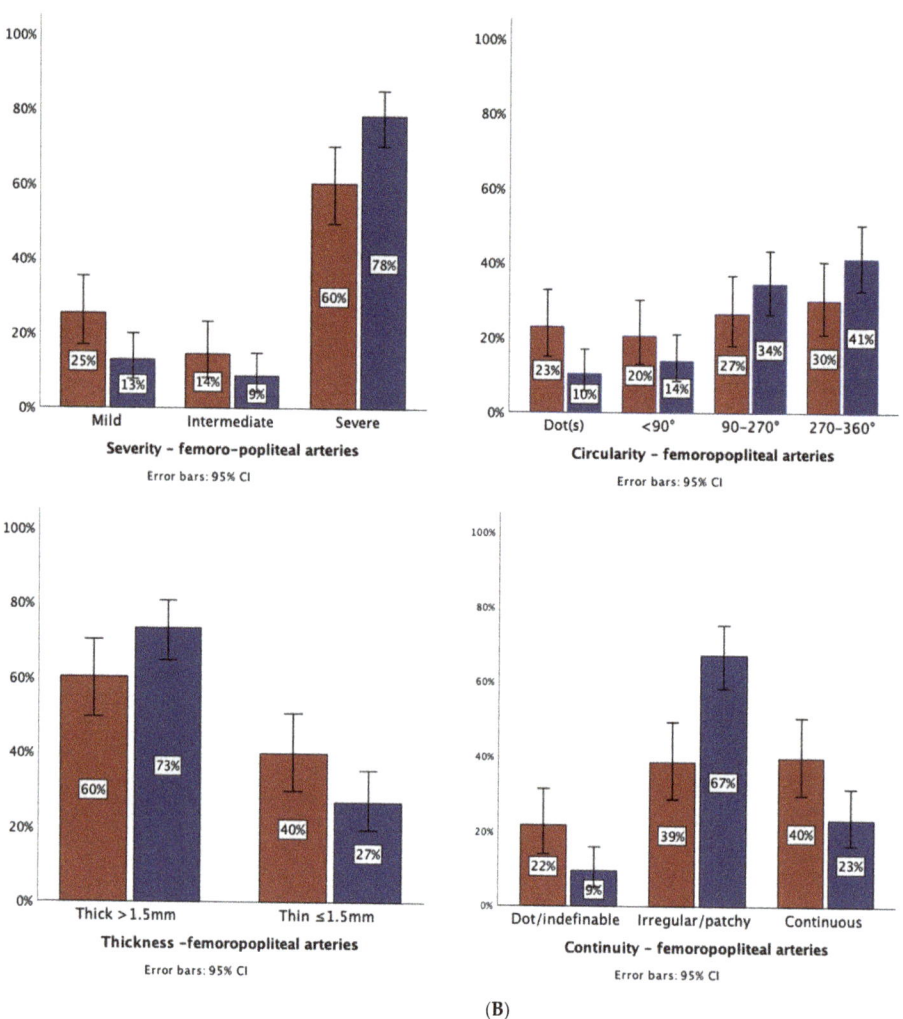

Figure 3. (**A**) CT calcification characteristics in the crural arteries as percentage of total number of age-matched patients. Red: non-PAD patients (n = 65). Blue: CLI patients (n = 115). (**B**) Severity, annularity, thickness, and continuity in the femoropopliteal arteries as percentage of total number of patients. Red: non-PAD patients (n = 83), blue: CLI patients (n = 116).

Table 2. Multivariate logistic regression analysis (sex-adjusted) was performed to determine the different calcification characteristics in the crural arteries associated to age-matched non-PAD (n = 65) and CLI patients (n = 115). The patients without calcifications were excluded from this analysis.

Variables in the Equation	OR	95% CI	Standard Error of the Mean	p-Value
Severity				
Mild	0.55	0.24–1.22	0.391	0.140
Intermediate	0.82	0.37–1.83	0.398	0.627
Severe	1.60	0.87–3.14	0.280	0.122

Table 2. *Cont.*

Variables in the Equation	OR	95% CI	Standard Error of the Mean	p-Value
Annularity				
Dot(s)	0.20	0.10–0.41	0.351	<0.005 *
<90°	1.20	0.84–4.69	0.430	0.121
90–270°	0.53	0.15–1.50	0.504	0.231
Complete annularity	2.92	1.55–5.54	0.304	0.001 *
Thickness				
Thick (≥1.5 mm)	1.08	0.58–1.98	0.273	0.820
Thin (<1.5 mm)	0.90	0.49–1.66	0.280	0.729
Continuity				
Irregular/patchy	1.50	0.79–2.84	0.305	0.212
Continuous	0.86	0.46–1.61	0.293	0.644

* = statistically significant p-value.

Table 3. Multivariate logistic regression analysis was performed to determine the different calcification characteristics in the femoropopliteal arteries correlated to age-matched non-PAD (n = 83) and CLI patients (n = 116). The patients without calcifications were excluded from this analysis.

Variables in the Equation	OR	95% CI	Standard Error of the Mean	p-Value
Severity				
Mild	0.44	0.21–0.91	0.366	0.028 *
Intermediate	0.56	0.23–1.36	0.398	0.200
Severe	2.40	1.29–4.48	0.280	0.006 *
Annularity				
Dot(s)	0.39	0.18–0.85	0.391	0.019 *
<90°	0.62	0.29–1.32	0.376	0.213
90–270°	1.46	0.79–2.71	0.306	0.232
Complete annularity	1.64	0.90–2.98	0.293	0.105
Thickness				
Thick (≥1.5 mm)	1.81	1.09–3.30	0.277	0.053
Thin (<1.5 mm)	0.55	0.30–1.01	0.293	0.053
Continuity				
Irregular/patchy	3.27	1.82–5.89	0.283	<0.005 *
Continuous	0.44	0.24–0.81	0.302	0.009 *

* = statistically significant p-value.

Next, the different calcification characteristics of annularity, thickness and continuity were compared between CLI and non-PAD patients and its results are schematically shown in Figure 4.

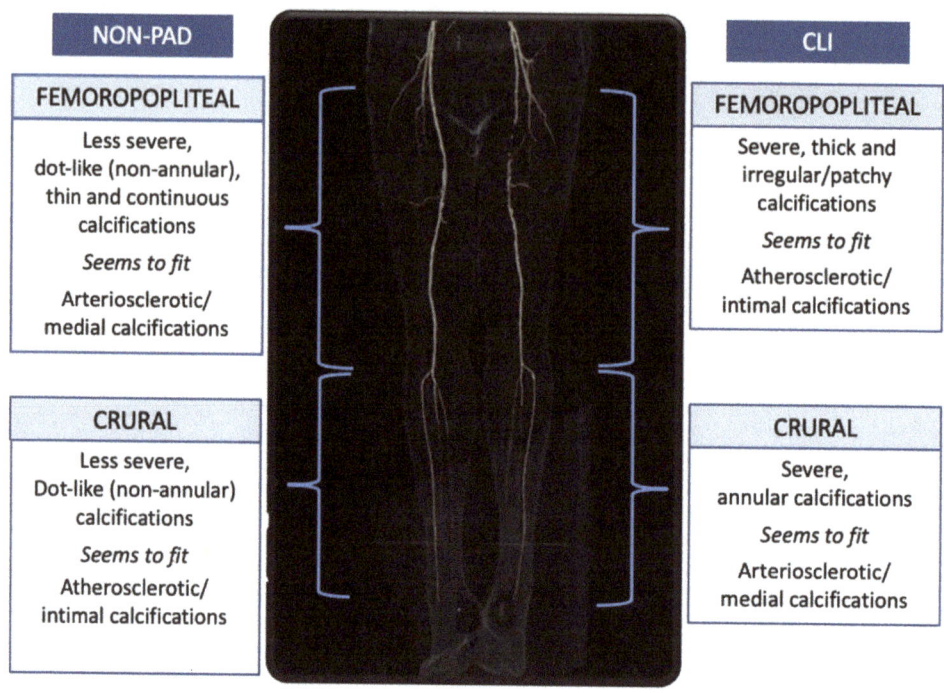

Figure 4. Schematic representation of the different calcification patterns between CLI and non-PAD patients.

In the crural arteries, CLI patients had significantly more complete annular calcifications (58.3% (67/115)) than in non-PAD patients (32.3%, 21/65, OR 2.92, 95% CI 1.55–5.44, $p = 0.001$). Dotted (non-annular) calcifications are more frequently found in non-PAD patients, with an OR of 0.20. No significant OR were found for all other calcification characteristics with respect to the crural arteries.

In the femoropopliteal arteries, CLI patients had irregular/patchy calcifications in 67.8% (78/116), significantly more than non-PAD patients with 38.6% (32/83), OR 3.27, 95% CI 1.82–5.89, $p < 0.005$). Moreover, CLI patients had significantly more thick calcifications in the femoropopliteal artery with 73.3% (85/116), compared to non-PAD patients with 60.2% (50/83, OR 1.81, 95% CI 1.09–3.30, $p = 0.05$). All other calcification characteristics the femoropopliteal arteries did not yield significant differences.

3.4. Sub Analyses CKD and DM

Since DM and CKD are present in a high percentage of CLI patients and have a substantially worse prognosis than patients without these characteristics, sub-analyses were performed to test the specific subcategories DM and CKD. However, the patient numbers of these sub-analyses were low (see baseline Table 1 for an overview of these numbers), so, p-values could not be calculated.

There were no substantial differences between patients with and without DM in non-PAD patients and those with CLI. In the CLI group with CKD, annularity was more frequent (65.4% vs. 54.3%) but the difference with non-CKD CLI patients was small.

4. Discussion

In this matched case-control study, the features of arterial calcifications in the arteries of the lower extremities between patients with CLI and non-PAD patients without known vascular disease were investigated using CT imaging.

The principal finding of this study is that in the crural arteries CLI patients have predominantly annular calcifications, while in non-PAD patients these calcifications are mainly dot-like. Second, almost all patients with CLI have calcifications in the femoropopliteal and crural arteries, while the controls without known vascular disease had any calcifications in less than two-thirds of the cases with a considerable difference between the femoropopliteal and crural arteries.

Annular calcifications are mainly found in the crural arteries of CLI patients have been more frequently related to medial arterial calcifications, while dot-like calcifications are mainly found in the crural arteries of non-PAD patients and seem related to atherosclerotic intimal calcifications. There are however no histologic-CT imaging correlation studies available for the crural arteries. However, a histologic-CT imaging study done in the intracranial internal carotid artery (carotid syphon) confirmed that annular calcifications are indeed more likely located in the medial layer of the arterial wall, while the dot-like ones were related to calcifications in atherosclerotic plaques [10].

Our findings are consistent with several histopathological studies showing that in the crural arteries, medial arterial calcifications play a prominent role in CLI patients. Soor et al. showed that the crural arteries in the majority of CLI patients contain medial calcifications (51–100% annularity) and do not have severe atherosclerosis [3]. O'Neill et al. found medial calcifications in 72% of the arteries of the amputation specimen, while atheromas were present in only 23% [26]. More recently, a histopathological post-mortem study analyzing especially CLI patients showed that medial calcifications occur significantly more frequently in the crural than in femoropopliteal arteries (OR 2.89, $p = 0.08$) [2]. These findings are quite different from the findings in the coronary arteries where medial calcifications are rarely found. In our cohort, only three patients had no crural vessel calcifications (2.5%) and only 2 patients (1.7%) had no femoropopliteal arterial calcifications. An occlusive thrombus and/or partially atheromatous wall changes may have played a role in these few patients with CLI.

Previous studies have shown that patients with medial calcifications have a poor prognosis [27–29]. Recently, we also showed that CLI patients with complete annular calcifications in the lower extremity had a significantly worse all-cause mortality compared to the group without complete annular calcifications [30]. Another study has shown that patients with a higher degree of annular calcification in the abdominal aorta is associated with a higher all-cause mortality (29).

It was recently suggested that medial calcification and atherosclerotic intimal disease can both be present in the arteries of the lower extremities in PAD patients, and that medial calcification prevents the arteries of the lower extremities from remodeling causing obstructive disease in PAD [31]. In our study, we were unable to demonstrate the presence of the two types due to the fact that when describing the characteristics, we always noted only the most common type. As a result, there was no room for less common calcifications. It may be that atherosclerotic disease could lead to much less severe obstructive disease only in the crural arteries, and the presence of both atherosclerotic and medial disease could lead to much more severe PAD.

In the femoropopliteal arteries of CLI patients we found remarkably severe, irregular/patchy, and thick calcifications, while in non-PAD patients, mild, thin, dot-like, and continuous calcifications are found. So, these findings are different from those in the crural arteries where in CLI patients annular medial type of calcifications were found and in non-PAD patients a dot-like atherosclerotic type. Calcification pattern differs in the different vascular territories.

We did not find a difference in calcification pattern between diabetic and non-diabetic patients in CLI and non-PAD patient groups. Such a difference was found in CKD patients but the difference was small and could not explain the high percentage of annular lesions. However, we should be careful with the interpretation since the numbers in this sub analysis were small.

Intimal calcifications are mainly related to atherosclerotic disease and medial calcifications are a metabolic disease due to an imbalance between pro- and anti-calcification agents. These two diseases therefore justify different therapeutic approaches. Intimal calcifications warrant more classical anti-atherosclerotic medication while medial calcification could be halted by calcification inhibitors such as etidronate. The recent TEMP trial was conducted in a group of PXE patients with severe medial calcified arteries [14,15]. After one year of treatment with etidronate, progressive calcification in the femoral arteries was stopped compared to controls, without significant side effects such as osteonecrosis being found. Therefore, we think that a similar study could be considered to perform in this severely affected patient group of CLI patients.

5. Strengths and Limitations

One of the major strengths is that this study compared arterial calcifications in patients with and without symptomatic peripheral vascular disease using CT. The use of CT makes prediction and longitudinal studies of PAD severity through calcification characteristics easier in the long term. A second important strength is that age has been corrected by means of case-matching. Age is a known important confounder of CLI research, and case-matching reduced the possibility of confounding.

However, the study also has its limitations. First, it remains difficult to measure an entire artery with an arbitrary three-, four-, or five-point score. This is certainly the case for CLI patients with a fair number of calcifications in the specific lower extremity arterial territory and therefore both (medial and intimal) patterns are often present. In this case, the most dominant characteristic was chosen to score.

Second, it is remarkable that of the patients without known PAD, there are relatively many patients with severe calcifications. This means that we may have chosen a too low cut-off point for severity of calcifications. Third, the CLI group underwent contrast enhanced CT and the non-PAD group unenhanced CT and therefore we might have underestimated the calcification burden in the CLI group and missed some thin annular calcifications because these may be less recognizable on CT with contrast than CT without contrast. If so, the reported association and findings could be stronger.

Finally, we cannot be completely sure that the non-PAD patients did not have any atherosclerotic disease since no angiograms were made and therefore the lumen was not examined. However, no clinical symptoms were present in these patients and therefore these patients were considered non-PAD patients.

6. Conclusions

This study shows that in the arteries of the lower extremities in CLI patients, any arterial calcification is almost always present. In non-PAD patients however, only two third of patients have any calcifications. Most calcifications are severe. In the crural arteries CLI patients have an annular type of calcifications as seen in medial calcifications, while non-PAD patients have a dot-like type of calcifications as seen in atherosclerotic disease. As medial calcifications are increasingly considered treatable, our findings may contribute to the development of a treatment strategy for these difficult-to-treat CLI patients.

Supplementary Materials: The following are available online at https://www.mdpi.com/article/10.3390/jpm11060493/s1, Table S1: Baseline variables of the sub populations with any calcifications of the initially age-matched CLI patients and the control non-PAD patients, Table S2: Baseline variables of the control group consisted of non-PAD patients, subdivided in patients with and without calcifications in the crural arteries, Table S3: Baseline variables of the control group consisted of non-PAD patients, subdivided in patients with and without calcifications in the femoropopliteal arteries, Table S4: Severity of calcifications in the crural arteries, stratified by age (decades). Table S5: Severity of calcifications in the femoropopliteal arteries, stratified by age (decades).

Author Contributions: L.C.D.K.: Conceptualization, Methodology, Formal analysis, Validation, Investigation, Writing—Original Draft, Writing—Review and Editing. R.A.P.T.: Methodology, Validation, Writing—Review and Editing, Supervision. H.T.C.V.: Writing—Review and Editing. W.P.T.M.M.: Conceptualization, Methodology, Investigation, Writing—Review and Editing, Supervision. H.v.O.: Conceptualization, Supervision. All authors have read and agreed to the published version of the manuscript.

Funding: The original PADI Trial received an unrestricted research grant from The Netherlands Society for Interventional Radiology. All authors of this current post hoc analysis declare that they have received no grants, contracts, or other forms of financial supports or relationships with the industry relevant to this paper. The PADI Imaging Trial was an investigator-initiated, non-funded study which received no specific grant from any funding agency in the public, commercial, or not-for-profit sectors.

Institutional Review Board Statement: These investigations were carried out following the rules of the Declaration of Helsinki of 1975. The medical ethical board of the participating centers approved the prospective PADI Imaging Trial (Unique identifier number: NL64059.098.17) and to re-use data from the PADI trial (ClinicalTrials.gov trial register Unique identifier number: NCT00471289) as a post hoc-analysis. Regarding the patients without PAD, the medical ethical board of the University Medical Center Utrecht (UMCU) waived review because of its non-invasive, retrospective character (study number: 17-897/C). This study was also approved by the ethical board of the Haga Teaching Hospital (study number: T18-003).

Informed Consent Statement: Written informed consent for the PADI Trial and PADI Imaging Trial was obtained in all participants.

Data Availability Statement: The data are not publicly available due to ongoing unpublished research.

Acknowledgments: We would like to thank the radiology technicians of the Haga Teaching Hospital and the UMC Utrecht for their work in collecting data.

Conflicts of Interest: The authors declare that there is no conflict of interest.

Abbreviations

CLI	Chronic limb-threatening ischemia
PAD	Peripheral arterial disease
Non-PAD	Patients without known peripheral arterial disease
OR	Odds ratio
CAD	Coronary artery disease
PADI Trial	Percutaneous transluminal Angioplasty and Drug-eluting stents for Infrapopliteal lesions in critical limb ischemia Trial
PADI Imaging Trial	Percutaneous transluminal Angioplasty and Drug-eluting stents for Infrapopliteal lesions in critical limb ischemia Imaging Trial
RCT	Randomized clinical trial
PTA	Percutaneous transluminal angioplasty
BMS	Bare metal stent
DES	Drug-eluting stent
DM	Diabetes mellitus
eGFR	Electronic glomerular filtration rate (mL/min/1.73 m^2)
BMI	Body-mass index

References

1. Kamenskiy, A.; Poulson, W.; Sim, S.; Reilly, A.; Luo, J.; MacTaggart, J. Prevalence of Calcification in Human Femoropopliteal Arteries and its Association with Demographics, Risk Factors, and Arterial Stiffness. *Arterioscler. Thromb. Vasc. Biol.* **2018**, *38*, e48–e57. [CrossRef]
2. Narula, N.; Dannenberg, A.J.; Olin, J.W.; Bhatt, D.L.; Johnson, K.W.; Nadkarni, G.; Min, J.; Torii, S.; Poojary, P.; Anand, S.S.; et al. Pathology of Peripheral Artery Disease in Patients With Critical Limb Ischemia. *J. Am. Coll. Cardiol.* **2018**, *72*, 2152–2163. [CrossRef] [PubMed]
3. Soor, G.S.; Vukin, I.; Leong, S.W.; Oreopoulos, G.; Butany, J. Peripheral vascular disease: Who gets it and why? A histomorphological analysis of 261 arterial segments from 58 cases. *Pathology* **2008**, *40*, 385–391. [CrossRef]

4. Chowdhury, M.M.; Makris, G.C.; Tarkin, J.M.; Joshi, F.R.; Hayes, P.D.; Rudd, J.H.; Coughlin, P.A. Lower limb arterial calcification (LLAC) scores in patients with symptomatic peripheral arterial disease are associated with increased cardiac mortality and morbidity. *PLoS ONE* **2017**, *12*, e0182952.
5. Kang, I.S.; Lee, W.; Choi, B.W.; Choi, D.; Hong, M.K.; Jang, Y.; Ko, Y.G. Semiquantitative assessment of tibial artery calcification by computed tomography angiography and its ability to predict infrapopliteal angioplasty outcomes. *J. Vasc. Surg.* **2016**, *64*, 1335–1343. [CrossRef] [PubMed]
6. Huang, C.L.; Wu, I.H.; Wu, Y.W.; Hwang, J.J.; Wang, S.S.; Chen, W.J.; Lee, W.J.; Yang, W.S. Association of lower extremity arterial calcification with amputation and mortality in patients with symptomatic peripheral artery disease. *PLoS ONE* **2014**, *9*, e90201 [CrossRef]
7. Lanzer, P.; Boehm, M.; Sorribas, V.; Thiriet, M.; Janzen, J.; Zeller, T.; St Hilaire, C.; Shanahan, C. Medial vascular calcification revisited: Review and perspectives. *Eur. Heart J.* **2014**, *35*, 1515–1525. [CrossRef]
8. Hendriks, E.J.; de Jong, P.A.; Beulens, J.W.; Mali, W.P.; van der Schouw, Y.T.; Beijerinck, D. Medial Arterial Calcification: Active Reversible Disease in Human Breast Arteries. *JACC Cardiovasc. Imaging* **2015**, *8*, 984–985. [CrossRef] [PubMed]
9. Hendriks, E.J.; de Jong, P.A.; van der Graaf, Y.; Mali, W.P.; van der Schouw, Y.T.; Beulens, J.W. Breast arterial calcifications: A systematic review and meta-analysis of their determinants and their association with cardiovascular events. *Atherosclerosis* **2015**, *239*, 11–20. [CrossRef]
10. Vos, A.; Van Hecke, W.; Spliet, W.G.; Goldschmeding, R.; Isgum, I.; Kockelkoren, R.; Bleys, R.L.; Mali, W.P.; de Jong, P.A.; Vink, A. Predominance of Nonatherosclerotic Internal Elastic Lamina Calcification in the Intracranial Internal Carotid Artery. *Stroke* **2016**, *47*, 221–223. [CrossRef]
11. Bostrom, K.; Watson, K.E.; Horn, S.; Wortham, C.; Herman, I.M.; Demer, L.L. Bone morphogenetic protein expression in human atherosclerotic lesions. *J. Clin. Investig.* **1993**, *91*, 1800–1809. [CrossRef]
12. McDougal, B.A.; Lukert, B.P. Resolution of breast pain and calcification with renal transplantation. *Arch. Intern. Med.* **1977**, *137*, 375–377. [CrossRef]
13. Han, K.H.; Hennigar, R.A.; O'Neill, W.C. The association of bone and osteoclasts with vascular calcification. *Vasc. Med.* **2015**, *20*, 527–533. [CrossRef]
14. Bartstra, J.W.; de Jong, P.A.; Kranenburg, G.; Wolterink, J.M.; Isgum, I.; Wijsman, A.; Wolf, B.; den Harder, A.M.; Willem, P.T.M.; Spiering, W. Etidronate halts systemic arterial calcification in pseudoxanthoma elasticum. *Atherosclerosis* **2020**, *292*, 37–41. [CrossRef] [PubMed]
15. Kranenburg, G.; de Jong, P.A.; Bartstra, J.W.; Lagerweij, S.J.; Lam, M.G.; Ossewaarde-van Norel, J.; Risseeuw, S.; van Leeuwen, R.; Imhof, S.M.; Verhaar, H.J.; et al. Etidronate for Prevention of Ectopic Mineralization in Patients With Pseudoxanthoma Elasticum. *J. Am. Coll. Cardiol.* **2018**, *71*, 1117–1126. [CrossRef] [PubMed]
16. Chowdhury, U.K.; Airan, B.; Mishra, P.K.; Kothari, S.S.; Subramaniam, G.K.; Ray, R.; Singh, R.; Venugopal, P. Histopathology and morphometry of radial artery conduits: Basic study and clinical application. *Ann. Thorac. Surg.* **2004**, *78*, 1614–1621. [CrossRef]
17. Spreen, M.I.; Martens, J.M.; Hansen, B.E.; Knippenberg, B.; Verhey, E.; van Dijk, L.C.; de Vries, J.P.P.; Vos, J.A.; de Borst, G.J.; Vonken, E.J.P.; et al. Percutaneous Transluminal Angioplasty and Drug-Eluting Stents for Infrapopliteal Lesions in Critical Limb Ischemia (PADI) Trial. *Circ. Cardiovasc. Interv.* **2016**, *9*, e002376. [CrossRef]
18. Spreen, M.I.; Martens, J.M.; Knippenberg, B.; van Dijk, L.C.; de Vries, J.P.P.; Vos, J.A.; de Borst, G.J.; Vonken, E.J.P.; Bijlstra, O.D.; Wever, J.J.; et al. Long-Term Follow-up of the PADI Trial: Percutaneous Transluminal Angioplasty Versus Drug-Eluting Stents for Infrapopliteal Lesions in Critical Limb Ischemia. *J. Am. Heart Assoc.* **2017**, *6*. [CrossRef]
19. Wakkie, T.; Konijn, L.C.D.; van Herpen, N.P.C.; Maessen, M.F.; Spreen, M.I.; Wever, J.J.; van Eps, R.G.S.; Veger, H.T.; van Dijk, L.C.; Willem, P.T.M.; et al. Cost-Effectiveness of Drug-Eluting Stents for Infrapopliteal Lesions in Patients with Critical Limb Ischemia: The PADI Trial. *Cardiovasc. Intervent. Radiol.* **2019**, *43*, 376–381. [CrossRef] [PubMed]
20. Konijn, L.C.D.; Wakkie, T.; Spreen, M.I.; De Jong, P.A.; Van Dijk, L.C.; Wever, J.J.; Veger, H.T.C.; Van Eps, R.G.S.; Mali, W.P.T.M.; Van Overhagen, H. 10-Year Paclitaxel Dose-Related Outcomes of Drug-Eluting Stents Treated Below the Knee in Patients with Chronic Limb-Threatening Ischemia (The PADI Trial). *Cardiovasc. Intervent. Radiol.* **2020**, *43*. [CrossRef]
21. Konijn, L.C.D.; van Overhagen, H.; Takx, R.A.P.; de Jong, P.A.; Veger, H.T.C.; Mali, W. CT calcification patterns of peripheral arteries in patients without known peripheral arterial disease. *Eur. J. Radiol.* **2020**, *128*, 108973. [CrossRef]
22. Levey, A.S.; Coresh, J.; Balk, E.; Kausz, A.T.; Levin, A.; Steffes, M.W.; Hogg, R.J.; Perrone, R.D.; Lau, J.; Eknoyan, G. National Kidney Foundation practice guidelines for chronic kidney disease: Evaluation, classification, and stratification. *Ann. Intern. Med.* **2003**, *139*, 137–147. [CrossRef]
23. Arvela, E.; Soderstrom, M.; Alback, A.; Aho, P.S.; Tikkanen, I.; Lepantalo, M. Estimated glomerular filtration rate (eGFR) as a predictor of outcome after infrainguinal bypass in patients with critical limb ischemia. *Eur. J. Vasc. Endovasc. Surg.* **2008**, *36*, 77–83. [CrossRef] [PubMed]
24. Kockelkoren, R.; Vos, A.; Van Hecke, W.; Vink, A.; Bleys, R.L.; Verdoorn, D.; Mali, W.P.T.M.; Hendrikse, J.; Koek, H.L.; De Jong, P.A.; et al. Computed Tomographic Distinction of Intimal and Medial Calcification in the Intracranial Internal Carotid Artery. *PLoS ONE* **2017**, *12*, e0168360. [CrossRef] [PubMed]
25. Kranenburg, G.; de Jong, P.A.; Mali, W.P.; Attrach, M.; Visseren, F.L.; Spiering, W. Prevalence and severity of arterial calcifications in pseudoxanthoma elasticum (PXE) compared to hospital controls. Novel insights into the vascular phenotype of PXE. *Atherosclerosis* **2017**, *256*, 7–14. [CrossRef]

26. O'Neill, W.C.; Han, K.H.; Schneider, T.M.; Hennigar, R.A. Prevalence of nonatheromatous lesions in peripheral arterial disease. *Arterioscler. Thromb. Vasc. Biol.* **2015**, *35*, 439–447. [CrossRef]
27. London, G.M.; Guerin, A.P.; Marchais, S.J.; Metivier, F.; Pannier, B.; Adda, H. Arterial media calcification in end-stage renal disease: Impact on all-cause and cardiovascular mortality. *Nephrol. Dial. Transplant.* **2003**, *18*, 1731–1740. [CrossRef]
28. Everhart, J.E.; Pettitt, D.J.; Knowler, W.C.; Rose, F.A.; Bennett, P.H. Medial arterial calcification and its association with mortality and complications of diabetes. *Diabetologia* **1988**, *31*, 16–23.
29. Lehto, S.; Niskanen, L.; Suhonen, M.; Ronnemaa, T.; Laakso, M. Medial artery calcification. A neglected harbinger of cardiovascular complications in non-insulin-dependent diabetes mellitus. *Arterioscler. Thromb. Vasc. Biol.* **1996**, *16*, 978–983. [CrossRef] [PubMed]
30. Konijn, L.C.D.; Takx, R.A.P.; de Jong, P.A.; Spreen, M.I.; Veger, H.T.C.; Mali, W.P.T.M.; van Overhagen, H. Arterial calcification and long-term outcome in chronic limb-threatening ischemia patients. *Eur. J. Radiol.* **2020**, *132*, 109305. [CrossRef] [PubMed]
31. Ho, C.Y.; Shanahan, C.M. Medial Arterial Calcification: An Overlooked Player in Peripheral Arterial Disease. *Arterioscler. Thromb. Vasc. Biol.* **2016**, *36*, 1475–1482. [CrossRef] [PubMed]

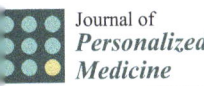

Article

Discriminating Reflux from Non-Reflux Diseases of Superficial Veins in Legs by Novel Non-Contrast MR with QFlow Technique

Yuan-Hsi Tseng [1,†], Chien-Wei Chen [2,3,†], Min Yi Wong [1,4], Teng-Yao Yang [5], Bor-Shyh Lin [4], Hua Ting [3] and Yao-Kuang Huang [1,*,‡]

1. Division of Thoracic and Cardiovascular Surgery, Chiayi Chang Gung Memorial Hospital, College of Medicine, Chia-Yi and Chang Gung University, Taoyuan 33302, Taiwan; 8802003@cgmh.org.tw (Y.-H.T.); mynyy001@gmail.com (M.Y.W.)
2. Department of Diagnostic Radiology, Chiayi Chang Gung Memorial Hospital, College of Medicine, Chia-Yi and Chang Gung University, Taoyuan 33302, Taiwan; chienwei33@gmail.com
3. Institute of Medicine, Chung Shan Medical University, Taichung 408, Taiwan; huating@csmu.edu.tw
4. Institute of Imaging and Biomedical Photonics, National Chiao Tung University, Tainan 300, Taiwan; borshyhlin@gmail.com
5. Department of Cardiology, Chiayi Chang Gung Memorial Hospital, College of Medicine, Chia-Yi and Chang Gung University, Taoyuan 33302, Taiwan; 2859@adm.cgmh.org.tw
* Correspondence: huang137@icloud.com
† Chen C.-W. and Tseng Y.-H. contributed equally to this article.
‡ Address reprint requests to: Department of Cardiovascular Surgery, Chia-Yi Chang Gung Memorial Hospital, West Section, Chia-Pu Rd., Putzu City 61363, Chiayi County, Taiwan.

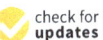

Citation: Tseng, Y.-H.; Chen, C.-W.; Wong, M.Y.; Yang, T.-Y.; Lin, B.-S.; Ting, H.; Huang, Y.-K. Discriminating Reflux from Non-Reflux Diseases of Superficial Veins in Legs by Novel Non-Contrast MR with QFlow Technique. *J. Pers. Med.* **2021**, *11*, 242. https://doi.org/10.3390/jpm11040242

Academic Editor: Pim A. de Jong

Received: 14 February 2021
Accepted: 22 March 2021
Published: 26 March 2021

Publisher's Note: MDPI stays neutral with regard to jurisdictional claims in published maps and institutional affiliations.

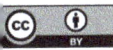

Copyright: © 2021 by the authors. Licensee MDPI, Basel, Switzerland. This article is an open access article distributed under the terms and conditions of the Creative Commons Attribution (CC BY) license (https://creativecommons.org/licenses/by/4.0/).

Abstract: Objectives: To find an objective diagnostic tool for the superficial veins in legs. **Methods**: This study included 137 patients who underwent TRANCE-MRI from 2017 to 2020 (IRB: 202001570B0). Among them, 53 with unilateral leg venous diseases underwent a QFlow scan and were classified into the reflux and non-reflux groups according to the status of the great saphenous veins. **Results**: The QFlow, namely stroke volume (SV), forward flow volume (FFV), mean flux (MF), stroke distance (SD), and mean velocity (MV) measured in the external iliac, femoral, popliteal, and great saphenous vein (GSV). The SV, FFV, SD, MF, SD, and MV in the GSV (morbid/non-morbid limbs) demonstrated a favorable ability to discriminate reflux from non-reflux in the ROC curve. The SD in the GSV and GSV/PV ratio ($p = 0.049$ and 0.047/cutoff = 86 and 117.1) and the MV in the EIV/FV ratio, GSV, and GSV/PV ratio ($p = 0.035$, 0.034, and 0.025/cutoff = 100.9, 86.1, and 122.9) exhibited the ability to discriminate between reflux and non-reflux group. The SD, MV, and FFV have better ability to discriminate a reflux from non-reflux group than the SV and MF. **Conclusions**: QFlow may be used to verify the reflux of superficial veins in the legs. An increasing GSV/PV ratio is a hallmark of reflux of superficial veins in the legs.

Keywords: MRI; non-contrast; venography; TRANCE; QFlow

1. Background

Patients were suspected as having a disease of venous origin when they came with tortuous varicose veins on calves, asymmetric swollen legs, and watery ulcers around the gaiter area of their feet. Venous diseases in those legs may be caused by superficial venous reflux from valvular dysfunction, occlusion of the deep venous system by thrombi, and compression of the pelvic mass. The resulting signs include spider veins, foot pigmentation, claudication, stasis ulcers, swollen limbs with deep vein thrombosis, and the fatal consequence of the pulmonary emboli [1–6]. Ultrasound examination (US) is the standard procedure for venous disease of the legs and could provide most information by experienced operators [7,8]. Few tools are available for objective venous evaluation in lower limbs. The venous system is not exactly enhanced by computed tomography (CT) venography, and high-quality enhancement requires specific access from the morbid limb. Compared with conventional angiography, most magnetic resonance venography (MRV) techniques that involve contrast media have been proven to be more sensitive towards the detection of lesions in vessels [9]. Triggered angiography non-contrast-enhanced (TRANCE) magnetic resonance imaging (MRI) can record differences in vascular signal intensity during the cardiac cycle for subsequent image subtraction and obtain vascular images without the use of contrast media (Figure 1). All images of the arterial systems are reconstructed by three-dimensional turbo spin-echo (TSE) at systolic and diastolic periods. During systole, arterial blood flows rapidly, and the arteries are black. In the diastole phase, blood flow in the arteries is slow, and the arteries are bright. Subtraction of the two-phased scans made up a 3D data set with only arteries (MRA). Another image of the venous systems (MRV) was evaluated by 3D TSE short tau inversion recovery (STIR) during the systolic period. STIR provides additional background suppression because the fat and bones are also suppressed. This technique was initially evaluated for pelvic vessels. Our clinical applications of this technique have innovated the anatomy of the whole venous system in legs since 2017 and further proven its efficiency in different venous scenarios thereafter [6,10,11]. TRANCE-MRI helps to not only exclude venous compression but also reveal the major tributaries, thus providing better guidance for venous ablation. In this study, we evaluated the possible correlation between reflux with ultrasound and morphologic changes from the TRANCE-MRI and studied the hemodynamic patterns obtained from QFlow analysis through TRANCE-MRI to help differentiate reflux in superficial veins further.

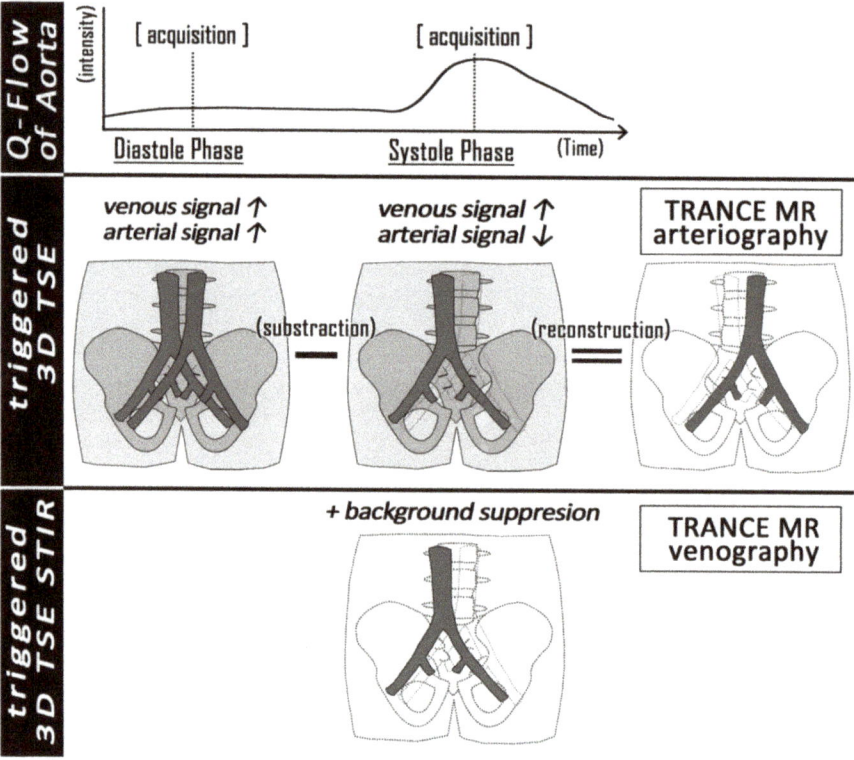

Figure 1. The principle of TRANCE-MRI: We use a peripheral pulse unit to identify the systolic and diastolic phases (**upper row**). The diastolic phase subtracting the systolic phase simulated arteriography (**middle row**). The systolic 3D TSE was further modified by background suppression (bone, soft tissue, and fat) to gain TRANCE-MR venography.

2. Methods

2.1. Patients

The study protocol was approved by the Institutional Review Board (IRB) of Chang Gung Memorial Hospital (IRB number: 202001570B0). The study recruited consecutive patients who underwent TRANCE-MRI for venous pathology in their legs at a tertiary hospital between April 2017 and September 2020. We analyzed their data to determine their clinical significance. All patients were suspected of having venous pathology in their legs. Patients were excluded if they exhibited poor compliance or had multiple comorbidities that made them unable to lie down for the 1 h TRANCE-MRI protocol. At first, 137 patients were enrolled for leg venous evaluation through TRANCE-MRI. Twelve patients were excluded for reasons including pregnancy, presence of non-MRI-compatible ferromagnetic implants, significant arrhythmia, and restless legs. The remaining 125 patients underwent anatomical evaluation through TRANCE-MRI. QFlow analysis and hemodynamic evaluation were performed in 53 patients with unilateral symptoms. These 53 patients were further categorized into the reflux and non-reflux groups according to the screening duplex and referral indication for TRANCE-MRI (Figure 2).

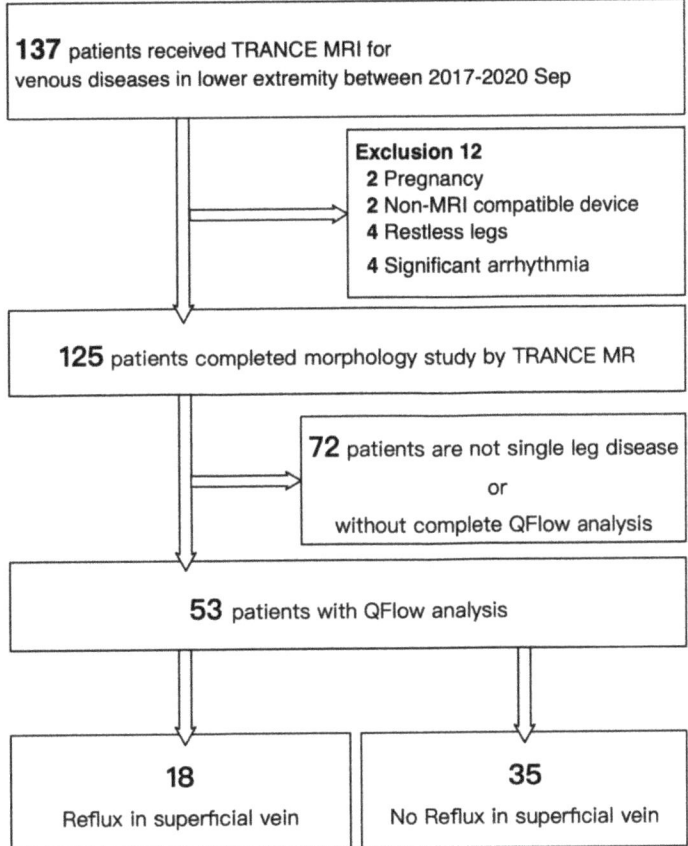

Figure 2. Flowchart of cohort selection.

All 53 patients received noninvasive color Doppler ultrasonography (US) for the venous status in their lower legs before the scheduled TRANCE-MRI. The duplex examination was performed in the supine position, and the femoral vein, great saphenous vein

(GSV), popliteal vein, and perforating vein in the calves were examined. Intra-abdominal and pelvic veins were not evaluated in all of the duplex examinations.

2.2. MRI Acquisition

MRI was performed using a 1.5 T MRI scanner (Philips Ingenia, Philips Healthcare, Best, The Netherlands) and a peripheral pulse unit trigger, with the patients in the supine position. All arterial system images were evaluated through a three-dimensional (3D) turbo spin-echo (TSE) technique during systole and diastole periods. TSE TRANCE imaging was executed using the following parameters: repetition time (TR), 1 beat; echo time (TE), shortest; flip angle, 90°; voxel size, $1.7 \times 1.7 \times 3$ mm^3; and field of view (FOV), 350×420. During systole, the arterial blood flow was relatively fast, which caused signal dephasing and lead to flow voids. Accordingly, when a systolic trigger was applied, the arteries would appear black. During diastole, the arterial blood flow was slow, and therefore, the signal was not dephased, and the arteries appeared bright on diastolic scans. Subtraction of the two-phased scans yielded a 3D data set of the arteries only. Other images of the venous systems were evaluated through 3D TSE short tau inversion recovery (STIR) during the systole period. TSE STIR TRANCE imaging was executed using the following parameters: TR, 1 beat; TE, 85; inversion recovery delay time, 160; voxel size, $1.7 \times 1.7 \times 4$ mm^3; and FOV, 360×320. STIR provides additional background suppression because the fat and bones are also suppressed. When a systolic trigger was applied, the arteries appear black. This imaging process yielded a 3D data set of the venous system, with no subtraction required. A quantitative flow scan was routinely performed to determine the appropriate trigger delay times for systolic and diastolic triggering. All images were acquired without the use of a gadolinium-based contrast medium. QFlow scans yielded multiple acquisitions within one cardiac cycle, resulting in multiple phases (Figure 3).

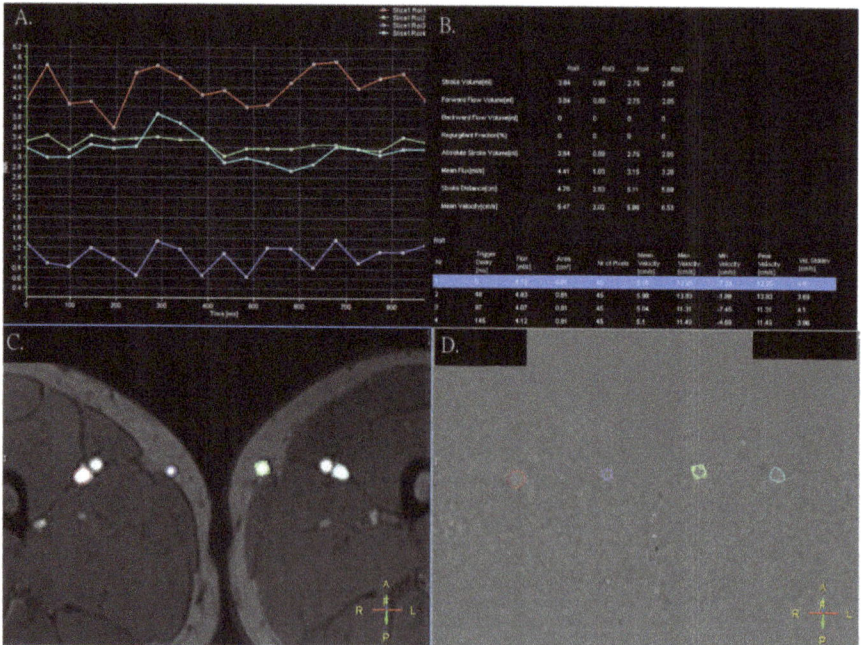

Figure 3. QFlow scanning through TRANCE-MRI including stroke volume (SV), forward flow volume (FFV), mean flux (MF), stroke distance (SD), and mean velocity (MV). (**A**) Two great saphenous veins and two popliteal veins with the flow sequence by time. (**B**) QFlow parameters with different trigger delays. (**C**) Areas of interest in both great saphenous and popliteal veins (blue: right side, normal GSV; green: left side, diseased GSV). (**D**) Image obtained during data acquisition.

QFlow analysis included the following parameters: stroke volume (SV), forward and backward flow volumes, flux, stroke distance (SD), mean velocity (MV), and vessel area. In this study, a postprocessing package was used to calculate quantitative information such as flow velocity and allow the visualization as 2D flow maps overlaid on anatomic references. The external iliac veins, femoral veins, popliteal veins, and greater saphenous veins were analyzed.

2.3. Statistical Analysis

The continuous variables (age and QFlow) were analyzed using an unpaired two-tailed Student's t test or one-way analysis of variance, and the discrete variables (sex, substance usage, comorbidities, and intervention history) were compared using a two-tailed Fisher's exact test. The QFlow parameters (including SV, forward flow volume (FFV), mean flux (MF), SD, and MV in each venous segment) and the obstructive venous diseases were evaluated using receiver operating characteristic (ROC) curve analysis. All statistical analyses were conducted using the STATA statistics/Data Analysis (version 8.0; Stata Corporation, College Station, TX, USA). The results are presented as means and standard deviations. Statistical significance was defined as $p < 0.05$.

3. Results

The demographic and medical data of the 53 patients, including regarding sex, age, substance use, and comorbidities, are summarized in Table 1.

Table 1. Clinical characteristics of the patients who underwent QFlow analysis by TRANCE-MRI by the presence of reflux in superficial veins.

Variable	Total (n = 53)	Reflux (n = 18)	No Reflux (n = 35)	p Value
Male sex	15 (28.3)	7 (38.9)	8 (22.9)	0.334
Age, year	59.7 ± 14.1	56.9 ± 12.9	61.1 ± 14.7	0.317
Substance use				
Smoking	10 (18.9)	5 (27.8)	5 (14.3)	0.279
Alcohol	3 (5.7)	1 (5.6)	2 (5.7)	1.000
Betel nuts	3 (5.7)	2 (11.1)	1 (2.9)	0.263
Comorbidities				
Hypertension	15 (28.3)	3 (16.7)	12 (34.3)	0.215
Diabetes	8 (15.1)	2 (11.1)	6 (17.1)	0.701
Coronary artery disease	1 (1.9)	0 (0.0)	1 (2.9)	1.000
Deep vein thrombosis	6 (11.3)	0 (0.0)	6 (17.1)	0.085
Cancer	8 (15.1)	1 (5.6)	7 (20.0)	0.240
Left leg involved	32 (60.4)	8 (44.4)	24 (68.6)	0.138
Chronic leg ulcer	8 (15.1)	5 (27.8)	3 (8.6)	0.104

Data are presented as a percentage or mean ± standard deviation.

The mean age in the cohort was 59.7 ± 14.1 years, and the majority were women (38/53, 71.7%). The patients were further divided into the patients with reflux in the great saphenous vein (reflux group) and patients without reflux in the great saphenous vein (non-reflux group) according to their presenting symptoms and duplex findings (Figure 4).

The two groups were similar in terms of age, sex, substance use, comorbidities, and co-existence of leg ulcers. QFlow analysis through TRANCE-MRI involved the evaluation of SV (mL), FFV (mL), MF (mL), SD (cm), and MV (cm) in the external iliac veins, femoral veins, popliteal veins, and GSVs in the 53 patients. The superficial veins in the non-reflux group were mostly in normal size, with competent valve function. To minimize individual bias in the QFlow analysis, we compared the morbid and non-morbid limbs of the same patients. The performance of the QFlow parameters (SV, FFV, MV, SD, and MV) in the discrimination of the reflux from non-reflux patients was assessed using the ratio of the morbid limb to normal limb in each venous segment (Table 2).

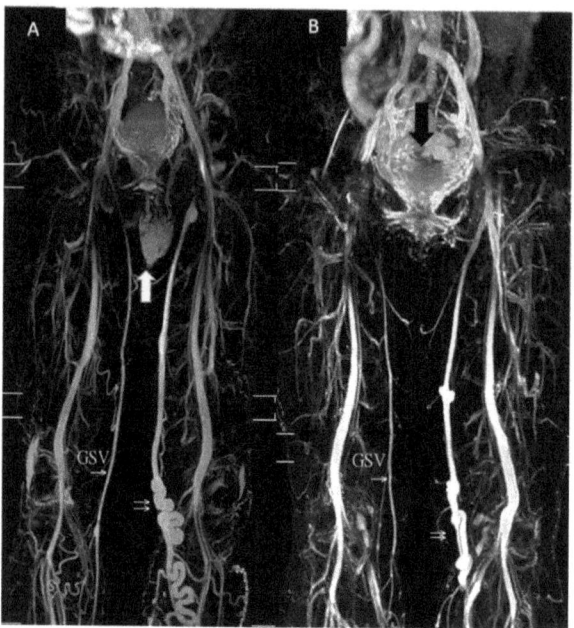

Figure 4. Typical patients with reflux in the great saphenous vein by TRANCE-MR. (**A**) A 56-year-old man with reflux of the left great saphenous vein. The white arrow indicates the testis. GSV: normal right great saphenous vein. The double arrow indicates the diseased great saphenous vein with its tributaries. (**B**) A 67-year-old woman also with reflux in the left great saphenous vein. The black arrow indicates the uterine. GSV: normal right side great saphenous vein. The double arrow indicates the diseased great saphenous vein with its tributaries.

The SV exhibited favorable discriminating ability for reflux in the GSV segment (AUC = 68.8%, 95% CI = 52.7–85%). The FFV had favorable discriminating ability for reflux in the GSV ratio (AUC = 74.9%, 95% CI = 58.2–86.5%) and GSV/PV ratio (AUC = 74%, 95% CI = 58.5–89.6%). The MF also effectively discriminated reflux from non-reflux in the GSV segment (AUC = 68.6%, 95% CI = 52.4–84.8%) and GSV/PV ratio (AUC = 66.7%, 95% CI = 50.4–83%). The SD demonstrated favorable discrimination performance for venous reflux in the EIV/FV ratio (AUC = 66.5%, 95% CI = 51.3–81.7%), GSV segment (AUC = 68.6%, 95% CI = 53.0–84.2%), and GSV/PV ratio (AUC = 66.8%, 95% CI = 53.0–84.7%). The MV demonstrated favorable discrimination performance for venous reflux in the EIV/FV ratio, (AUC = 67.8%, 95% CI = 52.5–83.1%), GSV segment, (AUC = 70%, 95% CI = 54.6–85.4%), and GSV/PV ratio (AUC = 71.2%, 95% CI = 55.7–86.7%). The SV exhibited a significant ability to discriminate between reflux and non-reflux venous diseases in the GSV segment ($p = 0.047$). The FFV in the GSV segment and GSV/PV ratio exhibited a significant ability to discriminate between reflux and non-reflux venous diseases ($p = 0.008$ and 0.011, respectively).

The MF in the GSV segment exhibited a significant ability to discriminate between reflux and non-reflux venous diseases ($p = 0.049$). The SD in the GSV and GSV/PV ratio exhibited a significant ability to discriminate between reflux and non-reflux venous diseases ($p = 0.049$ and 0.047, respectively, and cutoff = 86 and 117.1, respectively). Furthermore, the MV in the EIV/FV ratio, GSV segment, and GSV/PV ratio exhibited a significant ability to discriminate between reflux and non-reflux venous diseases ($p = 0.035, 0.034$, and 0.025, respectively, and cutoff = 100.9, 86.1, and 122.9, respectively). The SD, MV, and FFV have better ability to discriminate reflux from non-reflux venous diseases than the SV and MF by the QFlow analysis. The ROC curve of SD and MF is shown in Figure 5.

Table 2. The performance of QFlow parameters (the ratio of the morbid limb to normal limb) in discriminating reflux in superficial veins of legs.

Variable	Total (N = 53)	Reflux (n = 18)	No Reflux (n = 35)	p	AUC, % (95% CI) *	Cutoff #	Sensitivity, % (95% CI)	Specificity, % (95% CI)
SV								
EIV	100 (60, 124)	102 (78, 119)	82 (49, 132)	0.367	55.0 (37.3–72.7)	NA	NA	NA
FV	91 (60, 136)	101 (64, 165)	80 (52, 128)	0.237	57.1 (38.6–75.7)	NA	NA	NA
(EIV/FV) * 100	86 (58, 147)	99 (66, 147)	73 (53, 157)	0.419	60.7 (42.9–78.5)	NA	NA	NA
GSV	130 (72, 766)	276 (126, 875)	105 (59, 600)	0.047 *	68.8 (52.7–85.0) *	>108.6	85.7 (57.2–98.2)	53.3 (34.3–71.7)
PV	89 (53, 120)	78 (51, 207)	92 (53, 120)	0.851	52.9 (32.5–73.2)	NA	NA	NA
(GSV/PV) * 100	154 (79, 518)	257 (152, 563)	126 (61, 472)	0.087	66.2 (49.7–82.7)	NA	NA	NA
FFV								
EIV	92 (56, 121)	101 (70, 116)	84 (47, 132)	0.430	53.8 (36.2–71.4)	NA	NA	NA
FV	95 (64, 136)	101 (64, 165)	92 (58, 128)	0.320	56.7 (38.1–75.3)	NA	NA	NA
(EIV/FV) * 100	81 (49, 145)	99 (61, 147)	72 (45, 124)	0.348	58.6 (41.0–76.1)	NA	NA	NA
GSV	125 (81, 332)	276 (126, 821)	108 (64, 183)	0.008 *	74.9 (59.3–90.4) *	>114.3	85.7 (57.2–98.2)	60 (40.6–77.3)
PV	92 (63, 120)	78 (52, 207)	97 (71, 120)	0.693	55.0 (34.5–75.5)	NA	NA	NA
(GSV/PV) * 100	147 (73, 312)	260 (156, 563)	109 (63, 222)	0.011 *	74.0 (58.5–89.6) *	>222.0	71.4 (41.9–91.6)	76.7 (57.7–90.1)
MF								
EIV	100 (59, 124)	102 (70, 119)	82 (49, 133)	0.419	55.2 (37.6–72.8)	NA	NA	NA
FV	95 (64, 136)	102 (64, 164)	89 (59, 127)	0.302	57.6 (39.1–76.1)	NA	NA	NA
(EIV/FV) * 100	83 (55, 146)	96 (65, 147)	71 (53, 124)	0.338	61.2 (43.4–79.0)	NA	NA	NA
GSV	129 (67, 778)	276 (125, 847)	106 (60, 600)	0.049 *	68.6 (52.4–84.8) *	>109.3	85.7 (57.2–98.2)	53.3 (34.3–71.7)
PV	88 (61, 120)	77 (51, 209)	92 (65, 120)	0.778	53.8 (33.4–74.2)	NA	NA	NA
(GSV/PV) * 100	160 (80, 538)	257 (157, 569)	119 (61, 507)	0.078	66.7 (50.4–83.0) *	>136.5	78.6 (49.2–95.3)	60.0 (40.6–77.3)
SD								
EIV	98 (71, 123)	101 (74, 123)	88 (57, 128)	0.237	61.0 (43.0–78.9)	NA	NA	NA
FV	94 (76, 128)	94 (76, 128)	94 (70, 129)	0.910	53.8 (35.6–72.0)	NA	NA	NA
(EIV/FV) * 100	94 (64, 122)	106 (77, 163)	82 (51, 119)	0.051	66.5 (51.3–81.7) *	>101.0	61.1 (35.7–82.7)	68.6 (50.7–83.1)
GSV	126 (73, 423)	224 (118, 765)	93 (50, 365)	0.049 *	68.6 (53.0–84.2) *	>86	92.9 (66.1–99.8)	50.0 (31.3–68.7)
PV	91 (57, 119)	74 (53, 111)	98 (64, 120)	0.276	59.8 (38.8–80.7)	NA	NA	NA
(GSV/PV) * 100	135 (66, 333)	204 (133, 582)	112 (39, 318)	0.047 *	68.8 (53.0–84.7) *	>117.1	85.7 (57.2–98.2)	56.7 (37.4–74.5)
MV								
EIV	99 (71, 128)	101 (73, 151)	88 (57, 128)	0.176	61.0 (43.0–78.9)	NA	NA	NA
FV	94 (76, 128)	94 (76, 128)	94 (70, 129)	0.910	53.8 (35.6–72.0)	NA	NA	NA
(EIV/FV) * 100	94 (63, 129)	109 (77, 165)	82 (51, 119)	0.035 *	67.8 (52.5–83.1) *	>100.9	61.1 (35.7–82.7)	68.6 (50.7–83.1)
GSV	126 (73, 382)	300 (118, 768)	93 (56, 338)	0.034 *	70.0 (54.6–85.4) *	>86.1	92.3 (66.1–99.8)	50.0 (31.3–68.7)
PV	91 (57, 119)	74 (54, 111)	98 (64, 120)	0.276	59.8 (38.8–80.7)	NA	NA	NA
(GSV/PV) * 100	135 (66, 332)	206 (133, 585)	112 (40, 318)	0.025 *	71.2 (55.7–86.7) *	>122.9	85.7 (57.2–98.2)	60.0 (40.6–77.3)

Data are presented as median [25th percentile, 75th percentiles]; AUC, area under curve; CI, confidence interval; FFV, forward flow volume; MF, mean flux; MV, mean velocity; SD, stroke distance; SV, stroke volume; NA, not applicable; # Determined by the Youden index; * p value < 0.05.

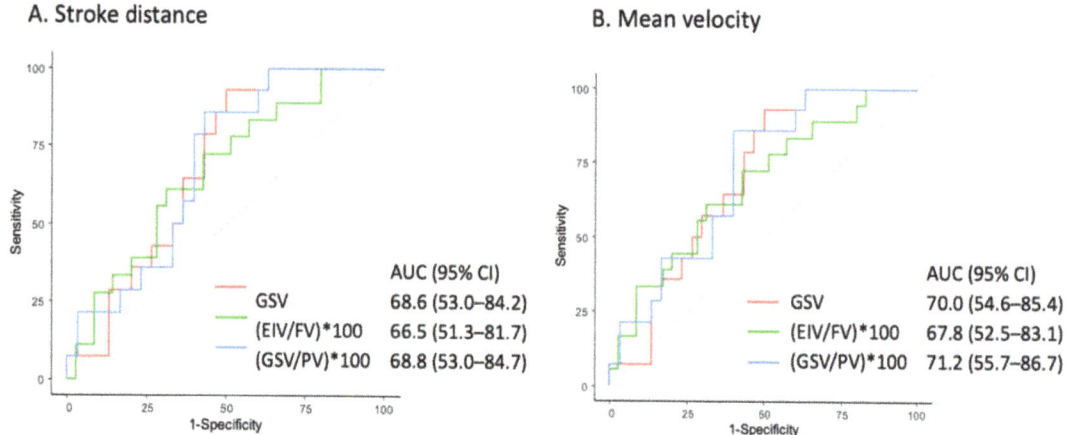

Figure 5. ROC examination of the QFlow parameters of (**A**) stroke distance and (**B**) mean velocity.

4. Discussion

Most patients with suspected venous diseases of the legs undergo air plethysmography (APG) and ultrasound examination (US) at the beginning of therapy. Air plethysmography is a non-invasive tool for quantifying venous reflux and obstruction by measuring volume changes in the leg. US, a rapid tool, could also provide additional information on active reflux and gravitational reflux through standing position by experienced operators. US is operator-dependent and lacking information of pelvic and abdominal areas. However, in many institutions, including ours, the duplex is performed exclusively in ultrasound centers and not done by the same physician in the clinic, which requires additional communication between staff to gain sufficient information.

Intravenous ultrasonography (IVUS) is a new imaging modality for diagnosing deep vein disease and is mostly guiding effective endovascular treatment in iliac and caval venous obstructive lesions [12,13]. However, IVUS is invasive and only provides details of the venous lumen without information of the superficial venous system. Venography was considered as standard for the detection of deep venous thrombosis and other venous occlusive diseases, but venography cannot display the superficial veins outside the drainage course of the contrast-media injection site. CT venography may be useful for the exclusion of pulmonary embolism in patients with signs of deep venous thrombosis in the legs; however, CT venography also requires the injection of contrast media in the morbid limb to achieve optimal venous imaging of the extremities, which can be dangerous for the diseased limb [14]. Magnetic resonance angiography (MRA) techniques for reconstructing vascular structures include time-of-flight (TOF), phase-contrast, and ECG-gated TSE MRA. The major disadvantage of TOF-MRV is that the FOV is small for each image obtained and that it requires considerable time to image the whole lower extremity. MRI with gadolinium-based contrast media is a relatively rapid method for imaging of the lower extremities [15,16]. Although MRI does not involve radiation exposure, the noniodinated contrast agents involved in the process have undesirable effects on the patients. For instance, nephrogenic systemic fibrosis is a dangerous condition caused by exposure to gadolinium-based contrast agents in patients with pre-existing impairment of kidney function and even in patients with normal renal function [17,18]. Phase-contrast MRI (PC-MRI) depends on phase shifts caused by blood flow. Thus, this technique permits the use of coronal or sagittal slice orientations with an FOV along the direction of the vessel of interest and can quantitatively measure the flow dynamics of the region of interest. Most studies have applied PC-MRA for evaluating central nervous system pathology including the hydrocephalus [19,20].

Imaging vascular structures of the whole lower extremity using traditional MRA techniques, such as TOF-MRA and PC-MRA, is time-consuming. The ECG-gated, multistep TSE technique (i.e., TRANCE-MRI) offers the possibility of imaging vascular structures of the whole lower extremity in a relatively short time in clinical settings. For ECG-gating, different imaging times are required for different flow characteristics, and therefore, the image quality can be optimized faster. Most related studies on non-contrast-enhanced MR have used this technique to evaluate arterial diseases [21–25]. Our team has innovated the use of TRANCE-MRI for obtaining more valuable information for the management of complicated lower venous diseases [4–6,11]. Moreover, experienced radiological teams may require an examination time of less than 30 min. Thus, 3D imaging of the morphology of the venous anatomy of the lower extremities, particularly low-flow superficial venous systems, is possible without the use of contrast media or radiation. TRANCE-MRI is not very expensive in our healthcare system (less than 250 USD/each examination) and has become one of the regular survey methods for venous diseases in our institution today (Video S1).

In contrast to a CT angiogram, TRANCE-MRI could be used to perform hemodynamic estimation. In this study, we further analyzed the QFlow data of the segmental leg veins. QFlow analysis through TRANCE-MRI involved the evaluation of SV (mL), FFV (mL), MF (mL), SD (cm), and MV (cm) in the external iliac veins, femoral veins, popliteal veins, and GSVs in the 53 patients with unilateral leg symptoms. Those results revealed that the MV and SD were more sensitive than SV and MF to the differentiation of reflux from non-reflux venous diseases in superficial veins.

QFlow hemodynamic patterns differ between reflux and non-reflux venous diseases mainly in terms of the GSV segment and GSV/PV ratio. In other words, a higher GSV/PV ratio (i.e., GSV/PV > 1 in TRANCE-MRI) is highly correlated to reflux in GSV. The differences were noted in all QFlow parameters, including SV, FFV, MF, SD, and MV. The MF in the GSV segment exhibited a significant ability to discriminate between reflux and non-reflux venous diseases ($p = 0.049$). The SD in the GSV segment and GSV/PV ratio exhibited a significant ability to discriminate between reflux and non-reflux venous diseases ($p = 0.049$ and 0.047, respectively, and cutoff = 86 and 117.1, respectively). The MV in the EIV/FV ratio, GSV segment, and GSV/PV ratio demonstrated a significant ability to discriminate between reflux and non-reflux venous diseases ($p = 0.035, 0.034$, and 0.025, respectively, and cutoff = 100.9, 86.1, and 122.9, respectively). Notably, the non-reflux venous group exhibited a higher EIV/FV ratio for MV. Obstructive venous diseases such as May–Thurner syndrome, external compression, and venous thrombosis account for at least part of the non-reflux venous leg diseases.

Study Limitations

The major limitations of this study are its non-randomized design and small sample size. Second, only patients with typical, unilateral leg disease were included. Third, the TRANCE-MR and US were performed in the supine position, without details of gravitational and muscular interactions. Retrograde flow is possibly not provoked during the TRANCE-MR examination and could be better reproduced by US in a standing position. However, this is the largest series to discuss the use of TRANCE-MRI as an imaging tool for venous diseases of the lower extremities. In addition to proving the morphological advantage and safety of TRANCE-MRI, this study is the first attempt to analyze QFlow in the clinical scenarios of the superficial venous reflux of the lower extremities.

5. Conclusions

TRANCE-MRI is a potential tool for verifying the characteristic ultrasound features of reflux venous diseases in the lower extremities. A higher GSV/PV ratio could be a hallmark in the QFlow study of reflux venous diseases in the legs through TRANCE-MRI.

6. Patents

This project is under the reviewing process in the Taiwan Intellectual property Office (No 109126307).

Supplementary Materials: The following are available online at https://www.mdpi.com/article/10.3390/jpm11040242/s1, Video S1: TRANCE-MRI for venous system in brief.

Author Contributions: Conception and design: Y.-K.H., C.-W.C.; Analysis and interpretation: Y.-H.T., Y.-K.H., C.-W.C., M.Y.W., H.T.; Data collection: C.-W.C., Y.-H.T., B.-S.L., T.-Y.Y.; Writing the article: Y.-K.H.; Statistical analysis: C.-W.C., M.Y.W.; Overall responsibility: Y.-K.H. and C.-W.C. All authors have read and agreed to the published version of the manuscript.

Funding: This study was supported by Chang Gung Memorial Hospital (Contract Nos. CORPG6G0009, CORPG6G0092, CORPG6D0292).

Institutional Review Board Statement: The study was conducted according to the guidelines of the Declaration of Helsinki, and approved by the Institutional Review Board of Chang Gung Memorial Hospital (IRB number: 202001570B0).

Informed Consent Statement: Informed consent was obtained from all subjects involved in the study.

Data Availability Statement: The data presented in this study are available on request from the corresponding author. The data are not publicly available due to ethical restrictions.

Acknowledgments: We acknowledge Raising Statistics Consultant Inc. for statistical analysis.

Conflicts of Interest: The authors declare no conflict of interest.

Abbreviations

3D	three-dimensional
CT	computed tomography
CTA	computed tomography angiography
DVT	deep venous thrombosis
EIV	external iliac vein
FFV	forward flow volume
FOV	field of view
FV	femoral vein
GSV	great saphenous vein
IR	inversion recovery
IRB	institutional review board
MF	mean flux
MRI	magnetic resonance imaging
MRV	magnetic resonance venography
MV	mean velocity
NSF	nephrogenic systemic fibrosis
PV	popliteal vein
ROC	receiver operating characteristic
SD	stroke distance
STIR	short tau inversion recovery
SV	stroke volume
TE	echo time
TOF	time-of-flight
TR	repetition time
TRANCE-MRI	triggered angiography non-contrast-enhanced MRI
TSE	turbo spin-echo
US	ultrasonography

References

1. Tassiopoulos, A.K.; Golts, E.; Oh, D.S.; Labropoulos, N. Current concepts in chronic venous ulceration. *Eur. J. Vasc. Endovasc. Surg.* **2000**, *20*, 227–232. [CrossRef]
2. Schleimer, K.; Barbati, M.E.; Grommes, J.; Hoeft, K.; Toonder, I.M.; Wittens, C.H.A.; Jalaie, H. Update on diagnosis and treatment strategies in patients with post-thrombotic syndrome due to chronic venous obstruction and role of endovenous recanalization. *J. Vasc. Surg. Venous Lymphat. Disord.* **2019**, *7*, 592–600. [CrossRef]
3. Bonkemeyer Millan, S.; Gan, R.; Townsend, P.E. Venous Ulcers: Diagnosis and Treatment. *Am. Fam. Physician* **2019**, *100*, 298–305.
4. Lin, B.S.; Chen, C.W.; Zhou, S.K.; Tseng, Y.H.; Wang, S.C.; Huang, Y.K. Evaluation of static ulcer on lower extremities using wireless wearable near-infrared spectroscopy device: Effect of deep venous thrombosis on TRiggered Angiography Non-Contrast-Enhanced sequence magnetic resonance imaging. *Phlebology* **2020**, 268355520935739. [CrossRef] [PubMed]
5. Kao, C.C.; Chen, C.W.; Tseng, Y.H.; Tsai, Y.H.; Wang, S.C.; Huang, Y.K. Non-contrast-enhanced magnetic resonance imaging: Objective figures in differentiation between acute and chronic deep venous thrombosis in the lower extremities. *Phlebology* **2020**, 268355520939375. [CrossRef] [PubMed]
6. Chen, C.W.; Tseng, Y.H.; Lin, C.C.; Kao, C.C.; Wong, M.Y.; Lin, B.S.; Huang, Y.K. Novel Diagnostic Options without Contrast Media or Radiation: Triggered Angiography Non-Contrast-Enhanced Sequence Magnetic Resonance Imaging in Treating Different Leg Venous Diseases. *Diagnostics* **2020**, *10*, 355. [CrossRef] [PubMed]
7. Coleridge-Smith, P.; Labropoulos, N.; Partsch, H.; Myers, K.; Nicolaides, A.; Cavezzi, A. Duplex ultrasound investigation of the veins in chronic venous disease of the lower limbs–UIP consensus document. Part I. Basic principles. *Eur. J. Vasc. Endovasc. Surg.* **2006**, *31*, 83–92. [CrossRef] [PubMed]
8. Marsden, G.; Perry, M.; Kelley, K.; Davies, A.H.; Guideline Development, G. Diagnosis and management of varicose veins in the legs: Summary of NICE guidance. *BMJ* **2013**, *347*, f4279. [CrossRef] [PubMed]
9. Asciutto, G.; Mumme, A.; Marpe, B.; Koster, O.; Asciutto, K.C.; Geier, B. MR venography in the detection of pelvic venous congestion. *Eur. J. Vasc. Endovasc. Surg.* **2008**, *36*, 491–496. [CrossRef] [PubMed]
10. Lee, Y.L.; Huang, Y.K.; Hsu, L.S.; Chen, P.Y.; Chen, C.W. The use of non-contrast-enhanced MRI to evaluate serial changes in endoleaks after aortic stenting: A case report. *BMC Med. Imaging* **2019**, *19*, 82. [CrossRef]
11. Huang, Y.K.; Tseng, Y.H.; Lin, C.H.; Tsai, Y.H.; Hsu, Y.C.; Wang, S.C.; Chen, C.W. Evaluation of venous pathology of the lower extremities with triggered angiography non-contrast-enhanced magnetic resonance imaging. *BMC Med. Imaging* **2019**, *19*, 96. [CrossRef]
12. Rossi, F.H.; Kambara, A.M.; Rodrigues, T.O.; Rossi, C.B.O.; Izukawa, N.M.; Pinto, I.M.F.; Thorpe, P.E. Comparison of computed tomography venography and intravascular ultrasound in screening and classification of iliac vein obstruction in patients with chronic venous disease. *J. Vasc. Surg. Venous Lymphat. Disord.* **2020**, *8*, 413–422. [CrossRef] [PubMed]
13. Montminy, M.L.; Thomasson, J.D.; Tanaka, G.J.; Lamanilao, L.M.; Crim, W.; Raju, S. A comparison between intravascular ultrasound and venography in identifying key parameters essential for iliac vein stenting. *J. Vasc. Surg. Venous Lymphat. Disord.* **2019**, *7*, 801–807. [CrossRef]
14. Goodman, L.R. Venous thromboembolic disease: CT evaluation. *Q. J. Nucl. Med.* **2001**, *45*, 302–310.
15. Gurel, K.; Gurel, S.; Karavas, E.; Buharalioglu, Y.; Daglar, B. Direct contrast-enhanced MR venography in the diagnosis of May-Thurner syndrome. *Eur. J. Radiol.* **2011**, *80*, 533–536. [CrossRef] [PubMed]
16. Ruehm, S.G.; Zimny, K.; Debatin, J.F. Direct contrast-enhanced 3D MR venography. *Eur. Radiol.* **2001**, *11*, 102–112. [CrossRef]
17. Alfano, G.; Fontana, F.; Ferrari, A.; Solazzo, A.; Perrone, R.; Giaroni, F.; Torricelli, P.; Cappelli, G. Incidence of nephrogenic systemic fibrosis after administration of gadoteric acid in patients on renal replacement treatment. *Magn. Reson. Imaging* **2020**, *70*, 1–4. [CrossRef] [PubMed]
18. Schieda, N.; Maralani, P.J.; Hurrell, C.; Tsampalieros, A.K.; Hiremath, S. Updated Clinical Practice Guideline on Use of Gadolinium-Based Contrast Agents in Kidney Disease Issued by the Canadian Association of Radiologists. *Can. Assoc. Radiol. J.* **2019**, *70*, 226–232. [CrossRef]
19. Ross, M.R.; Pelc, N.J.; Enzmann, D.R. Qualitative phase contrast MRA in the normal and abnormal circle of Willis. *AJNR Am. J. Neuroradiol.* **1993**, *14*, 19–25.
20. Forner Giner, J.; Sanz-Requena, R.; Florez, N.; Alberich-Bayarri, A.; Garcia-Marti, G.; Ponz, A.; Marti-Bonmati, L. Quantitative phase-contrast MRI study of cerebrospinal fluid flow: A method for identifying patients with normal-pressure hydrocephalus. *Neurologia* **2014**, *29*, 68–75. [CrossRef]
21. Gutzeit, A.; Sutter, R.; Froehlich, J.M.; Roos, J.E.; Sautter, T.; Schoch, E.; Giger, B.; Wyss, M.; Graf, N.; von Weymarn, C.; et al. ECG-triggered non-contrast-enhanced MR angiography (TRANCE) versus digital subtraction angiography (DSA) in patients with peripheral arterial occlusive disease of the lower extremities. *Eur. Radiol.* **2011**, *21*, 1979–1987. [CrossRef]
22. Suttmeyer, B.; Teichgraber, U.; Rathke, H.; Albrecht, L.; Guttler, F.; Schnackenburg, B.; Hamm, B.; de Bucourt, M. Initial experience with imaging of the lower extremity arteries in an open 1.0 Tesla MRI system using the triggered angiography non-contrast-enhanced sequence (TRANCE) compared to digital subtraction angiography (DSA). *Biomed. Tech.* **2016**, *61*, 383–392. [CrossRef] [PubMed]

23. Radlbauer, R.; Salomonowitz, E.; van der Riet, W.; Stadlbauer, A. Triggered non-contrast enhanced MR angiography of peripheral arteries: Optimization of systolic and diastolic time delays for electrocardiographic triggering. *Eur. J. Radiol.* **2011**, *80*, 331–335. [CrossRef] [PubMed]
24. Ohno, N.; Miyati, T.; Noda, T.; Alperin, N.; Hamaguchi, T.; Ohno, M.; Matsushita, T.; Mase, M.; Gabata, T.; Kobayashi, S. Fast Phase-Contrast Cine MRI for Assessing Intracranial Hemodynamics and Cerebrospinal Fluid Dynamics. *Diagnostics* **2020**, *10*, 241. [CrossRef]
25. Altaha, M.A.; Jaskolka, J.D.; Tan, K.; Rick, M.; Schmitt, P.; Menezes, R.J.; Wintersperger, B.J. Non-contrast-enhanced MR angiography in critical limb ischemia: Performance of quiescent-interval single-shot (QISS) and TSE-based subtraction techniques. *Eur. Radiol.* **2017**, *27*, 1218–1226. [CrossRef] [PubMed]

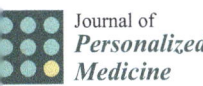

Article

Scoring Osteoarthritis Reliably in Large Joints and the Spine Using Whole-Body CT: OsteoArthritis Computed Tomography-Score (OACT-Score)

Willem Paul Gielis [1,2,*], Harrie Weinans [1], Frank J. Nap [3], Frank W. Roemer [4,5] and Wouter Foppen [2]

1. Department of Orthopaedics, University Medical Center Utrecht, Utrecht University, 3584 CX Utrecht, The Netherlands; h.h.weinans@umcutrecht.nl
2. Department of Radiology, University Medical Center Utrecht, Utrecht University, 3584 CX Utrecht, The Netherlands; W.Foppen@umcutrecht.nl
3. Department of Radiology, Central Military Hospital (CMH) Utrecht, 3584 CX Utrecht, The Netherlands; F.J.Nap-3@umcutrecht.nl
4. Department of Radiology, Friedrich-Alexander University Erlangen-Nürnberg & Universitätsklinikum Erlangen, 91054 Erlangen, Germany; Frank.Roemer@uk-erlangen.de
5. Department of Radiology, Boston University School of Medicine, Boston, MA 02118, USA
* Correspondence: w.p.gielis@umcutrecht.nl; Tel.: +31-88-755-9025

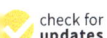

Citation: Gielis, W.P.; Weinans, H.; Nap, F.J.; Roemer, F.W.; Foppen, W. Scoring Osteoarthritis Reliably in Large Joints and the Spine Using Whole-Body CT: OsteoArthritis Computed Tomography-Score (OACT-Score). *J. Pers. Med.* **2021**, *11*, 5. https://dx.doi.org/10.3390/jpm11010005

Received: 26 October 2020
Accepted: 18 December 2020
Published: 22 December 2020

Publisher's Note: MDPI stays neutral with regard to jurisdictional claims in published maps and institutional affiliations.

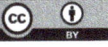

Copyright: © 2020 by the authors. Licensee MDPI, Basel, Switzerland. This article is an open access article distributed under the terms and conditions of the Creative Commons Attribution (CC BY) license (https://creativecommons.org/licenses/by/4.0/).

Abstract: A standardized method to assess structural osteoarthritis (OA) burden thorough the body lacks from literature. Such a method can be valuable in developing personalized treatments for OA. We developed a reliable scoring system to evaluate OA in large joints and the spine—the OsteoArthritis Computed Tomography (OACT) score, using a convenience sample of 197 whole-body low-dose non-contrast CTs. An atlas, containing example images as reference points for training and scoring, are presented. Each joint was graded between 0–3. The total OA burden was calculated by summing scores of individual joints. Intra- and inter-observer reliability was tested 25 randomly selected scans (N = 600 joints). Intra-observer reliability and inter-observer reliability between three observers was assessed using intraclass correlation coefficient (ICC) and square-weighted kappa statistics. The square-weighted kappa for intra-observer reliability for OACT-score at joint-level ranged from 0.79 to 0.95; the ICC for the total OA grade was 0.97 (95%-CI, 0.94 to 0.99). Square-weighted kappa for interobserver reliability ranged from 0.48 to 0.95; the ICC for the total OA grade was 0.95 (95%-CI, 0.90 to 0.98). The OACT score, a new reproducible CT-based grading system reflecting OA burden in large joints and the spine, has a satisfactory reproducibility. The atlas can be used for research purposes, training, educational purposes and systemic grading of OA on CT-scans.

Keywords: computed tomography; image analysis; osteoarthritis; reliability

1. Introduction

Osteoarthritis (OA) is a leading cause of disability worldwide, with the estimated socioeconomic burden being 1%–2.5% of the gross national product in Western countries [1]. Until now, the search for a disease modifying drug for OA has failed. A key factor for this failure is the use of a one-size-fits-all principle in the development and testing of potential treatments. End-stage osteoarthritis is a fairly uniform disease, but etiological pathways in early disease vary strongly. There is a desire to group OA patients into phenotypes, with the ultimate aim of finding the right treatment for the right patient [2]. The APPROACH study aims to describe these different phenotypes for knee OA and validate models to predict disease progression within these phenotypes [3]. This allows for more patient specific treatments and more efficient clinical trials. The APPROACH study includes knee specific parameters, including patient reported outcome measures (e.g., knee specific questionnaires), physical examination (e.g., knee range of motion), and imaging features (e.g., knee MRI). Additionally, more generic parameters are measured, such as general quality of life, physical performance (e.g., 40 m fast paced walk test) and biochemical marker levels in serum and urine. OA is often a polyarticular disease and the relationship between the latter parameters and knee OA will be heavily influenced by the overall OA burden in the body. However, there is no efficient and standardized method to assess this burden [4,5].

Radiography is widely used for visualizing and grading structural OA. However, it has limited sensitivity for detecting structural damage because of its projectile nature; repeatability is an also issue as positioning errors are common (e.g., wide variations in joint space measurements due to inconsistent flexion of the knee) [6]. Magnetic resonance imaging (MRI) is excellent for visualizing the different tissues within a joint, but it is expensive and time consuming; for example, to obtain good-quality MRI images of multiple joints, the patient would need to lie still for hours. However, CT has several advantages. It uses ionizing radiation to produce a three-dimensional (3D) tomographic images, without the projection limitations of radiography, and is known for its excellent visualization of bone. Advances, such as iterative reconstruction have substantially reduced exposure to ionizing radiation and scanning time [7,8]. Low-dose CT scans provide valuable information on the bony aspects of the joints, with a relatively high signal-to-noise ratio. Whole-body Low-dose CT (WBLDCT) scans, with a scan time of less than one minute and an effective radiation dose <3 mSv for a 70 kg adult male, are increasingly used for evaluation various conditions.

In this study, we aim to develop and describe a WBLDCT-based scoring system to quantify OA burden throughout the body. We believe that the score—the OsteoArthritis Computed Tomography (OACT) score—will be especially useful for research towards personalized OA treatments. We assess the inter- and intra-reader agreement of the new score and present an atlas, with extensive image examples, that can be used for training and educational purposes, for uniform grading of OA on CT-scans.

2. Materials and Methods

2.1. Study Sample and Image Acquisition

The scoring system was developed using a convenience sample of 197 WBLDCTs acquired for diagnosis or for attenuation correction in PET/CTs in the UMC Utrecht, Utrecht, The Netherlands, between June 2011 and November 2015; the scanning was performed as part of workup for suspected cancer and vascular or infectious disease. Scans were acquired in the supine position without any contrast enhancement, with 64×0.625-mm collimation, 120 kV, and dose modulation with a reference of 40 mAs; the estimated effective dose was <3.0 mSv for a 70-kg adult male. Reconstructions in the axial plane were made with 1-mm slices and 0.7-mm increments. Joints with metallic implants were excluded. This study was approved by the local institutional review board (protocol number 15/446-C), with waiver of the need for informed consent.

2.2. Image Assessment

The Picture Archiving and Communication System (PACS IDS7 19.3.12; SECTRA) was used to produce multiplanar view reconstructions. Using the 197 scans we created a feasible and reproducible system for grading the severity of OA in each of the major joints. Then, a reference atlas was composed that could be used to teach new readers the scoring definitions. Finally, we tested intra- and inter-observer reproducibility on a subset of 25 randomly selected scans (which included a total of 600 joints).

We aimed to grade all large synovial diarthrodial joints, intervertebral discs (IVD), and facet joints. The elbow was frequently positioned outside the field of view and was therefore excluded. Degenerative disc disease (DDD) of the IVD differs from OA, as IVDs are fibrocartilaginous and not synovial joints. However, the biochemical and radiological features of DDD closely resemble those of OA [4]. Many previous OA studies have assessed the lumbar spine but, as other researchers have suggested, DDD in the cervical and thoracic spine also needs to be considered [9,10]. We first performed a thorough literature search to locate CT-based scoring systems for OA of different joints. If no viable CT-based scoring system was found, we modified the standard radiography–based scores for use on CT images. If no viable scoring system was available for a joint, we developed a new system using the classic radiographic OA characteristics (joint space narrowing, osteophytosis, sclerosis, and subchondral cysts). Each joint was graded on a scale of 0 to 3; thus, four grades were possible. The goal was to develop a scoring system that could be used to score all joints in a single patient within 15 min. The process of development of the scoring system for each joint is described below. The scoring of each joint was discussed in multiple sessions between a group consisting of a MD researcher with 5 years of experiences in medical imaging of OA (WPG), a radiologist in training with a subspecialization in musculoskeletal radiology (WF), and a fellowship-trained musculoskeletal radiologist with 6 years of experience (FJN) and an associate professor, section chief of Musculo-Skeletal Research and attending Radiologist with extensive experience in developing radiologic scores (FWR) The supplementary atlas (Supplementary Materials), which contains extensive examples, can be used for training and also serves as a reference for scoring. Figure 1 presents an overview of the tibiofemoral joint, and Figure 2 shows different grades of tibiofemoral OA.

2.2.1. Upper Extremity
Acromioclavicular Joint

Our literature search located a single grading system for acromioclavicular joint degeneration [11]. Using 108 cadaveric joints, Stenlund et al. created a radiographic score that demonstrated satisfactory correlation with macroscopic morphological grade. However, this system was not tested for reproducibility. We used the radiographic characteristics identified by Sterlund et al. to create four grades (Table 1).

Glenohumeral Joint

We did not find a validated CT-based grading system for glenohumeral OA. Therefore, we based our score on the widely used and reliable system proposed by Samilson and Prieto that scores OA according to the size of inferior humeral osteophytes on radiographs (Table 1) [12,13]. As CT images offer 3D visualization of the joint, we considered osteophytes everywhere in the glenohumeral joint, i.e., inferior, anterior, and posterior humeral and glenoidal.

2.2.2. Spine
Degenerative Disc Disease

The system proposed by Lane et al. for grading degenerative disease of the thoracic and lumbar spine is convenient and reliable [14,15]. We modified it for use on CT images of the cervical, thoracic, and lumbar spine (Table 1). In addition to sclerosis, we considered endplate irregularity, which can be evaluated on CT, as a sign of disease involvement of cartilaginous and bony endplates. Extensive grading 21 spinal levels would be too time consuming, thus, a concise screening of the spine is performed to identify the two most affected levels within the cervical, thoracic, and lumbar regions. For these levels the extensive grading is performed. If these scores are low, this means that degenerative changes in the whole spinal region and therefore we expect limited impact on on systemic biomarker levels and quality of life measurements.

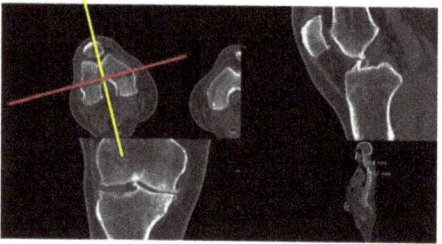

Figure 1. An example from the atlas showing the overview for scoring tibiofemoral osteoarthritis.

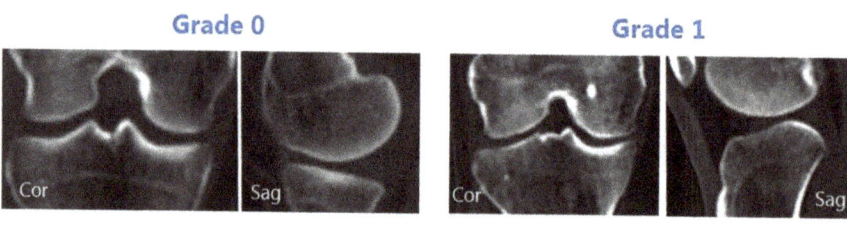

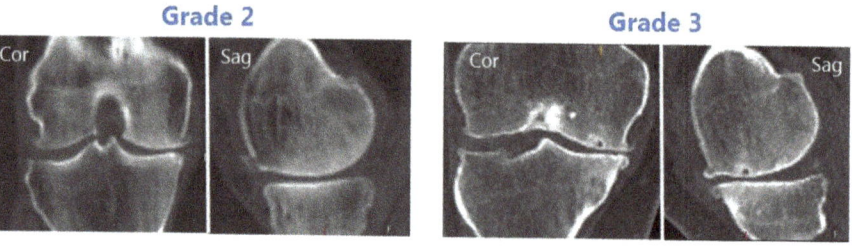

Figure 2. Example images from the atlas showing different grades of tibiofemoral osteoarthritis.

Table 1. Definition of OACT scores for individual joints.

	Acromioclavicular joint
0	No osteophytes or joint space narrowing (JSN)
1	Lipping and/or possible JSN
2	Definite osteophytes and/or JSN
3	Definite osteophytes and/or JSN and sclerosis and/or cysts and/or bony deformities
	Glenohumeral joint
0	No osteophytes or definite JSN
1	Osteophyte measured less than 3 mm
2	Osteophyte measured between 3 and 7 mm, slight joint irregularity
3	Osteophyte measured more than 7 mm, definite JSN and/or irregularity.
	Degenerative disc disease
0	Score 0–2 (Based on disc space narrowing, osteophytes, end plate regularity and sclerosis)
1	Score 3–5
2	Score 6–8
3	Score 9–10
	Facet joint
0	Normal facet joint space width (JSW) (2–4 mm)
1	Narrowing of facet JSW (<2 mm) and small osteophytes and/or mild hypertrophy of the articular process
2	Narrowing of facet JSW (<2 mm) and moderate osteophytes and/or moderate hypertrophy of the articular process and/or mild subarticulare bone erosions
3	Narrowing of facet JSW (<2 mm) and large osteophytes and/or severe hypertrophy of the articular process and/or severe subarticulare bone erosions and/or subchondral cysts
	Hip joint
0	Score 0–1 (Based on joint space narrowing, osteophytes, and cysts)
1	Score 2–3
2	Score 4–5
3	Score 6–7
	Tibiofemoral joint
0	Score 0–1 (Based on joint space narrowing, osteophytes, and cysts)
1	Score 2–3
2	Score 4–5
3	Score 6–7
	Patellofemoral joint
0	No osteophytes, joint space narrowing (JSN)/sclerosis
1	Small osteophyte/lipping and mild JSN, but no defined sclerosis
2	Moderate osteophytes, moderate JSN and possible sclerosis
3	Large osteophytes, (near) boney contact and defined sclerosis
	Ankle joint
0	No clinical evidence of OA; joint space integrity fully intact
1	Mild; osteophyte formation/lipping, possible joint space narrowing
2	Moderate; joint space narrowing evident, obvious osteophyte formation and some sclerosis/cystic changes
3	Severe; near absence of joint space, severe osteophyte/cyst formation, deformity of bone

All subscores are presented in the atlas.

Facet Joint OA

We incorporated the grading system created by Weishaupt et al. for the lumbar facet joint OA (an adaption of the original scoring system proposed by Pathria et al.) in our score, extending its application to the cervical and thoracic spine also [16,17].

We recommend the sagittal view for an easier, faster and more reproducible evaluation Only the two most affected levels within each region are extensively graded (Table 1).

2.2.3. Lower Extremity

Hip

Turmezei et al. published a CT grading system for hip OA [18]. This system is highly detailed and time-consuming. In our experience, it takes about 5–10 min for an experienced reader to score 2 hips. The learning curve was long for new readers. We did not find any other grading systems for hip OA on CT and modified the score of Turmezei et al. it to obtain a more straightforward four-grade score based on their principles (Table 1).

Knee—Tibiofemoral

We found no validated CT-based grading system for knee OA. A combination of characteristics of radiographic OA as described by Kellgren and Lawrence and, more recently, by Altman et al. (joint space narrowing, osteophytosis, and subchondral cysts) was used to create the four-grade score (Table 1) [19,20].

Knee—Patellofemoral

Scoring of patellofemoral joint OA was based on the grades described by Jones et al. [21] CT is acquired with extended knees, causing the patella to be located proximal to the femoral notch; in this position, it is difficult to accurately measure joint space narrowing. Therefore, we opted for a combined score that considered osteophytosis, sclerosis, and diminishment of the joint space (Table 1).

Ankle

The CT scoring system and atlas as published by Cohen et al. was used for grading ankle OA (Table 1) [22].

2.2.4. Total OA Grade

To test the eliability of a total score for OA in the large joints and the spine, a total OA score was calculated by summing the scores of the individual joints. Therefore, with each joint scored on a scale of 0–3, the total score could range from 0 to 72. (Table 1).

2.3. Testing Reproducibility

To test intra-observer reproducibility, a medical doctor and researcher with 4 years of experience (WPG) scored the same subset of 25 randomly selected WBLDCTs twice, with an interval of at least 1 week in between. To test inter-observer reproducibility, a radiologist in training, with a subspecialization in musculoskeletal radiology (WF) and a fellowship-trained musculoskeletal radiologist with 6 years of experience (FJN), scored the same random sample of 25 scans independently. The atlas was used as reference for the grading system. In accordance with the Guidelines for Reporting Reliability and Agreement Studies, reliability was tested using Cohen's kappa for binominal grade, squared weighted kappa for ordinal grade, and two-way intraclass correlation coefficient (ICC) for consistency for the total OA score [23,24]. Kappa values were interpreted according to Landis and Koch: i.e., 0–0.20 slight agreement; 0.21–0.40 fair agreement; 0.41–0.60 moderate agreement; 0.61–0.80 substantial agreement; 0.81–1 almost perfect agreement [25]. Agreement was tested using absolute agreement percentages for binominal and ordinal grades and Bland–Altman and Jones plots for continuous values [26,27]. All analyses were carried out in R version 3.4.4 (https://cran.r-project.org/) using the irr package, version 0.84.

3. Results

The 197 scans used for the development of the atlas were acquired from a sample comprising 43% males (85/197). The mean age (SD) of the patients was 54 (±15) years. Indications for scanning included vasculitis ($n = 106$), suspected infection ($n = 57$), and suspected malignancy ($n = 34$). The 25 scans included in the reliability analyses were from a patient subset that comprised 44% males (11/25). The mean age (SD) of the patients was 54 (±17) years. Indications for scanning were vasculitis ($n = 15$), suspected infection ($n = 8$), and suspected malignancy ($n = 2$). Within the test set, OA grades 0 to 3 were found in all joints, except for the hip and ankle, where only grades 0 to 2 were found (Table 2). Most joints were graded as having no OA or only mild OA, which is to be expected in a random sample of hospital. One ankle could not be scored due to beam-hardening artifacts caused by screws.

Table 2. Frequency of grades per joint ($n = 25$ patients).

Joint	0 (No)		1 (Mild)		2 (Moderate)		3 (Severe)	
Acromioclavicular, N(%)	24	(48)	10	(20)	5	(10)	11	(22)
Glenohumeral, N(%)	37	(74)	7	(14)	3	(6)	3	(6)
Intervertebral Disc, N(%)	48	(32)	47	(31)	33	(22)	22	(15)
Facet, N(%)	91	(61)	37	(25)	7	(5)	15	(10)
Hip, N(%)	33	(66)	13	(26)	4	(8)	0	(0)
Knee, N(%)	25	(50)	13	(26)	8	(16)	4	(8)
Patellofemoral, N(%)	25	(50)	15	(30)	5	(10)	5	(10)
Ankle[1], N(%)	26	(54)	19	(38)	4	(8)	0	(0)

[1] One ankle was not scored due to artefacts caused by screws; Scores presented are produced in the first scoring round by WPG.

3.1. Intra- and Interobserver Reliability for Total OA Grade

Intra-observer reliability for total OA grade was excellent, with an ICC of 0.97 (95% CI, 0.93 to 0.99). The Bland–Altman plot showed an even spread of errors between the first and second observation, with a mean error of −3.5 (SD, 3.4). Inter-observer reliability for total OA grade was also excellent, with an ICC of 0.94 (95% CI, 0.86 to 0.98). ICCs for inter-observer reliability were comparable between observer pairs of different proficiency levels, 0.95 between WPG and WF, 0.93 between WPG and FJN, and 0.97 between WF and FJN. The Jones plot showed an even spread of errors between all observers, with WF giving grades around the mean, FJN giving lower grades on average, and WPG giving higher grades on average (Figure 3).

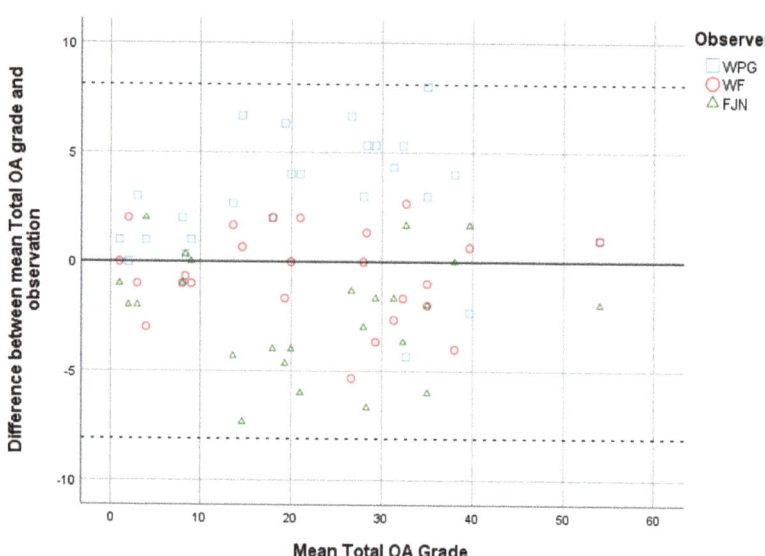

Figure 3. Jones plot depicting the difference between each observation of the different readers and the mean observed score for the total OA grade. The interrupted lines show the 95% limits of agreement.

3.2. Intra- and Interobserver Reliability for OACT Scores for Individual Joints

Intra-observer reliability of the OA grades for individual joints was substantial to almost perfect, with the kappa values ranging from 0.79 to 0.95 and absolute percentage agreement, ranging from 67% to 92% (Table 3). Inter-observer reliability of the OA grades for individual joints was moderate to almost perfect, with the kappa values ranging from 0.48 to 0.95 and absolute percentage agreement ranging from 36% to 90% (Table 3). Table A1 shows the intra- and inter-observer reliability for grading of individual OA characteristics (joint space narrowing, osteophytosis, and so on).

Table 3. Intra- and interobserver reliability as weighted kappa (percentage of absolute agreement) for OACT scores for individual joints.

Joints	Reader 1 (intra)	Reader 1 vs. Reader 2	Reader 1 vs. Reader 3	Reader 2 vs. Reader 3
Acromioclavicular	0.84 (80)	0.87 (74)	0.75 (62)	0.82 (68)
Glenohumeral	0.95 (92)	0.69 (72)	0.58 (38)	0.50 (48)
Intervertebral Disc	0.85 (67)	0.80 (61)	0.80 (68)	0.77 (53)
Facet	0.90 (85)	0.68 (64)	0.66 (57)	0.66 (57)
Hip	0.85 (88)	0.53 (68)	0.65 (64)	0.48 (64)
Knee	0.84 (72)	0.85 (68)	0.73 (50)	0.64 (36)
Patellofemoral	0.94 (88)	0.95 (90)	0.79 (60)	0.78 (64)
Ankle	0.79 (84)	0.74 (80)	0.56 (65)	0.49 (63)

Reader 1: Medical doctor and researcher; Reader 2: Radiologist in training with a subspecialization in musculoskeletal radiology; Reader 3: Fellowship-trained musculoskeletal radiologist with five years of experience.

4. Discussion

The OACT score described here—a new reproducible WBLDCT-based grading system for OA in large joints and the spine—was developed for research purposes. In this first step, we introduce the scoring methods and present a reference atlas with multiple example images. The atlas can be used as a reference for training new readers, educational purposes and systemic grading of OA on CT-scans. We demonstrated a satisfactory intra-observer reliability and decent inter-observer reliability. The use of WBLDCT for this goal is associated with short scanning time with comparatively low-level exposure to ionizing radiation (effective radiation dose <3 mSv for a 70-kg adult male). Furthermore, with this newly developed grading system, it is possible to reliably assess overall structural burden of OA in a patient within 15 min.

There is still no disease modifying drug for OA, mainly because drug development focused on finding a one-size-fits-all drug. Drug development and evaluation will have a higher chance of success if it is focused on specific structural phenotypes of OA. The selection criteria for these OA phenotypes has to be determined. The APPROACH study uses a combination of established and novel biomarkers to develop stratification models that can help select the appropriate therapy for each knee OA patient [3]. Many parameters, such as quality of life, physical performance and biochemical markers levels in serum or urine are affected by the disease burden of other joints [4,28–31]. These parameters potentially impact the efficacy of drug development and evaluation in OA. In the APPROACH study, the OACT score helps to phenotype OA patients and correct for confounding at the patient level when assessing the relation between systemic biomarkers, and e.g., knee OA. Besides structural progression, disease burden is an important marker for treatment success. Eventually the OACT-score will help improve patient selection for OA observational studies and clinical trials that include clinical outcome parameters. The clinical relevance needs to be established before clinical application may be considered. This has been the case for many other scoring-based assessment instrument in the field of OA that were primarily developed in the context of MRI evaluation [32,33]. Future studies should test the validity of the OACT-score against clinical outcome parameters and other biomarkers.

In our sample the total OACT score showed excellent intra- and inter-observer reliability (ICC, 0.97, and 0.94, respectively). To our knowledge, this is the first study test to reliability for an OA grade at patient level. However, we would like to stress that summing separate ordinal grades has limitations; for example, this would result in multiple low-grade joints being equivalent to a single high-grade joint. For future studies, the weighting factors for composing a total score, reflecting OA throughout the body, should be altered to the goal of the specific study. Systemic cartilage degradation markers or global quality of life measurements could be used to assess the influences of the different joints on the total OA burden in future studies. Adding the OA scores of the joints of the hands and feet would undoubtedly improve the value of the scoring system; however, we did not do so because of the variable positioning of the hands and feet in the CT images in our study. Validated radiographic scores for OA of the hands and feet could be used in combination with the OACT score for a more complete assessment of total OA burden in the body [34].

The reliability results are in the expected range for a semi-quantitative radiological score for OA. For the acromioclavicular joint, we found substantial to almost perfect reliability. No other CT-based study is available for comparison. For the glenohumeral joint, inter-observer reliability was moderate to substantial, while the intra-observer reliability was almost perfect. We expect the moderate intra-observer reliability to be caused by the high prevalence of no and mild glenohumeral OA, as this emphasizes the decision between the presence of no, or a small (<3 mm) osteophyte. Again, no CT-based studies are available for comparison. We found almost perfect intra-observer reliability and substantial to almost perfect inter-observer reliability for DDD. No CT-based studies are available for comparison. While, OA and DDD are different entities, the response to mechanical loading, symptoms and matrix degradation pattern are highly correlated [35]. Therefore, we chose to include DDD in our score. Based on the aim of their study, researcher may decide to in- or exclude DDD.

Pathria et al. tested the inter-observer reliability of their CT-based scoring system for facet joint OA and reported a kappa value of 0.46, while Weishaupt et al. reported a weighted kappa of 0.60 [16,17]; the overall percentage agreement was 63%, and 51%, respectively. These results were comparable to our results, where the weighted kappa values ranged from 0.66 to 0.68 and absolute percentage agreement ranged from 57% to 64%.

Turmezei et al. tested the reliability of their CT grading system for hip OA and reported a weighted kappa of 0.74 and 0.75 for intra- and inter-observer reliability, respectively. We simplified their scoring system to enhance grading speed and reliability for new readers and found a weighted kappa of 0.85 for intra-observer reliability and between 0.48 and 0.65 for inter-observer reliability. The lower inter-observer reliability in our study may be due to the very low prevalence of hip OA in our study population (8% with moderate OA or higher) compared to the study population of Turmezei et al., which was selected to include the full spectrum of hip OA.

For both patella and knee OA, we found almost perfect intra-observer reliability and substantial to almost perfect inter-observer reliability. For the ankle joint, we found moderate to substantial inter-observer agreement. Cohen et al. introduced an atlas for grading ankle osteoarthritis on CT and reported an ICC of 0.851 and unweighted kappa of 0.582 in a population of specifically selected scans. As such, a valid comparison with our results is not possible.

Our scoring system has several limitations. First, it does not consider OA in the elbows, hands, and feet. The elbow was not included in our score as it was positioned outside the field of view in a large number of scans. However, it should be noted that elbow OA is rare, with a prevalence of only ~2% [36]. Second, we used semi-quantitative grades. However, it must be noted that semi-quantitative grading enabled scoring a full WBLDCT in 15 min. Third, WBLDCT is obtained with the patient lying supine; assessment of joint space is influenced by the lack of weight bearing. The development of weight-bearing CT-scan will hopefully counter this problem in the near future. Fourth, WBLDCT can clearly visualize bony changes, but soft tissue degeneration (e.g., meniscal and capsule tears) will be missed. Fifth, concurrent pathology such as diffuse idiopathic skeletal hyperostosis may aggravate OA scores. Grading systems for such concurrent diseases could be used along with the OA scores to further characterize individuals [37–39]. Sixth, CT involves exposure to possibly harmful ionizing radiation. Due to technical advances, including iterative reconstruction, the effective radiation dose of the WBLDCT was around ≤ 3 mSv, which approximates one year of background radiation [40]. The exact risk for excess death by cancer to a given effective radiation dose is difficult to determine. Using the rule of 5% excess mortality per 1 Sv, each WBLDCT may be accompanied by a 0.00015% excess risk for cancer mortality [41]. Determining the sample size for a reproducibility study using weighted kappa statistics is not straightforward [24]. We deemed a sample of 25 as appropriate since this results in a minimum of 50 joints per analysis and a total time invested for training and scoring of ~10 h per reader. For the analysis of the total OA grade, only 25 cases were available, which partly explains the high standard deviations in the Bland–Altman and Jones plots.

5. Conclusions

To summarize, we introduce the OACT score, a WBLDCT-based reproducible grading system for large-joint OA burden in the body. The OACT score can be used as an outcome measure in OA research or to correct for the influence of total OA burden on patient reported outcomes and biochemical marker levels.

Supplementary Materials: The following are available online at https://www.mdpi.com/2075-4426/11/1/5/s1, The reference atlas is found in Appendix A.

Author Contributions: All authors contributed to the study design, interpretation of the data, and approved of the final version submitted for publication. W.P.G. and W.F. contributed to the first draft of the manuscript and formal analysis. F.J.N., H.W. and F.J.N. substantively reviewed and revised the manuscript. W.P.G., F.J.N., F.W.R. and W.F. developed the scoring system and contributed data acquisition for reproducibility testing. H.W. was responsible for resources and funding acquisition. All authors have read and agreed to the published version of the manuscript.

Funding: This work was supported by Reuma Nederland (LLP-22) and the APPROACH project. APPROACH has received support from the Innovative Medicines Initiative Joint Undertaking under

Grant Agreement n°115770, resources of which are composed of financial contribution from the European Union's Seventh Framework Programme (FP7/2007-2013) and EFPIA companies' in kind contribution. See www.imi.europa.eu.

Data Availability Statement: The data presented in this study are available on request from the corresponding author. The data are not publicly available due to ongoing unpublished research.

Acknowledgments: We would like to thank Chris van Kesteren for his work on the graphical abstract.

Conflicts of Interest: FWR is shareholder of Boston Imaging Core Lab (BICL), LLC., a company providing image assessment services to academia and the pharmaceutical industry. This did not impact any of the current findings.

Appendix A

Table A1. Intra- and interobserver reliability for grading of individual characteristics.

Intervertebral Disc Weighted Kappa (% agreement)	Reader 1 (intra)	Reader 1 vs. Reader 2	Reader 1 vs. Reader 3	Reader 2 vs. Reader 3
Disc space narrowing (0–3)	0.83 (65)	0.76 (57)	0.80 (63)	0.72 (50)
Osteophytes (0–3)	0.85 (73)	0.76 (65)	0.76 (51)	0.81 (65)
Sclerosis and/or end plate irregularity (0–1)	0.68 (84)	0.56 (79)	0.58 (79)	0.45 (72)
Hip Weighted kappa (% agreement)				
Joint space narrowing (0–3)	0.86 (82)	0.65 (64)	0.37 (64)	0.51 (54)
Osteophytes (0–3)	0.75 (80)	0.57 (72)	0.69 (74)	0.59 (70)
Cyst (0–1)	1.00 (100)	1.00 (100)	0.49 (96)	0.49 (96)
Tibiofemoral joint Weighted kappa (% agreement)				
Joint space narrowing (0–3)	0.77 (64)	0.63 (52)	0.74 (58)	0.45 (38)
Osteophytes (0–3)	0.90 (78)	0.90 (78)	0.85 (60)	0.86 (68)
Cyst (0–1)	0.81 (94)	0.38 (80)	0.31 (72)	0.44 (76)

Reader 1: Medical doctor and researcher; Reader 2: Radiologist in training with a subspecialization in musculoskeletal radiology; Reader 3: Fellowship-trained musculoskeletal radiologist with five years of experience.

References

1. Hunter, D.J.; Schofield, D.; Callander, E. The individual and socioeconomic impact of osteoarthritis. *Nat. Rev. Rheumatol.* **2014**, *10*, 437–441. [CrossRef]
2. Van Spil, W.E.; Kubassova, O.; Boesen, M.; Bay-Jensen, A.C.; Mobasheri, A. Osteoarthritis phenotypes and novel therapeutic targets. *Biochem. Pharmacol.* **2019**, *165*, 41–48. [CrossRef]
3. APPROACH Project. Available online: https://www.approachproject.eu (accessed on 8 March 2019).
4. Kraus, V.B.; Kepler, T.B.; Stabler, T.; Renner, J.; Jordan, J. First qualification study of serum biomarkers as indicators of total body burden of osteoarthritis. *PLoS ONE* **2010**, *5*, e9739. [CrossRef]
5. Meulenbelt, I.; Kloppenburg, M.; Kroon, H.M.; Houwing-Duistermaat, J.J.; Garnero, P.; Hellio-Le Graverand, M.-P.; DeGroot, J.; Slagboom, P.E. Clusters of biochemical markers are associated with radiographic subtypes of osteoarthritis (OA) in subject with familial OA at multiple sites. The GARP study. *Osteoarthr. Cartil.* **2007**, *15*, 379–385. [CrossRef]
6. Kinds, M.B.; Vincken, K.L.; Hoppinga, T.N.; Bleys, R.L.A.W.; Viergever, M.A.; Marijnissen, A.C.A.; Welsing, P.M.J.; Lafeber, F.P.J.G. Influence of variation in semiflexed knee positioning during image acquisition on separate quantitative radiographic parameters of osteoarthritis, measured by Knee Images Digital Analysis. *Osteoarthr. Cartil.* **2012**. [CrossRef]
7. Willemink, M.J.; Leiner, T.; de Jong, P.A.; de Heer, L.M.; Nievelstein, R.A.J.; Schilham, A.M.R.; Budde, R.P.J. Iterative reconstruction techniques for computed tomography part 2: Initial results in dose reduction and image quality. *Eur. Radiol.* **2013**, *23*, 1632–1642. [CrossRef] [PubMed]

8. Willemink, M.J.; de Jong, P.A.; Leiner, T.; de Heer, L.M.; Nievelstein, R.A.J.; Budde, R.P.J.; Schilham, A.M.R. Iterative reconstruction techniques for computed tomography Part 1: Technical principles. *Eur. Radiol.* **2013**, *23*, 1623–1631. [CrossRef] [PubMed]
9. Weiler, C.; Schietzsch, M.; Kirchner, T.; Nerlich, A.G.; Boos, N.; Wuertz, K. Age-related changes in human cervical, thoracal and lumbar intervertebral disc exhibit a strong intra-individual correlation. *Eur. Spine J.* **2012**, *21* (Suppl. 6), S810–S818. [CrossRef]
10. O'Neill, T.W.; McCloskey, E.V.; Kanis, J.a.; Bhalla, A.K.; Reeve, J.; Reid, D.M.; Todd, C.; Woolf, A.D.; Silman, A.J. The distribution, determinants, and clinical correlates of vertebral osteophytosis: A population based survey. *J. Rheumatol.* **1999**, *26*, 842–848. [PubMed]
11. Stenlund, B.; Marions, O.; Engström, K.F.; Goldie, I. Correlation of macroscopic osteoarthrotic changes and radiographic findings in the acromioclavicular joint. *Acta Radiol.* **1988**, *29*, 571–576. [CrossRef] [PubMed]
12. Elsharkawi, M.; Cakir, B.; Reichel, H.; Kappe, T. Reliability of radiologic glenohumeral osteoarthritis classifications. *J. Shoulder Elbow Surg.* **2013**, *22*, 1063–1067. [CrossRef] [PubMed]
13. Samilson, R.L.; Prieto, V. Dislocation arthropathy of the shoulder. *J. Bone Joint Surg. Am.* **1983**, *65*, 456–460. [CrossRef] [PubMed]
14. Lane, N.E.; Nevitt, M.C.; Genant, H.K.; Hochberg, M.C. Reliability of new indices of radiographic osteoarthritis of the hand and hip and lumbar disc degeneration. *J. Rheumatol.* **1993**, *20*, 1911–1918. [PubMed]
15. Kettler, A.; Wilke, H.-J. Review of existing grading systems for cervical or lumbar disc and facet joint degeneration. *Eur. Spine J.* **2006**, *15*, 705–718. [CrossRef] [PubMed]
16. Weishaupt, D.; Zanetti, M.; Boos, N.; Hodler, J. MR imaging and CT in osteoarthritis of the lumbar facet joints. *Skelet. Radiol.* **1999**, *28*, 215–219. [CrossRef]
17. Pathria, M.; Sartoris, D.J.; Resnick, D. Osteoarthritis of the facet joints: Accuracy of oblique radiographic assessment. *Radiology* **1987**, *164*, 227–230. [CrossRef]
18. Turmezei, T.D.; Fotiadou, A.; Lomas, D.J.; Hopper, M.a.; Poole, K.E.S. A new CT grading system for hip osteoarthritis. *Osteoarthr. Cartil.* **2014**, *22*, 1360–1366. [CrossRef]
19. Altman, R.D.; Gold, G.E. Atlas of individual radiographic features in osteoarthritis, revised. *Osteoarthr. Cartil.* **2007**, *15* (Suppl. A), A1–A56. [CrossRef]
20. Kellgren, J.H.; Lawrence, J.S. Radiological assessment of osteo-arthrosis. *Ann. Rheum. Dis.* **1957**, *16*, 494–502. [CrossRef]
21. Jones, A.C.; Ledingham, J.; Mcalindon, T.; Regan, M.; Hart, D.; Macmillan, P.J.; Doherty, M. Radiographic assessment of patellofemoral osteoarthritis. *Ann. Rheum. Dis.* **1993**, *52*, 655–658. [CrossRef]
22. Cohen, M.M.; Vela, N.D.; Levine, J.E.; Barnoy, E.A. Validating a New Computed Tomography Atlas for Grading Ankle Osteoarthritis. *J. Foot Ankle Surg.* **2014**, *54*, 207–213. [CrossRef] [PubMed]
23. Fleiss, J.L.; Cohen, J. The equivalence of weighted kappa and the intraclass correlation coefficient as measures of reliability. *Educ. Psychol. Meas.* **1973**, *33*, 613–619. [CrossRef]
24. Kottner, J.; Audigé, L.; Brorson, S.; Donner, A.; Gajewski, B.J.; Hróbjartsson, A.; Roberts, C.; Shoukri, M.; Streiner, D.L. Guidelines for Reporting Reliability and Agreement Studies (GRRAS) were proposed. *J. Clin. Epidemiol.* **2011**, *64*, 96–106. [CrossRef] [PubMed]
25. Landis, J.R.; Koch, G.G. The Measurement of Observer Agreement for Categorical Data. *Biometrics* **1977**, *33*, 159. [CrossRef]
26. Martin Bland, J.T.; Altman, D. Statistical methods for assessing agreement between two methods of clinical measurement. *Lancet* **1986**, *327*, 307–310. [CrossRef]
27. Jones, M.; Dobson, A.; O'Brian, S. A graphical method for assessing agreement with the mean between multiple observers using continuous measures. *Int. J. Epidemiol.* **2011**, *40*, 1308–1313. [CrossRef]
28. Mahir, L.; Belhaj, K.; Zahi, S.; Azanmasso, H.; Lmidmani, F.; El Fatimi, A. Impact of knee osteoarthritis on the quality of life. *Ann. Phys. Rehabil. Med.* **2016**, *59*, e159. [CrossRef]
29. Glazebrook, M.; Daniels, T.; Younger, A.; Foote, C.J.; Penner, M.; Wing, K.; Lau, J.; Leighton, R.; Dunbar, M. Comparison of Health-Related Quality of Life Between Patients with End-Stage Ankle and Hip Arthrosis. *J. Bone Jt. Surg.-Am. Vol.* **2008**, *90*, 499–505. [CrossRef]
30. Gautschi, O.P.; Smoll, N.R.; Corniola, M.V.; Joswig, H.; Chau, I.; Hildebrandt, G.; Schaller, K.; Stienen, M.N. Validity and reliability of a measurement of objective functional impairment in lumbar degenerative disc disease: The Timed Up and Go (TUG) test. *Neurosurgery* **2016**, *79*, 270–278. [CrossRef]
31. Dobson, F.; Hinman, R.S.; Hall, M.; Terwee, C.B.; Roos, E.M.; Bennell, K.L. Measurement properties of performance-based measures to assess physical function in hip and knee osteoarthritis: A systematic review. *Osteoarthr. Cartil.* **2012**, *20*, 1548–1562. [CrossRef]
32. Peterfy, C.G.; Guermazi, A.; Zaim, S.; Tirman, P.F.J.; Miaux, Y.; White, D.; Kothari, M.; Lu, Y.; Fye, K.; Zhao, S.; et al. Whole-organ magnetic resonance imaging score (WORMS) of the knee in osteoarthritis. *Osteoarthr. Cartil.* **2004**, *12*, 177–190. [CrossRef] [PubMed]
33. Hunter, D.J.; Guermazi, A.; Lo, G.H.; Grainger, A.J.; Conaghan, P.G.; Boudreau, R.M.; Roemer, F.W. Evolution of semi-quantitative whole joint assessment of knee OA: MOAKS (MRI Osteoarthritis Knee Score). *Osteoarthr. Cartil.* **2011**, *19*, 990–1002. [CrossRef] [PubMed]
34. Visser, A.W.; Bøyesen, P.; Haugen, I.K.; Schoones, J.W.; van der Heijde, D.M.; Rosendaal, F.R.; Kloppenburg, M. Radiographic scoring methods in hand osteoarthritis—A systematic literature search and descriptive review. *Osteoarthr. Cartil.* **2014**, *22*, 1710–1723. [CrossRef] [PubMed]

5. Rustenburg, C.M.E.; Emanuel, K.S.; Peeters, M.; Lems, W.F.; Vergroesen, P.-P.A.; Smit, T.H. Osteoarthritis and intervertebral disc degeneration: Quite different, quite similar. *JOR Spine* **2018**, *1*, e1033. [CrossRef] [PubMed]
6. Gramstad, G.D.; Galatz, L.M. Management of Elbow Osteoarthritis. *J. Bone Jt. Surg.* **2006**, *88*, 421–430. [CrossRef]
7. Kuperus, J.S.; Oudkerk, S.F.; Foppen, W.; Mohamed Hoesein, F.A.; Gielis, W.P.; Waalwijk, J.; Regan, E.A.; Lynch, D.A.; Oner, F.C.; de Jong, P.A.; et al. Criteria for Early-Phase Diffuse Idiopathic Skeletal Hyperostosis: Development and Validation. *Radiology* **2019**, *291*, 420–426. [CrossRef]
8. Meinberg, E.; Agel, J.; Roberts, C.; Karam, M.; Kellam, J. Fracture and Dislocation Classification Compendium—2018. *J. Orthop. Trauma* **2018**, *32*, S1–S10. [CrossRef]
9. Chanchairujira, K.; Chung, C.B.; Kim, J.Y.; Papakonstantinou, O.; Lee, M.H.; Clopton, P.; Resnick, D. Intervertebral Disk Calcification of the Spine in an Elderly Population: Radiographic Prevalence, Location, and Distribution and Correlation with Spinal Degeneration. *Radiology* **2004**, *230*, 499–503. [CrossRef]
10. Mettler, F.A.; Huda, W.; Yoshizumi, T.T.; Mahesh, M. Effective doses in radiology and diagnostic nuclear medicine: A catalog. *Radiology* **2008**, *248*, 254–263. [CrossRef]
11. Lin, E.C. Radiation risk from medical imaging. *Mayo Clin. Proc.* **2010**, *85*, 1142–1146. [CrossRef]

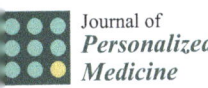

Article

Visceral Adipose Tissue and Different Measures of Adiposity in Different Severities of Diffuse Idiopathic Skeletal Hyperostosis

Netanja I. Harlianto [1,2,*], Jan Westerink [3], Wouter Foppen [1], Marjolein E. Hol [1], Rianne Wittenberg [4], Pieternella H. van der Veen [1], Bram van Ginneken [5], Jonneke S. Kuperus [2], Jorrit-Jan Verlaan [2], Pim A. de Jong [1], Firdaus A. A. Mohamed Hoesein [1] and on behalf of the UCC-SMART-Study Group [†]

1. Department of Radiology, University Medical Center Utrecht and Utrecht University, 3584 CX Utrecht, The Netherlands; W.Foppen@umcutrecht.nl (W.F.); M.E.Hol-6@umcutrecht.nl (M.E.H.); erika_vanderveen@hotmail.com (P.H.v.d.V.); P.deJong-8@umcutrecht.nl (P.A.d.J.); F.A.A.MohamedHoesein@umcutrecht.nl (F.A.A.M.H.)
2. Department of Orthopedic Surgery, University Medical Center Utrecht and Utrecht University, 3584 CX Utrecht, The Netherlands; J.S.Kuperus@umcutrecht.nl (J.S.K.); J.J.Verlaan@umcutrecht.nl (J.-J.V.)
3. Department of Vascular Medicine, University Medical Center Utrecht and Utrecht University, 3584 CX Utrecht, The Netherlands; J.Westerink-3@umcutrecht.nl
4. Department of Radiology, Netherlands Cancer Institute, 1066 CX Amsterdam, The Netherlands; Rianne_wittenberg@hotmail.com
5. Department of Medical Imaging, Radboud University Medical Center, 6525 GA Nijmegen, The Netherlands; bram.vanginneken@radboudumc.nl
* Correspondence: N.I.Harlianto@umcutrecht.nl
† Membership of the UCC-SMART-Study Group is provided in the Acknowledgments.

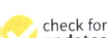

Citation: Harlianto, N.I.; Westerink, J.; Foppen, W.; Hol, M.E.; Wittenberg, R.; van der Veen, P.H.; van Ginneken, B.; Kuperus, J.S.; Verlaan, J.-J.; de Jong, P.A.; et al. Visceral Adipose Tissue and Different Measures of Adiposity in Different Severities of Diffuse Idiopathic Skeletal Hyperostosis. J. Pers. Med. 2021, 11, 663. https://doi.org/10.3390/jpm11070663

Academic Editor: Jasminka Ilich-Ernst

Received: 26 May 2021
Accepted: 13 July 2021
Published: 15 July 2021

Publisher's Note: MDPI stays neutral with regard to jurisdictional claims in published maps and institutional affiliations.

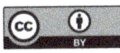

Copyright: © 2021 by the authors. Licensee MDPI, Basel, Switzerland. This article is an open access article distributed under the terms and conditions of the Creative Commons Attribution (CC BY) license (https://creativecommons.org/licenses/by/4.0/).

Abstract: Background: Diffuse idiopathic skeletal hyperostosis (DISH) is associated with both obesity and type 2 diabetes. Our objective was to investigate the relation between DISH and visceral adipose tissue (VAT) in particular, as this would support a causal role of insulin resistance and low grade inflammation in the development of DISH. Methods: In 4334 patients with manifest vascular disease, the relation between different adiposity measures and the presence of DISH was compared using z-scores via standard deviation logistic regression analyses. Analyses were stratified by sex and adjusted for age, systolic blood pressure, diabetes, non-HDL cholesterol, smoking status, and renal function. Results: DISH was present in 391 (9%) subjects. The presence of DISH was associated with markers of adiposity and had a strong relation with VAT in males (OR: 1.35; 95%CI: 1.20–1.54) and females (OR: 1.43; 95%CI: 1.06–1.93). In males with the most severe DISH (extensive ossification of seven or more vertebral bodies) the association between DISH and VAT was stronger (OR: 1.61; 95%CI: 1.31–1.98), while increased subcutaneous fat was negatively associated with DISH (OR: 0.65; 95%CI: 0.49–0.95). In females, increased subcutaneous fat was associated with the presence of DISH (OR: 1.43; 95%CI: 1.14–1.80). Conclusion: Markers of adiposity, including VAT, are strongly associated with the presence of DISH. Subcutaneous adipose tissue thickness was negatively associated with more severe cases of DISH in males, while in females, increased subcutaneous adipose tissue was associated with the presence of DISH.

Keywords: diffuse idiopathic skeletal hyperostosis; risk factors; adiposity; intra-abdominal fat

1. Introduction

Diffuse idiopathic skeletal hyperostosis (DISH) is a common condition characterized by abnormal hyperostosis with the formation of new bony bridges around ligaments, tendons, and joint capsules. DISH is most frequently present near the anterior longitudinal ligament of the spine but can also manifest in the peripheral skeleton [1]. The exact pathophysiology of DISH remains unclear, but various genetic, metabolic, and inflammatory pathways are likely involved [1]. DISH is more prevalent in older individuals, mostly affects males, and has been associated with several metabolic factors including obesity, hypertension, type 2 diabetes mellitus, and the metabolic syndrome [1–4]. Furthermore, individuals with DISH are more prone to spinal fractures and cardiovascular events such as stroke [1]. While usually asymptomatic, reported symptoms related to DISH include dysphagia, airway obstruction, and a reduced range of motion [1].

Abdominal obesity, also referred to as central or visceral obesity, is characterized by an increased volume of visceral adipose tissue (VAT) surrounding the intra-abdominal organs [5]. Abdominal obesity is an independent risk factor for cardiovascular disease, and has been related to different pathologies, including dyslipidemia, insulin resistance, cardiovascular disease, diabetes, and cancer [6,7]. VAT is known to produce various inflammatory cytokines and adipokines, the latter contributing to the development of insulin resistance in patients with increased depositions of VAT [8].

Different methods exist to quantify abdominal obesity. General obesity is most commonly quantified using body mass index (BMI), but BMI is limited in differentiating between lean and fat body mass. More accurate approximations of VAT include indirect anthropometric measurements with the waist circumference and waist-to-hip ratio, or direct measurements with ultrasonography or computed tomography (CT) imaging [9].

Previous studies have shown that obesity is associated with both DISH and cardiovascular disease [1,3], however, it is unknown how obesity leads to a higher prevalence of DISH. Moreover, the adiposity measurement showing the strongest relation with DISH is also not known. A strong relation between markers of adiposity with the closest approximation of visceral adiposity may suggest a causal role of insulin resistance and low grade inflammation in the pathogenesis of DISH. Therefore, in the present study we aimed to investigate the relation between DISH and different measurements of adiposity, including VAT. The secondary aim was to compare the relation between adiposity measurements and different severities of DISH, to analyze how the extent of ossification relates to each measure of adiposity.

2. Materials and Methods

2.1. Study Population

Patients enrolled in the Second Manifestations of ARTerial disease (UCC-SMART) study, an ongoing prospective cohort study of the University Medical Center Utrecht, with a patient population between 18 and 79 years with either manifest or risk factors for vascular disease were included. All patients provided written informed consent at inclusion. The UCC-SMART study is in accordance with the declaration of Helsinki and has been approved by our institutional review board (NL45885.041.13). Patients underwent extensive vascular screening: patients were asked to complete a health questionnaire covering medical history, risk factors, smoking and drinking habits, and prescribed drugs. A standardized diagnostic protocol was followed consisting of a physical examination and laboratory testing in a fasting state. A more detailed description of the UCC-SMART study protocol has been published previously [10]. We identified all patients from the UCC-SMART cohort who received a digital chest radiograph within three months of inclusion, resulting in 4791 available patients. Of this population, 88 patients were subsequently excluded due to technical image deficiencies ($n = 44$), only the frontal radiograph being available ($n = 34$), and poor image quality ($n = 10$). For the current study, we also excluded patients enrolled before May 2000 as visceral fat measurements were not regularly performed before that date. In the end, 4334 patients were available for inclusion (Figure 1).

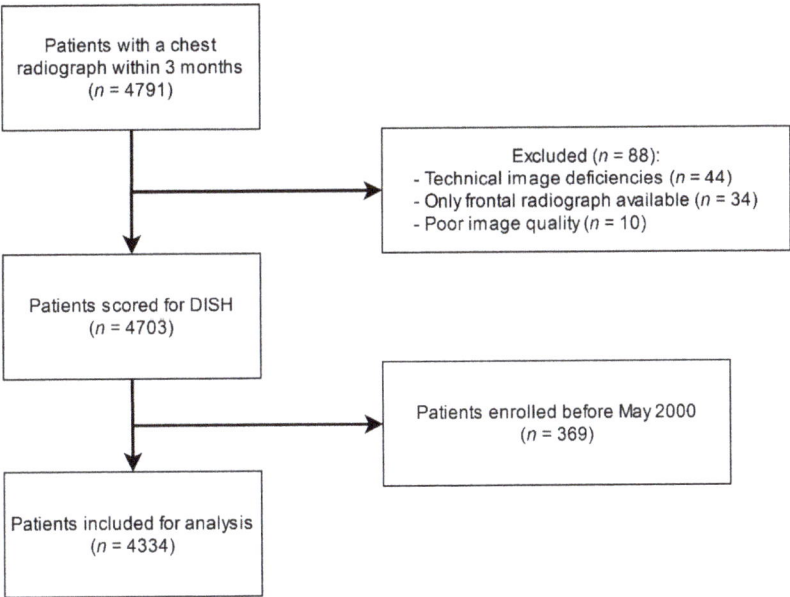

Figure 1. Flow chart of patient selection.

2.2. Assessment of DISH

Using the Resnick criteria [11], chest radiographs were assessed for the presence of DISH. These classification criteria include the presence of ossification of at least four contiguous vertebrae, (relative) preservation of the intervertebral disc height, and the absence of apophyseal joint bony ankylosis or sacroiliac joint erosion. The chest radiographs were scored by a group of six readers from the department of Radiology of our institution, all of whom were certified to read chest radiographs independently (entrusted professional activity level 4 or 5). To analyze the extent of anterolateral ossification in relation to the markers of adiposity, the severity of DISH was also scored depending on the number of involved vertebral bodies with adjacent bony bridges. Although no standardized criteria have been validated for scoring different severities of DISH, we classified the severity of DISH as the following: grade 1 DISH indicated flowing bridging osteophytes of 4 adjacent vertebral bodies; grade 2 DISH indicated flowing bridging osteophytes of 5 or 6 vertebral bodies; and grade 3 DISH indicated flowing bridging osteophytes of 7 or more vertebral bodies.

2.3. Measurements of Adiposity Markers

Body mass index (BMI) was calculated by dividing the weight by the squared height (kg/m^2). Waist circumference was measured halfway between the lower rib and the iliac crest in the standing position. Hip circumference was measured at the level of the greater trochanter in the standing position. The waist-to-hip ratio was calculated using the waist circumference divided by the hip circumference. To measure subcutaneous and intra-abdominal fat, B-mode ultrasound of the abdomen was obtained and performed by well-trained registered vascular technologists in a certified vascular laboratory. Measurements were made with the patient in supine position using an ATL HDI 3000 (Philips Medical Systems, Eindhoven, The Netherlands) with a C4-2 transducer without prior bowel preparation. Good reproducible results (interobserver coefficient of variation of 5.4%) and a strong association (Pearson's correlation coefficient of 0.81, $p < 0.001$) were found when comparing ultrasonographic measurements with a subset of CT scans for intra-abdominal fat in our cohort [12]. Adhering to a strict protocol, measurements were performed using electronic calipers at the end of a quiet inspiration, applying minimal pressure without displacement or compression of the abdominal cavity. The transducer was placed in a straight line drawn between the left and right midpoints of the lower rib and the iliac crest. Three different measurements at three different positions were performed. Subcutaneous fat was measured as the distance between the linea alba and the skin. Intra-abdominal fat was measured as the distance between the peritoneum and the lumbar spine or psoas muscles. The contribution of VAT to total abdominal fat (VAT%) was calculated as [100 × VAT ÷ (VAT + SAT)] to evaluate the impact of an increased VAT, independent of other adipose tissue locations or height.

2.4. Statistics

Categorical variables were expressed using frequencies and percentages, and normally distributed continuous variables using the mean and standard deviation. Positively skewed data were transformed using logarithmic transformation. Univariate and multivariate logistic regression analyses were performed for each of the population characteristics with the presence or absence of DISH as outcome, adjusted for age and sex. Risk was calculated using odds ratios (OR) with 95% confidence intervals (95% CI). Specifically for the adiposity measurements, data were transformed using z-scores for a per standard deviation (SD) analysis using a stepwise adjusted approach including confounder selection based upon literature and etiologic considerations with sex-stratification. In addition to the crude analysis, two models were used: model two was adjusted for age, and model three additionally adjusted for cardiovascular risk factors such as renal function calculated with the Chronic Kidney Disease Epidemiology Collaboration equation (CKD-EPI) [13], systolic blood pressure, diabetes, smoking status, and non-high density lipoprotein (HDL) cholesterol. Missing data (1%) were imputed using multiple imputation based on the Markov Chain Monte Carlo method ($n = 10$ and 40 iterations) and estimates for statistical inference were pooled according to Rubin's Rules [14]. Significance was set at $p < 0.05$. Data analysis was performed using R, version 3.6.3 (R Foundation for Statistical Computing, Vienna, Austria) using the mice package [15].

3. Results

3.1. Baseline Characteristics

A total of 4334 patients were included, of whom 391 (9.0%) satisfied the criteria for DISH. A total of 146 patients were classified as grade 1 DISH, 131 as grade 2 DISH, and 114 as grade 3 DISH. Population characteristics are summarized in Table 1. Compared to patients without DISH, subjects with DISH were older (67 vs. 59 years) and more often male (85.7% vs. 68.4%). Furthermore, DISH subjects had significantly more metabolic syndrome (66% vs. 52%) and diabetes (30% vs. 20%). All adiposity measurements except subcutaneous fat were increased in patients with DISH when compared with patients without DISH.

Table 1. Baseline patient characteristics.

Variable	Total Group (n = 4334)	No DISH (n = 3943)	Total DISH (n = 391)	Grade 1 DISH (n = 146)	Grade 2 DISH (n = 131)	Grade 3 DISH (n = 114)
Age (years), mean (SD)	58.5 (±11.3)	57.8 (±11.3)	66.1 (±7.7)	65.2 (±8)	65.6 (±7.6)	68 (±7)
Sex (male), %	70.0%	68.4%	85.7%	80.1%	87.8%	83%
Diabetes, %	19.3%	18.3%	29.4%	25.3%	32.1%	31.6%
Glucose (mmol/L), mean (SD)	6.3 (±1.7)	6.3 (±1.7)	6.6 (±1.5)	6.5 (±1.4)	6.8 (±1.6)	6.6 (±1.3)
HbA1c (%), mean (SD)	5.9 (±0.9)	5.9 (±1)	6 (±0.8)	5.9 (±0.7)	6.1 (±0.9)	5.8 (±1)
CKD EPI (mL/min/1.73 m^2), mean (SD)	78.5 (±19)	79.1 (±19.1)	73 (±17.5)	73.4 (±17.9)	74.1 (±17.3)	71.3 (±17.2)
Systolic blood pressure (mmHg), mean (SD)	140.9 (±21.7)	140.5 (±21.6)	145.8 (±22.2)	144.8 (±22.8)	143.4 (±21.1)	149.9 (±22)
Diastolic blood pressure (mmHg), mean (SD)	83.2 (±12.7)	83.3 (±12.8)	82.4 (±12.1)	83.1 (±12.7)	80.7 (±11.4)	83.5 (±11.9)
Hypertension, % #	24.6%	24.1%	30.2%	29%	23.1%	40.3%

Table 1. Cont.

Variable	Total Group (n = 4334)	No DISH (n = 3943)	Total DISH (n = 391)	Grade 1 DISH (n = 146)	Grade 2 DISH (n = 131)	Grade 3 DISH (n = 114)
Pulse pressure (mmHg), mean (SD)	57.8 (±15.3)	57.2 (±15.2)	63.4 (±16)	61.8 (±15.3)	62.6 (±16.6)	66.4 (±15.7)
HDL-cholesterol (mmol/L), mean (SD)	1.3 (±0.4)	1.3 (±0.4)	1.2 (±0.3)	1.2 (±0.3)	1.2 (±0.4)	1.2 (±0.3)
LDL-cholesterol (mmol/L), mean (SD)	2.8 (±1.1)	2.8 (±1)	2.7 (±1.1)	2.8 (±1.2)	2.7 (±0.9)	2.6 (±1)
Triglycerides (mmol/L), mean (SD) [&]	0.94 (±0.37)	0.92 (±0.36)	0.93 (±0.34)	0.96 (±0.46)	0.93 (±0.31)	0.98 (±0.32)
Non-HDL cholesterol (mmol/L), mean (SD)	3.6 (±1.2)	3.6 (±1.2)	3.5 (±1.3)	3.6 (±1.5)	3.4 (±1.2)	3.4 (±1.1)
hsCRP (mg/L), mean (SD) [&]	1.24 (±0.78)	1.23 (±0.78)	1.29 (±0.77)	1.25 (±0.72)	1.26 (±0.79)	1.36 (±0.80)
Metabolic syndrome, % [#]	53.3%	52.2%	65.9%	63.7%	63.3%	68.4%
Smoking (current vs. former), % [#]	72.7%	72.3%	77.0%	75.1%	78.5%	79.6%
Packyears, mean (SD)	17.3 (±19.5)	17.2 (±19.4)	18.6 (±20.2)	18 (±20.5)	19 (±19.5)	19 (±20.6)
Drinking (current vs. former), % [#]	80.9%	80.4%	86.2%	83.4%	89.2%	87.7%
History of cerebral vascular disease, % [#]	15.7%	15.2%	14.1%	15.1%	10.7%	16.7%
History of coronary artery disease (%) [#]	50.5%	49.5%	59.8%	56.2%	64.1%	59.6%
History of peripheral artery disease, % [#]	9.1%	9.2%	7.9%	8.9%	7.6%	7%
History of abdominal aortic aneurysm, % [#]	5.3%	4.9%	8.7%	8.2%	8.4%	9.6%
Weight (kg), mean (SD)	82.7 (±15.8)	82.1 (±15.8)	88.2 (±15.4)	87.5 (±15.6)	87.8 (±14.7)	89.4 (±15.9)
BMI (kg/m^2), mean (SD)	27.1 (±4.5)	26.9 (±4.4)	27.8 (±4.5)	28.8 (±4.5)	28.5 (±4.7)	29 (±4.4)
Waist circumference (cm), mean (SD)	95.5 (±13.1)	94.9 (±8.7)	102 (±12.2)	101.1 (±12.7)	101.5 (±11.2)	103.6 (±12.7)
Waist-to-hip ratio, mean (SD)	0.92 (±0.09)	0.91 (±0.09)	0.96 (±0.07)	0.94 (±0.08)	0.95 (±0.06)	0.97 (±0.08)
Subcutaneous fat (cm), mean (SD)	2.4 (±1.2)	2.4 (±1.2)	2.1 (±1.3)	2.3 (±1.5)	2.2 (±1.1)	1.8 (±0.9)
Visceral fat (cm), mean (SD)	9 (±2.7)	8.9 (±2.6)	10.1 (±2.8)	9.8 (±2.8)	9.9 (±2.7)	10.7 (±2.9)

[#] Percentages were calculated after excluding missing cases from the denominator; [&] Log-transformed; Data are displayed using number (percentage) for categorical variables and mean (±standard deviation) for normally continuous data. BMI: body mass index; hsCRP: high sensitivity c-reactive protein; CKD-EPI: Chronic Kidney Disease Epidemiology Collaboration; HDL: high density lipoprotein; LDL: low density lipoprotein.

3.2. Risk Factors for DISH

Results of logistic regression analyses are listed in Table 2. After adjusting for age and sex, DISH was significantly associated with presence of metabolic syndrome (OR 1.78 (95%CI: 1.43–2.24)), the presence of diabetes (OR 1.50 (95%CI: 1.18–1.91)), and glucose (per 1 mmol/L) (OR 1.10 (95%CI: 1.04–1.17)). Systolic blood pressure (per 1 mmHg), the presence of hypertension, and pulse pressure (per 1 mmHg) were also associated with DISH, whereas diastolic blood pressure was not. Regarding blood lipid profile, DISH was associated with HDL-cholesterol.

Table 2. Risk factor analysis for the DISH group.

Variable	Units	Univariate Model		Age + Sex Adjusted	
		OR (95%CI)	p-Value	OR (95%CI)	p-Value
Age *	+1 year	1.09 (1.08–1.10)	<0.001	1.09 (1.08–1.11)	<0.001
Sex [#]	Male vs. female	2.78 (2.08–3.7)	<0.001	2.86 (2.13–3.85)	<0.001
Diabetes	Present vs. absent	1.72 (1.36–2.16)	<0.001	1.50 (1.18–1.91)	<0.001
Glucose	+1 mmol/L	1.1 (1.05–1.16)	<0.001	1.1 (1.04–1.17)	<0.001
HbA1c	+1%	1.14 (1.03–1.27)	0.01	1.13 (0.99–1.27)	0.06
CKD-EPI	+1 mL/min/1.73 m^2	0.98 (0.98–0.99)	<0.001	1.0 (0.99–1.01)	0.20
Systolic blood pressure	+1 mmHg	1.01 (1.00–1.02)	<0.001	1.01 (1.00–1.01)	0.008
Diastolic blood pressure	+1 mmHg	0.99 (0.99–1.00)	0.21	1.00 (0.99–1.01)	0.55
Hypertension	Present vs. absent	1.36 (1.09–1.72)	0.007	1.43 (1.13–1.82)	0.003
Pulse pressure	+1 mmHg	1.02 (1.02–1.03)	<0.001	1.01 (1.00–1.02)	0.001
HDL-cholesterol	+1 mmol/L	0.66 (0.49–0.88)	0.005	0.68 (0.49–0.94)	0.02
LDL-cholesterol	+1 mmol/L	0.92 (0.83–1.01)	0.08	1.05 (0.93–1.18)	0.43

Table 2. Cont.

Variable	Units	Univariate Model		Age + Sex Adjusted	
		OR (95%CI)	p-Value	OR (95%CI)	p-Value
Triglycerides &	+1 log(1 mmol/L)	1.05 (0.88–1.27)	0.58	1.33 (1.08–1.63)	0.006
Non HDL-cholesterol	+1 mmol/L	0.94 (0.86–1.02)	0.14	1.11 (1.01–1.22)	0.03
hsCRP &	+1 log(1 (mg/L)	1.07 (0.97–1.19)	0.18	1.05 (0.95–1.17)	0.30
Metabolic syndrome	Present vs. absent	1.69 (1.36–2.11)	<0.001	1.78 (1.43–2.24)	<0.001
Smoking	Current vs. former	1.31 (1.02–1.68)	0.03	1.03 (0.79–1.34)	0.82
Packyears	+1 packyear	1.00 (0.99–1.01)	0.15	1.00 (0.99–1.00)	0.38
Drinking	Current vs. former drinker	1.54 (1.14–2.09)	0.004	1.12 (0.81–1.54)	0.51
History of cerebral vascular disease	Yes vs. no	0.92 (0.67–1.22)	0.56	0.79 (0.57–1.06)	0.13
History of coronary artery disease	Yes vs. no	1.52 (1.23–1.88)	<0.001	0.91 (0.72–1.14)	0.39
History of peripheral artery disease	Yes vs. no	0.85 (0.57–1.22)	0.4	0.74 (0.49–1.08)	0.13
History of abdominal aortic aneurysm	Yes vs. no	1.84 (1.24–2.66)	0.002	1.02 (0.67–1.49)	0.94

* Sex adjusted; # Age adjusted; & Log-transformed. OR: odds ratio; CI: confidence interval; BMI: body mass index; hsCRP: high sensitivity c-reactive protein; CKD-EPI: Chronic Kidney Disease Epidemiology Collaboration; HDL: high density lipoprotein; LDL: low density lipoprotein.

3.3. Intra-Abdominal Fat Measurements and Adiposity Markers in Relation to DISH in Males

Results of adiposity measurements with an increase of 1 SD in relation to the presence of DISH in males are listed in Table 3. In the crude analysis, the presence of DISH was associated with the adiposity measures weight, BMI, waist circumference, subcutaneous fat, VAT, and VAT%. After full adjustments, the significant adiposity markers were weight (OR 1.56; 95%CI: 1.36–1.79), BMI (OR 1.58; 95%CI: 1.28–1.94), waist circumference (OR 1.45; 95%CI: 1.15–1.82), and VAT (OR 1.35; 95%CI: 1.20–1.54). An increase of 1 SD of subcutaneous fat, the waist-to-hip ratio, or VAT% was not significantly associated with the presence of DISH. In general, the adiposity measures weight, BMI, waist circumference, and VAT were significant for all grades of DISH in crude and full adjusted analyses. In the most severe DISH group, the relation between VAT and the presence of DISH became stronger (OR 1.61; 95%CI: 1.31–1.98). Moreover, in this group with most severe DISH, 1 SD increase in subcutaneous fat was negatively associated with the presence of DISH (OR 0.65; 95%CI: 0.49–0.95), whereas VAT% was positively associated with the presence of DISH (OR 1.80; 95%CI: 1.25–2.68). These relations for subcutaneous fat and VAT% were not observed in the groups with grade 1 or grade 2 DISH.

Table 3. Adiposity measurements per SD with different severities of DISH as outcome in males.

	Model	Total DISH	Grade 1 DISH	Grade 2 DISH	Grade 3 DISH
		OR (95%CI)	OR (95%CI)	OR (95%CI)	OR (95%CI)
Weight (kg), per SD increase	1	1.24 (1.10–1.39) a	1.26 (1.05–1.51) a	1.16 (0.96–1.41) a	1.30 (1.07–1.58) a
	2	1.59 (1.39–1.81) a	1.53 (1.26–1.87) a	1.44 (1.17–1.77) a	1.81 (1.45–2.25) a
	3	1.56 (1.36–1.79) a	1.54 (1.26–1.89) a	1.40 (1.14–1.74) a	1.73 (1.39–2.17) a
BMI (kg/m²), per SD increase	1	1.39 (1.20–1.60) a	1.38 (1.12–1.70) a	1.27 (1.05–1.54) a	1.44 (1.14–1.83) a
	2	1.60 (1.31–1.94) a	1.51 (1.14–2.00) a	1.41 (1.10–1.79) a	1.71 (1.17–2.51) a
	3	1.58 (1.28–1.94) a	1.53 (1.13–2.09) *	1.38 (1.08–1.77) a	1.66 (1.16–2.39) a
Waist circumference (cm), per SD increase	1	1.44 (1.20–1.71) a	1.41 (1.16–1.73) a	1.33 (1.07–1.66) a	1.53 (1.15–2.04) a
	2	1.47 (1.18–1.83) a	1.43 (1.14–1.79) a	1.35 (1.05–1.75) a	1.59 (1.10–2.29) a
	3	1.45 (1.15–1.82) a	1.44 (1.13–1.83) a	1.32 (1.01–1.72) a	1.53 (1.07–2.18) a
Waist-to-hip ratio, per SD increase	1	1.40 (0.97–2.01)	1.37 (1.02–1.84) a	1.27 (0.90–1.79)	1.54 (0.89–2.66)
	2	1.32 (0.94–1.87)	1.30 (0.98–1.74)	1.20 (0.86–1.69)	1.48 (0.86–2.53)
	3	1.29 (0.92–1.82)	1.30 (0.97–1.76)	1.16 (0.83–1.63)	1.42 (0.85–2.36)
Subcutaneous fat (cm), per SD increase	1	0.81 (0.68–0.95) a	0.90 (0.71–1.14)	0.96 (0.76–1.21)	0.53 (0.37–0.76) a
	2	0.95 (0.81–1.10)	1.02 (0.81–1.29)	1.10 (0.87–1.38)	0.64 (0.44–0.94) a
	3	0.95 (0.82–1.11)	1.02 (0.81–1.28)	1.10 (0.88–1.37)	0.65 (0.49–0.95) a

Table 3. Cont.

	Model	Total DISH OR (95%CI)	Grade 1 DISH OR (95%CI)	Grade 2 DISH OR (95%CI)	Grade 3 DISH OR (95%CI)
VAT (cm), per SD increase	1	1.37 (1.22–1.54) [a]	1.30 (1.08–1.56) [a]	1.24 (1.03–1.51) [a]	1.64 (1.35–1.97) [a]
	2	1.38 (1.22–1.56) [a]	1.29 (1.07–1.57) [a]	0.24 (1.02–1.51) [a]	1.68 (1.38–2.05) [a]
	3	1.35 (1.20–1.54) [a]	1.30 (1.06–1.59) [a]	1.21 (0.98–1.49)	1.61 (1.31–1.98) [a]
VAT%, per SD increase	1	1.39 (1.18–1.65)	1.25 (0.99–1.59)	1.10 (0.87–1.40)	2.19 (1.55–3.10) [a]
	2	1.21 (1.02–1.43) [a]	1.11 (0.87–1.42)	0.97 (0.76–1.23)	1.87 (1.30–2.66) [a]
	3	1.18 (0.99–1.39)	1.10 (0.86–1.41)	0.94 (0.74–1.20)	1.80 (1.25–2.68) [a]

Model 1: DISH crude; Model 2: adjusted for age; Model 3: adjusted for age, systolic blood pressure, diabetes, non-HDL cholesterol, smoking status, and renal function. [a] $p < 0.05$, SD: standard deviation; OR: odds ratio; CI: confidence interval; BMI: body mass index; VAT: visceral adipose tissue; VAT%: visceral adipose tissue in relation to total abdominal fat.

3.4. Intra-Abdominal Fat Measurements and Adiposity Markers in Relation to DISH in Females

Table 4 lists the results of adiposity measures in females in relation to the presence of DISH. The presence of DISH was related to the markers weight (OR 1.52; 95%CI: 1.20–1.94), BMI (OR 1.55; 95%CI: 1.28–1.89), waist circumference (OR 1.54; 95%CI: 1.06–2.24), and VAT (OR 1.71; 95%CI: 1.33–2.19). After adjusting for cardiovascular risk factors, the relation between the presence of DISH and waist circumference became attenuated (OR 1.39; 95%CI: 0.89–2.16), while an increase by 1 SD of subcutaneous fat was associated with the presence of DISH (OR 1.43; 95%CI: 1.14–1.80). The adiposity markers weight (OR 1.75; 95%CI: 1.29–2.38), BMI (OR 1.66; 95%CI: 1.30–2.13), and VAT (OR 1.43; 95%CI: 1.06–1.93) remained significantly associated after full adjustment. For the different Grades of DISH, the adiposity measures weight and BMI were significant for all grades of DISH in crude and full adjusted analyses.

Table 4. Adiposity measurements per SD with different severities DISH as outcome in females.

	Model	Total DISH OR (95%CI)	Grade 1 DISH OR (95%CI)	Grade 2 DISH OR (95%CI)	Grade 3 DISH OR (95%CI)
Weight (kg), per SD increase	1	1.52 (1.20–1.94) [a]	1.36 (0.97–1.91)	1.71 (1.15–2.54) [a]	1.57 (0.96–2.58)
	2	1.94 (1.46–2.57) [a]	1.68 (1.14–2.47) [a]	2.20 (1.39–3.49) [a]	2.21 (1.20–4.04) [a]
	3	1.75 (1.29–2.38) [a]	1.59 (1.04–2.43) [a]	1.84 (1.11–3.04) [a]	2.08 (1.08–4.03) [a]
BMI (kg/m^2), per SD increase	1	1.55 (1.28–1.89) [a]	1.42 (1.09–1.84) [a]	1.66 (1.20–2.29) [a]	1.57 (1.08–2.30) [a]
	2	1.13 (1.08–1.20) [a]	1.60 (1.18–2.16) [a]	1.93 (1.34–2.80) [a]	1.97 (1.24–3.17) [a]
	3	1.66 (1.30–2.13) [a]	1.55 (1.11–2.16) [a]	1.72 (1.16–2.55) [a]	1.89 (1.12–3.17) [a]
Waist circumference (cm), per SD increase	1	1.54 (1.06–2.24) [a]	1.37 (0.89–2.10)	1.69 (1.10–2.59) [a]	1.68 (0.91–3.11)
	2	1.54 (0.99–2.38)	1.33 (0.82–2.18)	1.69 (1.05–2.72) [a]	1.69 (0.80–3.61)
	3	1.39 (0.89–2.16)	1.24 (0.71–2.18)	1.44 (0.89–2.31)	1.62 (0.74–3.53)
Waist-to-hip ratio, per SD increase	1	1.31 (0.83–2.06)	1.05 (0.64–1.73)	1.44 (0.87–2.40)	1.57 (0.72–3.49)
	2	1.15 (0.76–1.75)	0.86 (0.47–1.57)	1.33 (0.81–2.18)	1.47 (0.64–3.39)
	3	1.03 (0.65–1.64)	0.77 (0.38–1.60)	1.15 (0.67–1.99)	1.48 (0.60–3.60)
Subcutaneous fat (cm), per SD increase	1	1.21 (0.97–1.52)	1.34 (1.04–1.74) [a]	1.21 (0.72–2.04)	0.81 (0.44–1.48)
	2	1.44 (1.15–1.81) [a]	1.58 (1.20–2.10) [a]	1.39 (0.85–2.29)	0.94 (0.49–1.81)
	3	1.43 (1.14–1.80) [a]	1.55 (1.16–2.08) [a]	1.48 (0.90–2.44)	0.93 (0.47–1.82)
VAT (cm), per SD increase	1	1.71 (1.33–2.19) [a]	1.47 (1.04–2.05)	2.08 (1.35–3.19) [a]	1.72 (1.02–2.88) [a]
	2	1.63 (1.24–2.13) [a]	1.36 (0.94–1.98)	2.05 (1.31–3.22) [a]	1.66 (0.93–2.97)
	3	1.43 (1.06–1.93) [a]	1.26 (0.84–1.92)	1.61 (0.97–2.65)	1.46 (0.78–2.75)
VAT%, per SD increase	1	1.21 (0.91–1.61)	0.98 (0.69–1.40)	2.07 (1.35–3.19) [a]	1.75 (0.94–3.26)
	2	1.10 (1.06–1.13) [a]	0.80 (0.55–1.17)	1.19 (0.61–2.35)	1..46 (0.75–2.83)
	3	0.90 (0.67–1.22)	0.76 (0.51–1.14)	0.97 (0.50–1.89)	1.36 (0.69–2.72)

Model 1: DISH crude; Model 2: adjusted for age; Model 3: adjusted for age, systolic blood pressure, diabetes, non-HDL cholesterol, smoking status, and renal function. [a] $p < 0.05$, SD: standard deviation; OR: odds ratio; CI: confidence interval; BMI: body mass index; VAT: visceral adipose tissue; VAT%: visceral adipose tissue in relation to total abdominal fat.

4. Discussion

In the current study, we aimed to assess the relation between different severities of DISH and various measurements of adiposity in both males and females with a high risk for cardiovascular disease. We found that, in males, all adiposity markers except for subcutaneous fat and the waist-to-hip ratio were associated with the presence of DISH. When analyzing the group with the most severe DISH, the relation between VAT and the presence of DISH became stronger. Moreover, increased subcutaneous fat was negatively associated with cases of DISH with extensive ossification, reinforcing the importance of adipose tissue distribution in the pathogenesis of DISH.

In females, the adiposity markers we identified with the presence of DISH were weight, BMI, subcutaneous fat, and VAT. Waist circumference was not associated with the presence of DISH, which was the case for males, whereas in female DISH patients increased subcutaneous fat was positively associated with the presence of DISH.

The risk factors we identified for DISH in our cohort also strongly relate to the presence of VAT and obesity [16] showing the probable causal relation between VAT and insulin resistance. The formation of bone in DISH is potentially linked with metabolic derangements via the insulin-like growth factor-I pathway, which is able to induce proliferation in chondrocytes and osteoblasts [17].

The prevalence of DISH in our cohort was 9.0% and our data confirm previously observed associations between DISH and BMI [3,18–21], diabetes [3,19–21], waist circumference [5,18,22], metabolic syndrome [5,18], systolic blood pressure [18,23], and hypertension [5,18]. A higher level of HDL-cholesterol was significantly associated with the presence of DISH in our study, whereas other cohorts did not find this relation [5,18]. These risk factors are described to strongly relate to excess levels of VAT and the presence of insulin resistance [16]. In line with previous work, no association was found between DISH and hsCRP [18]. As our patient population had increased risk for cardiovascular disease, a large portion of our cohort was treated with statin therapy for cardiovascular risk management. The use of statins is associated with a reduction in levels of hsCRP [24], which may explain why no significant difference was observed for hsCRP between the groups with and without DISH in our cohort.

Our results show that the presence of DISH is associated with VAT, which is in accordance with Lantsman et al. [25] and Okada et al. [26], who measured VAT in DISH patients using CT imaging. In the study by Okada and colleagues, the area of VAT was significantly increased in DISH patients ($130.7 \pm SD\ 58.2\ cm^2$ vs. $89.0 \pm SD\ 48.1\ cm^2$).

Interestingly, females with DISH had both increased subcutaneous fat and VAT in our cohort. Contrarily in males, an increased VAT was linked with DISH while increased subcutaneous fat was not. When estimating the percentage of VAT in relation to total abdominal fat, no association was found between VAT% and DISH for both sexes. This might be explained by the poor reliability of using adiposity measurements with ultrasound as proxies for VAT accumulation in relation to total abdominal fat. Ideally, CT-based segmentations in the coronal plane are preferred as this can more accurately measure the total area of visceral fat in relation to the total area of abdominal fat. To minimize this discrepancy, our measurements adhered to a strict protocol, and the estimations were averaged over multiple measurements of the same patient.

Although other adiposity markers had stronger observed associations with DISH compared to VAT in our study, our results still indicate that one SD increase of VAT is associated with a 35% and 43% increase in risk for DISH in males and females, respectively. VAT is known to increase with older age, and a higher percentage of VAT is found in men [27,28]. Furthermore, it is now well established that VAT produces different adipokines and inflammatory molecules including leptin, adiponectin, tumor necrosis factor-α, and interleukin-6. In the literature, few studies have reported these adipokines in relation to DISH. Visceral obesity results in lower levels of adiponectin [29], which was reported for DISH in two studies [30,31]. Moreover, increased levels of leptin [31,32] and visfatin [30] were also observed in DISH patients. Both leptin and adiponectin are known to influence bone metabolism and bone homeostasis [31,33]. An adequate explanation for the role of these adipokines in the pathogenesis of DISH remains to be determined. Recently, Mader et al. [34] reviewed the involvement of a possible inflammatory component in DISH, and concluded that local inflammation, prior to or as a consequence of metabolic derangements, could play a crucial role in the development of DISH. Our results support the notion that research on VAT and inflammation should be further (re)explored in patients with DISH.

Strengths and Limitations

The strengths of our study are the relatively large sample size of our prospective cohort, with extensive and accurate information on a broad array of cardiovascular risk factors. Moreover, we studied the relative importance of adiposity measurements and corrected for confounders, which has not been reported previously in DISH.

Our study, however, also has limitations. Visceral and subcutaneous fat measured with ultrasonography have been reported to be prone to measurement variability. However, an interobserver coefficient of variation of 5.4% was found for our cohort, indicating good measurement reliability [12]. Secondly, the Resnick criteria for DISH are arbitrary and some milder forms or earlier stages of DISH will be misclassified. This can result in some underestimation of the associations. Finally, the cross-sectional design of our study should warrant a cautious approach when drawing causal etiological conclusions.

5. Conclusions

To summarize, measurements of adiposity, including visceral adipose tissue thickness, were associated with the presence of DISH in both males and females. Subcutaneous adipose tissue thickness was negatively associated in males with most severe DISH. In females, subcutaneous adipose tissue was positively associated with the presence of DISH. Our research supports further investigation into the role of visceral adipose tissue and insulin resistance in the pathogenesis of DISH.

Author Contributions: Conceptualization, N.I.H., J.W. and P.A.d.J.; methodology, N.I.H. and J.W.; software, N.I.H.; validation, N.I.H. and J.W.; formal analysis, N.I.H.; visualization, N.I.H.; data curation, UCC-SMART-Study Group, F.A.A.M.H., P.A.d.J., W.F., M.E.H., R.W., P.H.v.d.V., and B.v.G.; writing—original draft preparation, N.I.H., J.W., P.A.d.J., and F.A.A.M.H.; writing—review and editing, N.I.H., J.W., W.F., M.E.H., R.W., P.H.v.d.V., B.v.G., J.S.K., J.-J.V., P.A.d.J., and F.A.A.M.H.; supervision, J.W., P.A.d.J., J.-J.V., and F.A.A.M.H.; project administration, N.I.H. All authors have read and agreed to the published version of the manuscript.

Funding: The UCC-SMART study was financially supported by a grant from the University Medical Center Utrecht. The funders had no role in the study design, data collection and analysis, decision to publish, or preparation of the manuscript.

Institutional Review Board Statement: The UCC-SMART study was conducted according to the guidelines of the Declaration of Helsinki and approved by the Institutional Review of the University Medical Center Utrecht (NL45885.041.13).

Informed Consent Statement: Informed consent was obtained from all subjects involved in the study.

Data Availability Statement: The informed consent that was signed by the study participants is not compliant with publishing individual data in an open access institutional repository or as supporting information files with the published paper. However, a data request can be sent to the SMART Steering Committee at uccdatarequest@umcutrecht.nl.

Acknowledgments: We gratefully acknowledge the contribution of the research nurses; R. van Petersen; B. van Dinther and the Members of the Utrecht Cardiovascular Cohort-Second Manifestations of ARTerial disease-Study Group (UCC-SMART-Study Group); F.W. Asselbergs and H.M. Nathoe, Department of Cardiology; G.J. de Borst, Department of Vascular Surgery; M.L. Bots and M.I. Geerlings, Julius Center for Health Sciences and Primary Care; M.H. Emmelot, Department of Geriatrics; P.A. de Jong and T. Leiner, Department of Radiology; A.T. Lely, Department of Obstetrics and Gynecology; N.P. van der Kaaij, Department of Cardiothoracic Surgery; L.J. Kappelle and Y.M. Ruigrok,

Department of Neurology; M.C. Verhaar, Department of Nephrology; F.L.J. Visseren and J. Westerink, Department of Vascular Medicine, University Medical Center Utrecht and Utrecht University.

Conflicts of Interest: The authors declare no conflict of interest. The funders had no role in the design of the study; in the collection, analyses, or interpretation of data; in the writing of the manuscript; or in the decision to publish the results.

References

1. Mader, R.; Verlaan, J.J.; Buskila, D. Diffuse idiopathic skeletal hyperostosis: Clinical features and pathogenic mechanisms. *Nat. Rev. Rheumatol.* **2013**, *9*, 741–750. [CrossRef]
2. Kiss, C.; Szilágyi, M.; Paksy, A.; Poór, G. Risk factors for diffuse idiopathic skeletal hyperostosis: A case-control study. *Rheumatol. (Oxf.)* **2002**, *41*, 27–30. [CrossRef] [PubMed]
3. Zincarelli, C.; Iervolino, S.; Di Minno, M.N.; Miniero, E.; Rengo, C.; Di Gioia, L.; Vitale, D.; Nicolino, A.; Furgi, G.; Pappone, N. Diffuse idiopathic skeletal hyperostosis prevalence in subjects with severe atherosclerotic cardiovascular diseases. *Arthritis Care Res. (Hoboken)* **2012**, *64*, 1765–1769. [CrossRef]
4. Mader, R.; Novofestovski, I.; Adawi, M.; Lavi, I. Metabolic syndrome and cardiovascular risk in patients with diffuse idiopathic skeletal hyperostosis. *Semin. Arthritis Rheum.* **2009**, *38*, 361–365. [CrossRef] [PubMed]
5. Fox, C.S.; Massaro, J.M.; Hoffmann, U.; Pou, K.M.; Maurovich-Horvat, P.; Liu, C.Y.; Vasan, R.S.; Murabito, J.M.; Meigs, J.B.; Cupples, L.A.; et al. Abdominal visceral and subcutaneous adipose tissue compartments: Association with metabolic risk factors in the Framingham Heart Study. *Circulation* **2007**, *116*, 39–48. [CrossRef] [PubMed]
6. Ritchie, S.A.; Connell, J.M. The link between abdominal obesity, metabolic syndrome and cardiovascular disease. *Nutr. Metab. Cardiovasc. Dis.* **2007**, *17*, 319–326. [CrossRef]
7. Oh, T.H.; Byeon, J.S.; Myung, S.J.; Yang, S.K.; Choi, K.S.; Chung, J.W.; Kim, B.; Lee, D.; Byun, J.H.; Jang, S.J.; et al. Visceral obesity as a risk factor for colorectal neoplasm. *J. Gastroenterol. Hepatol.* **2008**, *23*, 411–417. [CrossRef]
8. Foster, M.T.; Pagliassotti, M.J. Metabolic alterations following visceral fat removal and expansion: Beyond anatomic location. *Adipocyte* **2012**, *1*, 192–199. [CrossRef]
9. Shuster, A.; Patlas, M.; Pinthus, J.H.; Mourtzakis, M. The clinical importance of visceral adiposity: A critical review of methods for visceral adipose tissue analysis. *Br. J. Radiol.* **2012**, *85*, 1–10. [CrossRef] [PubMed]
10. Simons, P.C.; Algra, A.; van de Laak, M.F.; Grobbee, D.E.; van der Graaf, Y. Second manifestations of ARTerial disease (SMART) study: Rationale and design. *Eur. J. Epidemiol.* **1999**, *15*, 773–781. [CrossRef]
11. Resnick, D.; Niwayama, G. Radiographic and pathologic features of spinal involvement in diffuse idiopathic skeletal hyperostosis (DISH). *Radiology* **1976**, *119*, 559–568. [CrossRef]
12. Stolk, R.P.; Wink, O.; Zelissen, P.M.; Meijer, R.; van Gils, A.P.; Grobbee, D.E. Validity and reproducibility of ultrasonography for the measurement of intra-abdominal adipose tissue. *Int. J. Obes. Relat. Metab. Disord.* **2001**, *25*, 1346–1351. [CrossRef]
13. Levey, A.S.; Stevens, L.A.; Schmid, C.H.; Zhang, Y.L.; Castro, A.F., III; Feldman, H.I.; Kusek, J.W.; Eggers, P.; Van Lente, F.; Greene, T.; et al. A new equation to estimate glomerular filtration rate. *Ann. Intern. Med.* **2009**, *150*, 604–612. [CrossRef]
14. Rubin, D.B. Inference and missing data. *Biometrika* **1976**, *63*, 581–592. [CrossRef]
15. van Buuren, S.; Groothuis-Oudshoorn, C.G.M. Mice: Multivariate imputation by chained equations. *R. J. Stat. Softw.* **2011**, *45*. [CrossRef]
16. Després, J.P. Cardiovascular disease under the influence of excess visceral fat. *Crit. Pathw. Cardiol.* **2007**, *6*, 51–59. [CrossRef] [PubMed]
17. Denko, C.W.; Boja, B.; Moskowitz, R.W. Growth promoting peptides in osteoarthritis and diffuse idiopathic skeletal hyperostosis–insulin, insulin-like growth factor-I, growth hormone. *J. Rheumatol.* **1994**, *21*, 1725–1730.
18. Pariente-Rodrigo, E.; Sgaramella, G.A.; Olmos-Martínez, J.M.; Pini-Valdivieso, S.F.; Landeras-Alvaro, R.; Hernández, J.L. Relationship between diffuse idiopathic skeletal hyperostosis, abdominal aortic calcification and associated metabolic disorders: Data from the Camargo Cohort. *Med. Clin. (Barc.)* **2017**, *149*, 196–202. [CrossRef] [PubMed]
19. Katzman, W.B.; Huang, M.H.; Kritz-Silverstein, D.; Barrett-Connor, E.; Kado, D.M. Diffuse idiopathic skeletal hyperostosis (DISH) and impaired physical function: The rancho bernardo study. *J. Am. Geriatr. Soc.* **2017**, *65*, 1476–1481. [CrossRef]
20. Kagotani, R.; Yoshida, M.; Muraki, S.; Oka, H.; Hashizume, H.; Yamada, H.; Enyo, Y.; Nagata, K.; Ishimoto, Y.; Teraguchi, M.; et al. Prevalence of diffuse idiopathic skeletal hyperostosis (DISH) of the whole spine and its association with lumbar spondylosis and knee osteoarthritis: The ROAD study. *J. Bone Min. Metab.* **2015**, *33*, 221–229. [CrossRef]
21. Fujimori, T.; Watabe, T.; Iwamoto, Y.; Hamada, S.; Iwasaki, M.; Oda, T. Prevalence, concomitance, and distribution of ossification of the spinal ligaments: Results of whole spine CT scans in 1500 Japanese patients. *Spine* **2016**, *41*, 1668–1676. [CrossRef]
22. Mader, R.; Novofastovski, I.; Rosner, E.; Adawi, M.; Herer, P.; Buskila, D. Nonarticular tenderness and functional status in patients with diffuse idiopathic skeletal hyperostosis. *J. Rheumatol.* **2010**, *37*, 1911–1916. [CrossRef]
23. Holton, K.F.; Denard, P.J.; Yoo, J.U.; Kado, D.M.; Barrett-Connor, E.; Marshall, L.M.; Osteoporotic Fractures in men (MrOS) Study Group. Diffuse idiopathic skeletal hyperostosis and its relation to back pain among older men: The MrOS study. *Semin. Arthritis Rheum.* **2011**, *41*, 131–138. [CrossRef]
24. Asher, J.; Houston, M. Statins and C-reactive protein levels. *J. Clin. Hypertens. (Greenwich)* **2007**, *9*, 622–628. [CrossRef]

25. Dan, L.C.; Herman, A.; Verlaan, J.J.; Stern, M.; Mader, R.; Eshed, I. Abdominal fat distribution in diffuse idiopathic skeletal hyperostosis and ankylosing spondylitis patients compared to controls. *Clin. Radiol.* **2018**, *73*, e15–e910.e20.
26. Okada, E.; Ishihara, S.; Azuma, K.; Michikawa, T.; Suzuki, S.; Tsuji, O.; Nori, S.; Nagoshi, N.; Yagi, M.; Takayama, M.; et al. Metabolic syndrome is a predisposing factor for diffuse idiopathic skeletal hyperostosis. *Neurospine* **2020**, *18*, 109–116. [CrossRef]
27. Onat, A.; Avci, G.S.; Barlan, M.M.; Uyarel, H.; Uzunlar, B.; Sansoy, V. Measures of abdominal obesity assessed for visceral adiposity and relation to coronary risk. *Int. J. Obes. Relat. Metab. Disord.* **2004**, *28*, 1018–1025. [CrossRef]
28. Seidell, J.C.; Oosterlee, A.; Deurenberg, P.; Hautvast, J.G.; Ruijs, J.H. Abdominal fat depots measured with computed tomography: Effects of degree of obesity, sex, and age. *Eur. J. Clin. Nutr.* **1988**, *42*, 805–815.
29. Kwon, H.; Kim, D.; Kim, J.S. Body fat distribution and the risk of incident metabolic syndrome: A longitudinal cohort study. *Sci. Rep.* **2017**, *7*, 10955. [CrossRef]
30. Tenti, S.; Palmitesta, P.; Giordano, N.; Galeazzi, M.; Fioravanti, A. Increased serum leptin and visfatin levels in patients with diffuse idiopathic skeletal hyperostosis: A comparative study. *Scand. J. Rheumatol.* **2017**, *46*, 156–158. [CrossRef]
31. Mader, R.; Novofastovski, I.; Schwartz, N.; Rosner, E. Serum adiponectin levels in patients with diffuse idiopathic skeletal hyperostosis (DISH). *Clin. Rheumatol.* **2018**, *37*, 2839–2845. [CrossRef]
32. Shirakura, Y.; Sugiyama, T.; Tanaka, H.; Taguchi, T.; Kawai, S. Hyperleptinemia in female patients with ossification of spinal ligaments. *Biochem. Biophys. Res. Commun.* **2000**, *267*, 752–755. [CrossRef] [PubMed]
33. Upadhyay, J.; Farr, O.M.; Mantzoros, C.S. The role of leptin in regulating bone metabolism. *Metabolism* **2015**, *64*, 105–113. [CrossRef] [PubMed]
34. Mader, R.; Pappone, N.; Baraliakos, X.; Eshed, I.; Sarzi-Puttini, P.; Atzeni, F.; Bieber, A.; Novofastovski, I.; Kiefer, D.; Verlaan, J.-J.; et al. Diffuse idiopathic skeletal hyperostosis (DISH) and a possible inflammatory component. *Curr. Rheumatol. Rep.* **2021**, *23*, 6. [CrossRef] [PubMed]

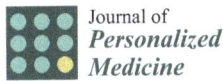

Article

Evaluation of Scalability and Degree of Fine-Tuning of Deep Convolutional Neural Networks for COVID-19 Screening on Chest X-ray Images Using Explainable Deep-Learning Algorithm

Ki-Sun Lee [1,*,†], Jae Young Kim [1,†], Eun-tae Jeon [1], Won Suk Choi [2], Nan Hee Kim [3] and Ki Yeol Lee [4]

1. Medical Science Research Center, Ansan Hospital, Korea University College of Medicine, Ansan si 15355, Korea; jaykim830@gmail.com (J.Y.K.); gksmfskdls@gmail.com (E.-t.J.)
2. Division of Infectious Diseases, Department of Internal Medicine, Ansan Hospital, Korea University College of Medicine, Ansan si 15355, Korea; cmcws@hanmail.net
3. Division of Endocrinology and Metabolism, Department of Internal Medicine, Ansan Hospital, Korea University College of Medicine, Ansan si 15355, Korea; nhkendo@gmail.com
4. Department of Radiology, Ansan Hospital, Korea University College of Medicine, Ansan si 15355, Korea; kiylee@korea.ac.kr
* Correspondence: kisuns@gmail.com
† These authors are co-first authors.

Received: 22 October 2020; Accepted: 30 October 2020; Published: 7 November 2020

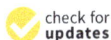

Abstract: According to recent studies, patients with COVID-19 have different feature characteristics on chest X-ray (CXR) than those with other lung diseases. This study aimed at evaluating the layer depths and degree of fine-tuning on transfer learning with a deep convolutional neural network (CNN)-based COVID-19 screening in CXR to identify efficient transfer learning strategies. The CXR images used in this study were collected from publicly available repositories, and the collected images were classified into three classes: COVID-19, pneumonia, and normal. To evaluate the effect of layer depths of the same CNN architecture, CNNs called VGG-16 and VGG-19 were used as backbone networks. Then, each backbone network was trained with different degrees of fine-tuning and comparatively evaluated. The experimental results showed the highest AUC value to be 0.950 concerning COVID-19 classification in the experimental group of a fine-tuned with only 2/5 blocks of the VGG16 backbone network. In conclusion, in the classification of medical images with a limited number of data, a deeper layer depth may not guarantee better results. In addition, even if the same pre-trained CNN architecture is used, an appropriate degree of fine-tuning can help to build an efficient deep learning model.

Keywords: COVID-19; chest X-ray; deep learning; convolutional neural network; Grad-CAM

1. Introduction

CORONAVIRUS disease (COVID-19) has quickly become a global pandemic since it was first reported in December 2019, reaching approximately 21.3 million confirmed cases and 761,799 deaths as of 16 August 2020 [1]. Due to the highly infectious nature and unavailability of appropriate treatments and vaccines for the virus, early screening of COVID-19 is crucial to prevent the spread of the disease by the timely isolation of susceptive individuals and the proper allocation of limited medical resources.

Currently, reverse transcription polymerase chain reaction (RT-PCR) was introduced as the gold standard screening method for COVID-19 [2]. However, since the overall positive rate of RT-PCR, using nasal and throat swabs, is reported to be 60–70% [3], there is a risk that a false-negative patient may again act as another source of infection in a healthy community. Conversely, there have been reports of high sensitivity to COVID-19 screening in radiological tests such as chest computed tomography or chest X-ray (CXR) [3–5]. According to the reports on CXR characteristics of patients confirmed as the COVID-19 case, it demonstrated multi-lobar involvement and peripheral airspace opacities, which was most frequently demonstrated as ground-glass [6]. However, in the early stages of COVID-19, this ground-glass pattern may appear at the edges of the lung vessels, or as asymmetric diffused airspace opacities [7], it can be difficult to visually detect the characteristic patterns of COVID-19 from X-rays. Therefore, considering the fact that the number of suspected patients increases exponentially in contrast to the limited number of highly trained radiologists, the diagnostic supporting procedures, using an automated screening algorithm with a producing objective, reproducible, and scalable results, can speed up earlier precise diagnosis.

In recent years, deep learning (DL) technology, a specific field of artificial intelligence (AI) technology, has made remarkable advances in medical image analysis and diagnosis, and is considered to be a potentially powerful tool to solve such problems [8,9]. Despite the lack of available published data to date, DL approaches for the diagnosis of COVID-19 from CXR have been actively studied [10–17]. Because the available data are limited, previous research has focused on creating a new DL architecture based on deep convolutional neural networks (CNNs) for providing effective diagnosis algorithms. However, previous studies have focused only on the efficacy of the newly created network through comparison between different CNNs, so the effect of the layer depth, called scalability, and degree of fine-tuning of transfer learning with CNN has not been comparatively studied. Therefore, the main objective of this study was to further investigate the effect of layer depth on the same CNN architecture, and the degree of fine-tuning of transfer learning with the same CNN at the same hyper-parameters. Furthermore, by employing the gradient-weighted class activation map (Grad-CAM) [18,19], this study provided a visual interpretation explaining the feature characteristic region that the DL model has the most influence on classification prediction.

2. Materials and Methods

2.1. Experimental Design

The overall experimental steps and experimental groups used in this study are shown in Figure 1. The experiment consisted of 12 experimental subgroups. To evaluate the scalability of the same CNN architecture, the experiment consisted of two main groups according to the layer depths of each CNN. Each CNN main group is divided into 6 subgroups according to the degree of fine-tuning.

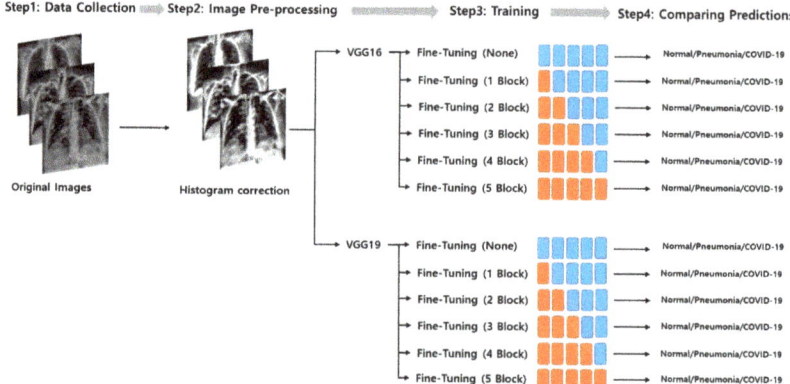

Figure 1. The experiment consists of a total of 12 experimental subgroups. It is largely divided into two main groups according to the layer depths, and each convolutional neural network (CNN) subgroup is divided into 6 subgroups according to the degree of fine-tuning.

2.2. Datasets

The datasets used for classification are described in Table 1. Several publicly available image data repositories have been used to collect COVID-19 chest-ray images. Normal and pneumonia samples were extracted from the open source NIH chest X-ray dataset used for the Radiological Society of North America (RSNA) pneumonia detection challenge [20]. The total dataset was curated into three classes: normal, pneumonia, and COVID-19. Since the balance of data for each class is a very important factor in classification analysis, this study randomly extracted the images of other classes according to the number of COVID-19 images that can be obtained as much as possible.

Table 1. Description of datasets for COVID-19 classification.

Class	Reference	Samples
Normal	RSNA pneumonia detection challenge [20]	607
Pneumonia	RSNA pneumonia detection challenge [20]	607
COVID-19	COVID-19 image data collection [21]	468
	Figure 1 COVID-19 Chest X-ray [22]	35
	Actualmed COVID-19 Chest X-rays [23]	58
	COVID-19 Radiography Database [24]	46
Total		1821

The entire dataset was combined with 607 COVID-19 image data publicly shared at the time of the study, as well as 607 normal and 607 pneumonia chest radiographs randomly extracted from the RSNA Pneumonia Detection Challenge dataset, resulting in 1821 data being combined. In the case of the COVID-19 dataset, four public datasets were used, and only one image was used when the source of the image was duplicated. In the public datasets used in the experiment, patient information was de-identified or not provided.

The entire collected dataset was randomly divided into a training and testing ratio of 80:20 for each class, and training data were also randomly divided by a training and validation ratio of 80:20 for use in the 5-fold cross validation.

2.3. Image Preprocessing

Because the image data used in this experiment were collected from multiple centers, most of the images have different contrast and dimensions. Therefore, all images used in this study required contrast correction through the histogram equalization technique and resizing to a uniform size before the experiment. In this study, preprocessing was performed using the contrast limited adaptive histogram equalization (CLAHE) technique [25], which has been adopted in previous studies related to lung segmentation and pneumonia classification [26–28]. Figure 2 shows sample images with CXR contrast corrected using the CLAHE technique. For the consistency of image analysis, each image was resized to a uniform size of 800 × 800.

2.4. Convolutional Neural Networks

This study employed two different deep CNNs as backbone networks: VGG-16 and VGG-19. VGG [29] is a pre-trained CNN, from the Visual Geometry Group, Department of Engineering Science, University of Oxford. The numbers 16 and 19 represent the number of layers with trainable weights of VGG networks. VGG architecture had been widely adopted and recognized as a state of the art in both general and medical image classification tasks [30]. Since VGG-16 and VGG-19 have the same neural network architecture but different layer depths, a comparative evaluation of performance according to the degree of layer depths can be performed under the same architectural condition.

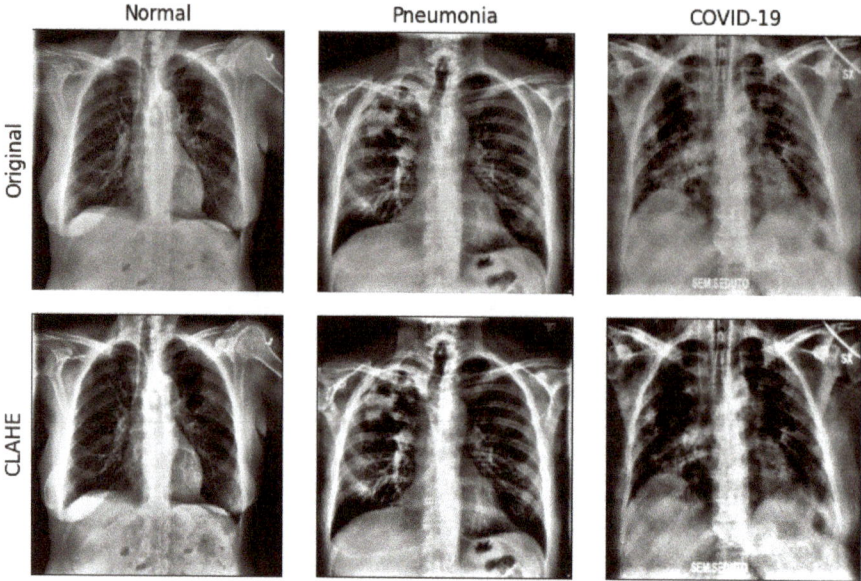

Figure 2. Sample images after applying contrast correction by contrast limited adaptive histogram equalization (CLAHE) and the semantic segmentation of lung on original chest X-ray (CXR) images.

2.5. Fine-Tuning

When the training dataset is relatively small, transferring a network pre-trained on a large annotated dataset and fine-tuning it for a specific task can be an efficient way to achieve acceptable accuracy and less training time [31]. Although the classification of diseases from CXR images differs from object classification and natural images, they can share similar learned features [32]. During the fine-tuning of transfer learning with deep CNNs, model weights were initialized based on pre-training on a general image dataset, except that some of the last blocks were unfrozen so that their weights were updated in each training step. In this study, the VGG-16 and VGG-19, used in this study as a backbone neural network, consist of 5 blocks regardless of the network layer depth. Therefore, fine-tuning was performed in a total of 6 steps in a manner that was unfrozen sequentially from 0 to 5 blocks starting from the last block, depending on how many blocks were unfrozen. As a result, VGG-16 and VGG-19 were used as backbone networks, and each deep CNN was divided into 6 subgroups according to the degree of fine-tuning. Figure 3 shows the schematic diagrams of the layer composition and the degree of fine-tuning of VGG-16 and VGG-19.

2.6. Training

The 1458 images selected as the training dataset were randomly divided into five folds. This was done to perform 5-fold cross validation to evaluate the model training, while avoiding overfitting or bias [33–35]. Within each fold, the dataset was partitioned into independent training and validation sets using an 80 to 20% split. The selected validation set was a completely independent fold from the other training folds and was used to evaluate the training status during the training. After one model training step was completed, the other independent fold was used as a validation set and the previous validation set was reused as part of the training set to evaluate the model training. An overview of the 5-fold cross validation performed in this study is presented in Figure 4. As an additional method to prevent overfitting, drop out was applied to the last fully connected layers, and early stopping was also applied by monitoring the validation loss at each epoch.

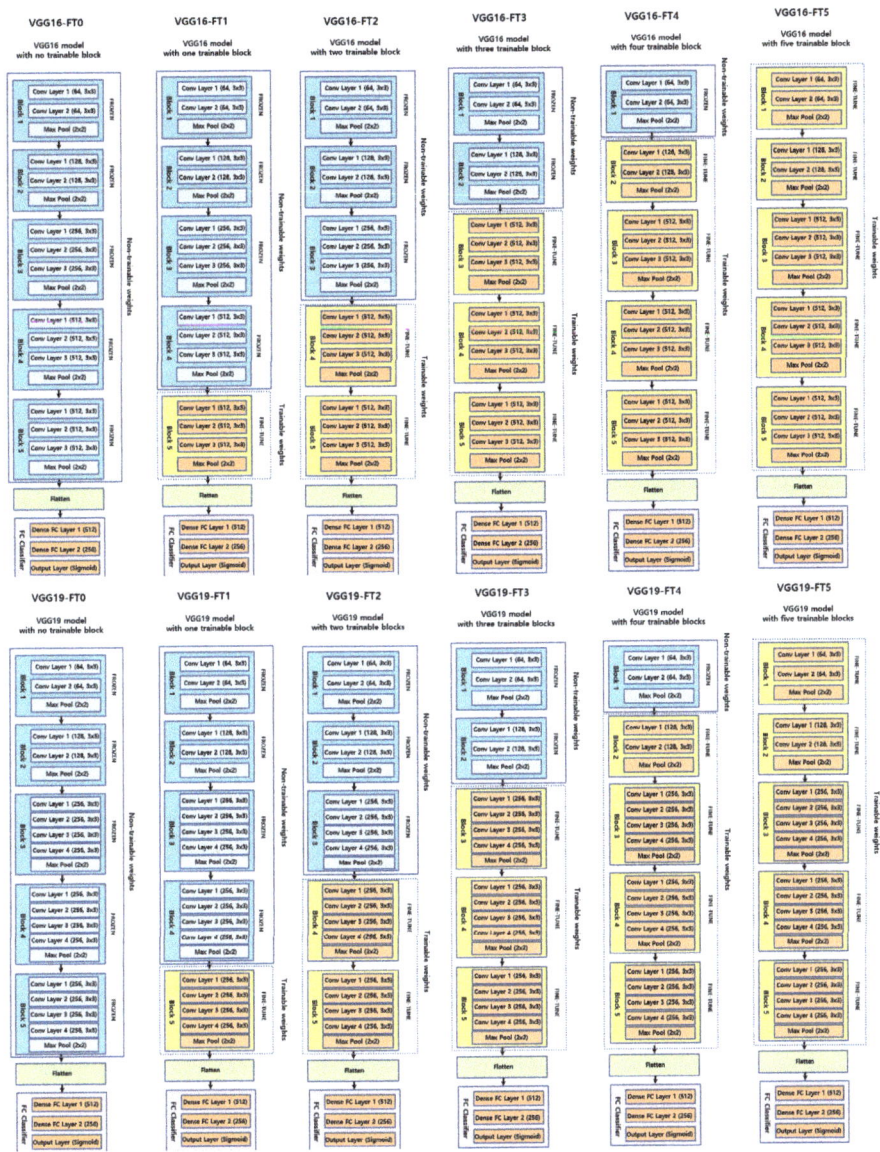

Figure 3. Schematic diagram of 12 experimental groups according to the degree of fine-tuning in the VGG-16 (**top**) and VGG-19 (**bottom**) backbone neural networks.

The above training process was repeated for all 24 experimental groups (Figure 1). All deep CNN models were trained and evaluated on an NVIDIA DGX Station™ (NVIDIA Corp., Santa Clara, CA, USA) with an Ubuntu 18 operating system, 256 GB system memory, and four NVIDIA Telsa V100 GPU. The building, training, validation, and prediction of DL models were performed using the Keras [36] library and TensorFlow [37] backend engine. The initial training rate of each model was 0.00001. A ReduceLROn-Plateau method was employed because it reduces the learning rate when it stops improving the training performance. The RMSprop algorithm was used as the solver.

After training all the 5-fold deep CNN models, the best model was identified by testing with the test dataset.

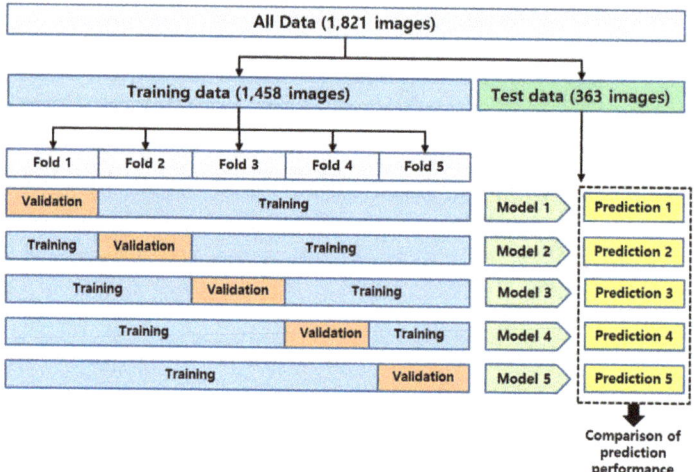

Figure 4. The overview of the 5-fold cross validation applied in this study.

2.7. Performance Evaluation

To comprehensively evaluate the screening performance on the test dataset, the accuracy, sensitivity, specificity, receiver operating characteristic (ROC) curve, and precision recall (PR) curve were calculated. The accuracy, sensitivity, and specificity score can be calculated as follows:

$$\text{Accuracy} = \frac{TP + TN}{TP + TN + FN + FP}$$

$$\text{Sensitivity} = \frac{TP}{TP + FN}$$

$$\text{Specificity} = \frac{TN}{TN + FP}.$$

TP and FP are the number of correctly and incorrectly predicted images, respectively. Similarly, TN and FN represent the number of correctly and incorrectly predicted images, respectively. The area under the ROC curve (AUC) was also calculated in this study.

2.8. Interpretation of Model Prediction

Because it is difficult to know the process of how deep CNNs make predictions, DL models have often been referred to as non-interpretable black boxes. To determine the decision-making process of the model, and which features are most important for the model to screen COVID-19 in CXR images, this study employed the gradient-weighted class activation mapping technique (Grad-CAM) [18,19] so that the most significant regions for screening COVID-19 in CXR images were highlighted.

3. Results

3.1. Classification Performance

Table 2 summarizes the classification performance of the three classes, normal (N), pneumonia (P), and COVID-19 (C), for each experimental group.

Table 2. Performance metrics of experimental groups where N, P and C are normal, pneumonia and COVID-19, respectively.

CNN Models	Number of Fine-Tuning Blocks		Accuracy	Specificity	Sensitivity	AUC
VGG-16	0	N	0.871	0.909	0.793	0.851
		P	0.832	0.814	0.868	0.841
		C	0.906	0.883	0.752	0.868
	1	N	0.873	0.884	0.851	0.868
		P	0.884	0.913	0.826	0.870
		C	0.945	0.979	0.876	0.928
	2	N	0.901	0.930	0.842	0.886
		P	0.909	0.921	0.884	0.903
		C	0.959	0.975	0.925	0.950
	3	N	0.884	0.888	0.876	0.882
		P	0.884	0.909	0.835	0.872
		C	0.939	0.983	0.851	0.917
	4	N	0.901	0.934	0.835	0.884
		P	0.862	0.847	0.893	0.870
		C	0.928	0.988	0.810	0.899
	5	N	0.873	0.905	0.810	0.857
		P	0.796	0.748	0.893	0.820
		C	0.857	0.992	0.587	0.789
VGG-19	0	N	0.873	0.971	0.678	0.824
		P	0.804	0.777	0.860	0.818
		C	0.904	0.938	0.835	0.886
	1	N	0.893	0.913	0.851	0.882
		P	0.857	0.893	0.785	0.836
		C	0.926	0.950	0.876	0.913
	2	N	0.882	0.909	0.826	0.868
		P	0.868	0.905	0.793	0.849
		C	0.937	0.950	0.909	0.930
	3	N	0.879	0.897	0.843	0.870
		P	0.847	0.876	0.777	0.826
		C	0.920	0.959	0.843	0.901
	4	N	0.860	0.872	0.835	0.853
		P	0.840	0.876	0.769	0.822
		C	0.915	0.963	0.818	0.890
	5	N	0.862	0.864	0.860	0.862
		P	0.835	0.888	0.727	0.808
		C	0.912	0.955	0.826	0.890

Compared with all the tested deep CNN models, the fine-tuned with two blocks of the VGG-16 (VGG16-FT2) model achieved the highest performance in terms of the COVID-19 classification of accuracy (95.9%), specificity (97.5%), sensitivity (92.5%), and AUC (0.950). For all the tested deep CNNs, fine-tuning the last two convolutional blocks presented a higher classification performance compared to the fine-tuning of the other number of convolutional blocks. In addition, the case of all untrainable convolutional blocks without fine-tuning, regardless of the scalability of the backbone network, showed the lowest classification. Generally, the fine-tuned models using VGG16 as a backbone architecture were better than those using VGG19.

Figure 5 shows how the number of fine-tuned deep CNN blocks influences the classification performance in terms of the accuracy of COVID-19 screening. In this figure, the classification performance was not proportionately dependent on the degree of fine-tuning with the base model. There was a decrease in classification accuracy when more than three convolutional blocks of all deep CNNs were used. In addition, regardless of the number of fine-tuned blocks, the VGG19 models with more convolutional layers had lower classification accuracy than the VGG16 models. The confusion matrix and ROC of VGG16-FT2 achieving the highest performance in multi-class classification are presented in Figures 6 and 7.

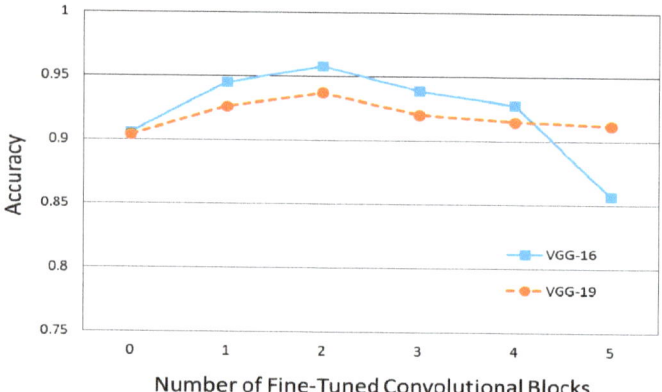

Figure 5. COVID-19 classification performance versus the number of fine-tuned convolutional blocks.

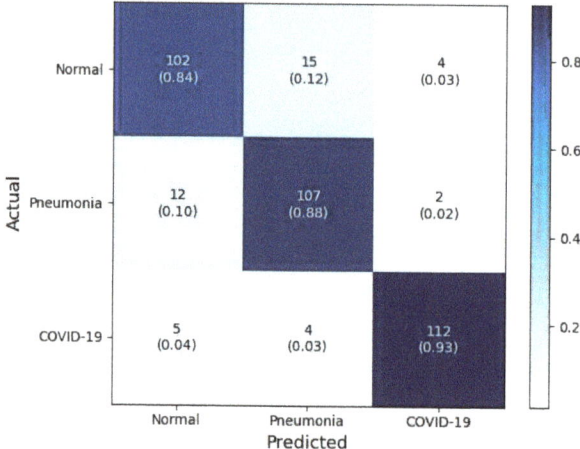

Figure 6. Confusion matrix of the best performed classification model (VGG16-FT2) in this study.

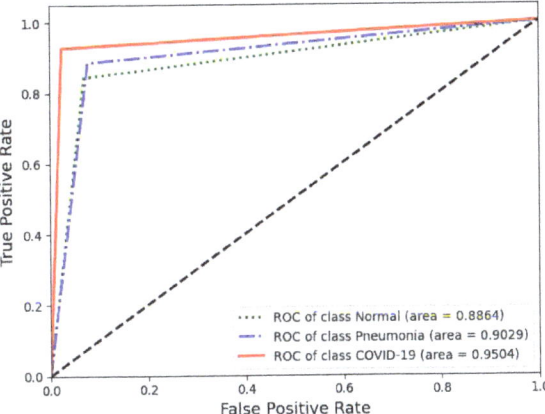

Figure 7. Receiver operating characteristics (ROC) curve of the best performing classification model (VGG16-FT2) in this study.

3.2. Interpretation of Model Decision Using Grad-CAM

Figures 8–10 show examples of a visualized interpretation of predictions using deep CNN models in this study. In each example, the color heat map presented which areas were most affected by the classification of the deep CNN model.

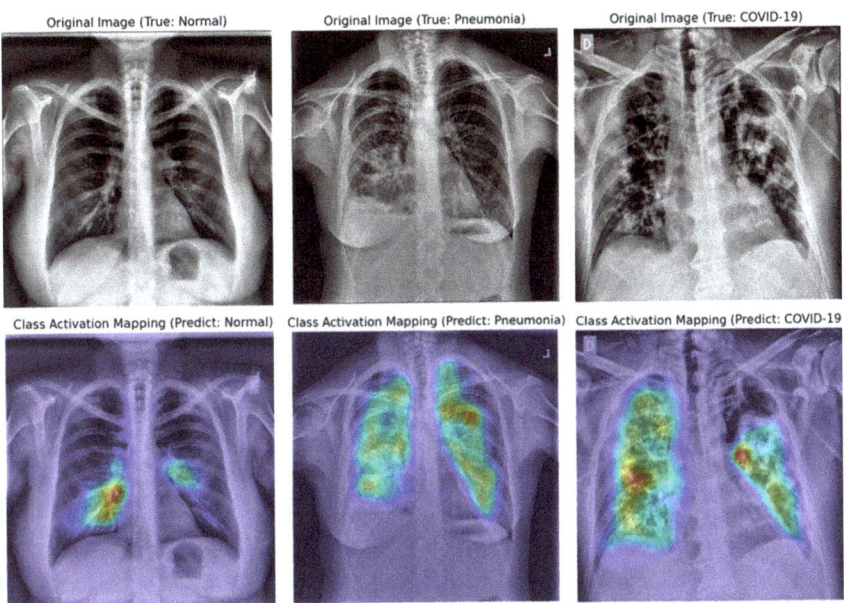

Figure 8. Samples of original and gradient-weighted class activation mapping technique (Grad-CAM) images were correctly predicted by the best performing classification model (VGG16-FT2) in this study.

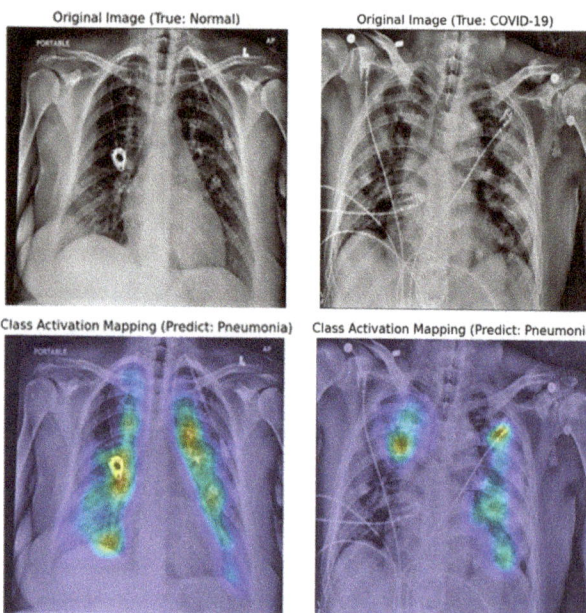

Figure 9. Original and Grad-CAM sample images presumed to be misclassified according to the wrong reason by the best performing classification model in this study (VGG16-FT2).

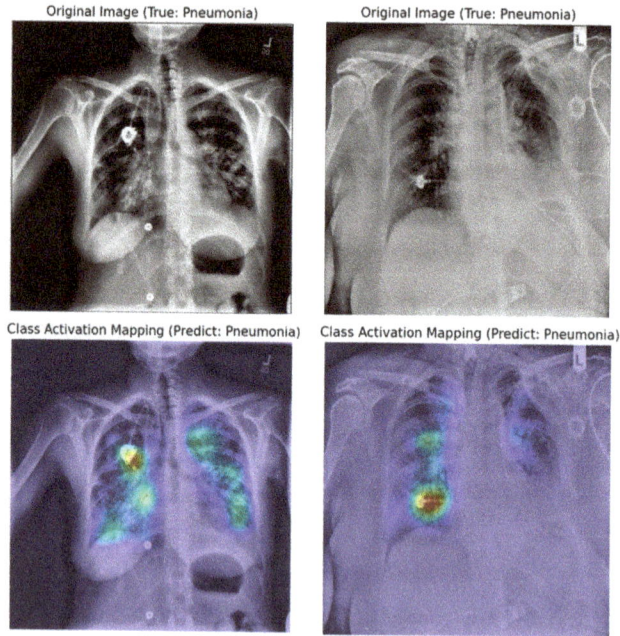

Figure 10. Original and Grad-CAM sample images presumed to be correctly classified according to the wrong reason by the best performing classification model in this study (VGG16-FT2).

Figure 8 shows representative examples of correctly classified cases for each of the three classes (normal, pneumonia, and COVID-19) in the VGG16-TF2 experimental group that showed the highest classification performance. Through the Grad-CAM result in Figure 8, it is possible to identify the significant region where the difference in CXR image features of each of the three classes is made. Figures 9 and 10 show representative examples of wrong and right classifications based on the wrong reasons. In most cases where classification has occurred based on the wrong reason, there is a foreign body in the chest cavity of the CXR image.

4. Discussion

In addition to the long-term sustainability of the COVID-19 pandemic and symptom similarity with other pneumonia diseases, the limited medical resources and lack of expert radiologists have greatly increased the importance of screening for COVID-19 from CXR images for the right concentration of medical resources and isolation of potential patients. To overcome these limitations, various cutting-edge artificial intelligence (AI) technologies have been applied to screen COVID-19 from various medical data. Accordingly, until recently, numerous new DL models, such as COVID-Net [10], Deep-COVID [16], CVDNet [38], and Covid-resnet [13], to classify COVID-19 through publicly shared CXR images have been proposed, or mutual comparison studies through the transfer learning of various pre-trained DL models have been presented [39,40]. These previous papers showed high accuracy of more than 95%. However, most of them performed transfer learning but did not mention the specific degree of fine-tuning. It is also rare to have a qualitative evaluation. As a result, it is often difficult to reproduce a similar degree of accuracy with the same pre-trained DL model. Therefore, in the present study, the effects of the degree of fine-tuning and layer depths on deep CNNs for the screening performance of COVID-19 from CXR images were evaluated. Furthermore, these influences were visually interpreted using the Grad-CAM technique.

4.1. Scalability of Deep CNN

It is known that the VGG architecture used as the deep CNN backbone network in this experiment does not leverage residual principles, has a lightweight design, and low architectural diversity, so it is convenient to fine-tune [10]. In particular, the VGG-16 and VGG-19 used in this study have the same architecture with five convolutional blocks; however, the depth of the layers of VGG-19 is deeper than that of VGG-16 (Figure 3).

According to Table 2 and Figure 5, the overall classification performance of VGG-16 was higher than that of VGG-19, regardless of the fine-tuning degree. These results are similar to the fact that the latest deep neural networks do not guarantee higher accuracy in the classification of medical images such as CXR images, as in other previous research papers [39]. It can be considered that in the case of medical images requiring less than 10 classifications, deep CNNs with low scalability can show better performance, unlike the classification of general objects that require more than 1000 classifications.

4.2. Degree of Fine-Tuning of Deep CNN

In general, the deep CNN model learned from pre-trained deep neural networks on a large natural image dataset which could be used to classify common images but cannot be well utilized for specific classifying tasks of medical images. However, according to a previous study that described the effects and mechanisms of fine-tuning on deep CNNs, when certain convolutional blocks of a deep CNN model were fine-tuned, the deep CNN model could be further specialized for specific classifying tasks [32,41]. More specifically, the earlier layers of a deep CNN contain generic features that should be useful for many classification tasks; however, later layers progressively contain more specialized features to the details of the classes contained in the original dataset. Using this property, when the parameters of the early layers are preserved and that in later layers are updated during the training of new datasets, the deep CNN model can be effectively used in new classification tasks. In conclusion, fine-tuning uses the parameters learned from a previous training of the network on a large dataset, and then adjusts the parameters in later layers from the new dataset, improving the performance and accuracy in the new classification task.

As far as the authors know, there has been no previous research paper evaluating the accuracy of COVID-19 screening according to the degree of fine-tuning. According to Figure 5, regardless of the scalability of VGG, classification accuracy increases as the degree of fine-tuning increases; however, the fine-tuning of more than a certain convolutional block (more than 3 blocks in this experiment) decrease the classification accuracy. Therefore, it seems necessary to find the appropriate degree of fine-tuning by judging the degree of fine-tuning in the transfer learning by a hyper-parametric variable such as batch-size or learning rate in DL.

4.3. Visual Interpretation Using Grad-CAM

Grad-CAM uses the gradient information flowing into the last convolutional layer of the deep CNN to understand the significance of each neuron for making decisions [18]. In this experiment, a qualitative evaluation of classification adequacy was performed using the Grad-CAM technique. In the case of the deep CNN model, which showed the best classification as shown in Figure 8, image feature points for each class were specified within the lung cavity in CXR images. However, as shown in Figure 9, if there is a foreign substance in the lung cavity in a CXR image, it can be classified incorrectly. Moreover, even if a CXR image is correctly classified, it can be classified for an incorrect reason as shown in Figure 10. In the CXR image analysis using the DL algorithm, the implanted port catheter and pacemaker or defibrillator generator have shown similar results to the previous studies that interfere with the performance of the DL algorithm by causing false positives or false negatives [42]. This shows the pure function of the Grad-CAM technique and suggests candidate areas to be excluded through image preprocessing for areas or foreign body subjects that affect classification accuracy improvement on the image.

5. Conclusions

This experiment showed the appropriate transfer learning strategy of a deep CNN to screen for COVID-19 in CXR images as follows. In using the deep CNNs for COVID-19 screening in CXR images, it is not always guaranteed to achieve cutting-edge results, increasing their complexity and layer depth. In addition, when applying transfer learning to a deep CNN for classification, an appropriate degree of fine-tuning is required, and this must also be treated as an important hyper-parametric variable that affects the accuracy of DL. In particular, in the case of image classification using DL, it is also necessary to qualitatively evaluate a classification as to whether an appropriate classification has occurred based on the correct reason, using visual interpretation methods such as the Grad-CAM technique.

Author Contributions: Conceptualization, K.-S.L., J.Y.K., W.S.C., N.H.K. and K.Y.L.; data curation, K.-S.L., J.Y.K. and E.-t.J.; formal analysis, K.-S.L., J.Y.K. and E.-t.J.; funding acquisition, K.-S.L.; investigation, K.-S.L., J.Y.K. and K.Y.L.; methodology, K.-S.L. and E.-t.J.; project administration, K.-S.L. and N.H.K.; resources, N.H.K.; software, K.-S.L. and E.-t.J.; supervision, K.-S.L., J.Y.K. and W.S.C.; validation, J.Y.K., W.S.C., N.H.K. and K.Y.L.; visualization, K.-S.L.; writing—original draft, K.-S.L.; writing—review and editing, K.-S.L., W.S.C., N.H.K. and K.Y.L. All authors have read and agreed to the published version of the manuscript.

Funding: This work was supported by the National Research Foundation of Korea under Grant NRF-2019R1I1A1 A01062961 and a Korea University Ansan Hospital Grant O2000301.

Conflicts of Interest: The authors declare no conflict of interest. The funders had no role in the design of the study; in the collection, analyses, or interpretation of data; in the writing of the manuscript, or in the decision to publish the results.

References

1. World Health Organization. *Coronavirus Disease (COVID-19): Situation Report, 182*; World Health Organization: Geneva, Switzerland, 2020.

2. Wang, W.; Xu, Y.; Gao, R.; Lu, R.; Han, K.; Wu, G.; Tan, W. Detection of SARS-CoV-2 in different types of clinical specimens. *JAMA* **2020**, *323*, 1843–1844. [CrossRef] [PubMed]
3. Yang, Y.; Yang, M.; Shen, C.; Wang, F.; Yuan, J.; Li, J.; Zhang, M.; Wang, Z.; Xing, L.; Wei, J. Laboratory diagnosis and monitoring the viral shedding of 2019-nCoV infections. *MedRxiv* **2020**. [CrossRef]
4. Kanne, J.P.; Little, B.P.; Chung, J.H.; Elicker, B.M.; Ketai, L.H. *Essentials for Radiologists on COVID-19: An Update—Radiology Scientific Expert Panel*; Radiological Society of North America: Oak Brook, IL, USA, 2020.
5. Ai, T.; Yang, Z.; Hou, H.; Zhan, C.; Chen, C.; Lv, W.; Tao, Q.; Sun, Z.; Xia, L. Correlation of chest CT and RT-PCR testing in coronavirus disease 2019 (COVID-19) in China: A report of 1014 cases. *Radiology* **2020**, *296*, 200642. [CrossRef] [PubMed]
6. Kong, W.; Agarwal, P.P. Chest imaging appearance of COVID-19 infection. *Radiol. Cardiothorac. Imaging* **2020**, *2*, e200028. [CrossRef]
7. Rodrigues, J.; Hare, S.; Edey, A.; Devaraj, A.; Jacob, J.; Johnstone, A.; McStay, R.; Nair, A.; Robinson, G. An update on COVID-19 for the radiologist—A British society of Thoracic Imaging statement. *Clin. Radiol.* **2020**, *75*, 323–325. [CrossRef]
8. Zhou, S.K.; Greenspan, H.; Shen, D. *Deep Learning for Medical Image Analysis*; Academic Press: Cambridge, MA, USA, 2017.
9. Shen, D.; Wu, G.; Suk, H.-I. Deep learning in medical image analysis. *Annu. Rev. Biomed. Eng.* **2017**, *19*, 221–248. [CrossRef] [PubMed]
10. Wang, L.; Wong, A. COVID-Net: A Tailored Deep Convolutional Neural Network Design for Detection of COVID-19 Cases from Chest X-ray Images. *arXiv* **2020**, arXiv:2003.09871.
11. Narin, A.; Kaya, C.; Pamuk, Z. Automatic detection of coronavirus disease (covid-19) using X-ray images and deep convolutional neural networks. *arXiv* **2020**, arXiv:2003.10849.
12. Hemdan, E.E.-D.; Shouman, M.A.; Karar, M.E. Covidx-net: A framework of deep learning classifiers to diagnose covid-19 in X-ray images. *arXiv* **2020**, arXiv:2003.11055.
13. Farooq, M.; Hafeez, A. Covid-resnet: A deep learning framework for screening of covid19 from radiographs. *arXiv* **2020**, arXiv:2003.14395.
14. Afshar, P.; Heidarian, S.; Naderkhani, F.; Oikonomou, A.; Plataniotis, K.N.; Mohammadi, A. Covid-caps: A capsule network-based framework for identification of covid-19 cases from X-ray images. *arXiv* **2020**, arXiv:2004.02696. [CrossRef] [PubMed]
15. Oh, Y.; Park, S.; Ye, J.C. Deep learning covid-19 features on cxr using limited training data sets. *IEEE Trans. Med Imaging* **2020**, *39*, 2688–2700. [CrossRef] [PubMed]
16. Minaee, S.; Kafieh, R.; Sonka, M.; Yazdani, S.; Jamalipour Soufi, G. Deep-COVID: Predicting COVID-19 from chest X-ray images using deep transfer learning. *Med. Image Anal.* **2020**, *65*, 101794. [CrossRef] [PubMed]
17. Apostolopoulos, I.D.; Mpesiana, T.A. Covid-19: Automatic detection from X-ray images utilizing transfer learning with convolutional neural networks. *Phys. Eng. Sci. Med.* **2020**, *43*, 635–640. [CrossRef]
18. Selvaraju, R.R.; Cogswell, M.; Das, A.; Vedantam, R.; Parikh, D.; Batra, D. Grad-cam: Visual explanations from deep networks via gradient-based localization. In Proceedings of the IEEE International Conference on Computer Vision, Venice, Italy, 22–29 October 2017; pp. 618–626.
19. Chattopadhay, A.; Sarkar, A.; Howlader, P.; Balasubramanian, V.N. Grad-cam++: Generalized gradient-based visual explanations for deep convolutional networks. In Proceedings of the 2018 IEEE Winter Conference on Applications of Computer Vision (WACV), Lake Tahoe, NV, USA, 12–15 March 2018; pp. 839–847.
20. Radiological Society of North America. *RSNA Pneumonia Detection Challenge*; Radiological Society of North America: Oak Brook, IL, USA, 2018.
21. Cohen, J.P.; Morrison, P.; Dao, L. COVID-19 image data collection. *arXiv* **2020**, arXiv:2003.11597.
22. Chung, A. Figure 1 COVID-19 Chest X-ray Data Initiative. 2020. Available online: https://github.com/agchung/Figure1-COVID-chestxray-dataset (accessed on 4 May 2020).
23. Chung, A. Actualmed COVID-19 Chest X-ray Data Initiative. 2020. Available online: https://github.com/agchung/Actualmed-COVID-chestxray-dataset (accessed on 6 May 2020).
24. Rahman, T.; Chowdhury, M.; Khandakar, A. *COVID-19 Radiography Database*; Kaggle: San Francisco, CA, USA, 2020.
25. Stark, J.A. Adaptive image contrast enhancement using generalizations of histogram equalization. *IEEE Trans. Image Process.* **2000**, *9*, 889–896. [CrossRef] [PubMed]

26. Ferreira, J.R.; Cardenas, D.A.C.; Moreno, R.A.; de Sá Rebelo, M.d.F.; Krieger, J.E.; Gutierrez, M.A. Multi-View Ensemble Convolutional Neural Network to Improve Classification of Pneumonia in Low Contrast Chest X-ray Images. In Proceedings of the 2020 42nd Annual International Conference of the IEEE Engineering in Medicine & Biology Society (EMBC), Montreal, QC, Canada, 20–24 July 2020; pp. 1238–1241.
27. Ntirogiannis, K.; Gatos, B.; Pratikakis, I. A combined approach for the binarization of handwritten document images. *Pattern Recognit. Lett.* **2014**, *35*, 3–15. [CrossRef]
28. Singh, R.K.; Pandey, R.; Babu, R.N. COVIDScreen: Explainable deep learning framework for differential diagnosis of COVID-19 using chest X-Rays. *Res. Sq.* **2020**. [CrossRef]
29. Simonyan, K.; Zisserman, A. Very deep convolutional networks for large-scale image recognition. *arXiv* **2014**, arXiv:1409.1556.
30. Litjens, G.; Kooi, T.; Bejnordi, B.E.; Setio, A.A.A.; Ciompi, F.; Ghafoorian, M.; Van Der Laak, J.A.; Van Ginneken, B.; Sánchez, C.I. A survey on deep learning in medical image analysis. *Med. Image Anal.* **2017**, *42*, 60–88. [CrossRef]
31. Yosinski, J.; Clune, J.; Bengio, Y.; Lipson, H. How transferable are features in deep neural networks? In Proceedings of the Advances in Neural Information Processing Systems (NIPS 2014), Montreal, QC, Canada, 8–13 December 2014; pp. 3320–3328.
32. Pan, S.J.; Yang, Q. A survey on transfer learning. *IEEE Trans. Knowl. Data Eng.* **2009**, *22*, 1345–1359. [CrossRef]
33. Stone, M. Cross-validatory choice and assessment of statistical predictions. *J. R. Stat. Soc. Ser. B Methodol.* **1974**, *36*, 111–133. [CrossRef]
34. Cawley, G.C.; Talbot, N.L. On over-fitting in model selection and subsequent selection bias in performance evaluation. *J. Mach. Learn. Res.* **2010**, *11*, 2079–2107.
35. Steyerberg, E.W.; Harrell, F.E. Prediction models need appropriate internal, internal–external, and external validation. *J. Clin. Epidemiol.* **2016**, *69*, 245–247. [CrossRef]
36. Chollet, F. Keras: The python deep learning library. *ascl*, 2018; ascl: 1806.1022.
37. Abadi, M.; Agarwal, A.; Barham, P.; Brevdo, E.; Chen, Z.; Citro, C.; Corrado, G.S.; Davis, A.; Dean, J.; Devin, M. Tensorflow: Large-scale machine learning on heterogeneous distributed systems. *arXiv* **2016**, arXiv:1603.04467.
38. Ouchicha, C.; Ammor, O.; Meknassi, M. CVDNet: A novel deep learning architecture for detection of coronavirus (Covid-19) from chest X-ray images. *ChaosSolitons Fractals* **2020**, *140*, 110245. [CrossRef]
39. Bressem, K.K.; Adams, L.; Erxleben, C.; Hamm, B.; Niehues, S.; Vahldiek, J. Comparing Different Deep Learning Architectures for Classification of Chest Radiographs. *arXiv* **2020**, arXiv:2002.08991.
40. Marques, G.; Agarwal, D.; de la Torre Díez, I. Automated medical diagnosis of COVID-19 through EfficientNet convolutional neural network. *Appl. Soft Comput.* **2020**, *96*, 106691. [CrossRef]
41. Tajbakhsh, N.; Shin, J.Y.; Gurudu, S.R.; Hurst, R.T.; Kendall, C.B.; Gotway, M.B.; Liang, J. Convolutional neural networks for medical image analysis: Full training or fine tuning? *IEEE Trans. Med. Imaging* **2016**, *35*, 1299–1312. [CrossRef]
42. Singh, R.; Kalra, M.K.; Nitiwarangkul, C.; Patti, J.A.; Homayounieh, F.; Padole, A.; Rao, P.; Putha, P.; Muse, V.V.; Sharma, A. Deep learning in chest radiography: Detection of findings and presence of change. *PLoS ONE* **2018**, *13*, e0204155. [CrossRef] [PubMed]

Publisher's Note: MDPI stays neutral with regard to jurisdictional claims in published maps and institutional affiliations.

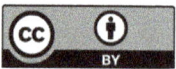

© 2020 by the authors. Licensee MDPI, Basel, Switzerland. This article is an open access article distributed under the terms and conditions of the Creative Commons Attribution (CC BY) license (http://creativecommons.org/licenses/by/4.0/).

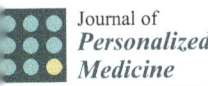

Article

Towards Personalised Contrast Injection: Artificial-Intelligence-Derived Body Composition and Liver Enhancement in Computed Tomography

Daan J. de Jong [1], Wouter B. Veldhuis [1], Frank J. Wessels [1], Bob de Vos [2], Pim Moeskops [2] and Madeleine Kok [1,*]

1. Department of Radiology, University Medical Center Utrecht, Heilberglaan 100, 3584 CX Utrecht, The Netherlands; d.j.dejong4@students.uu.nl (D.J.d.J.); W.Veldhuis@umcutrecht.nl (W.B.V.); f.j.wessels-3@umcutrecht.nl (F.J.W.)
2. Quantib-U, Padualaan 8, 3584 CH Utrecht, The Netherlands; b.devos@quantib.com (B.d.V.); p.moeskops@quantib.com (P.M.)
* Correspondence: m.kok-16@umcutrecht.nl; Tel.: +31-88-75555-55

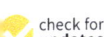

Citation: de Jong, D.J.; Veldhuis, W.B.; Wessels, F.J.; de Vos, B.; Moeskops, P.; Kok, M. Towards Personalised Contrast Injection: Artificial-Intelligence-Derived Body Composition and Liver Enhancement in Computed Tomography. *J. Pers. Med.* **2021**, *11*, 159. https://doi.org/10.3390/jpm11030159

Academic Editors: Pim A. de Jong, Wouter Foppen and Nelleke Tolboom

Received: 12 December 2020
Accepted: 18 February 2021
Published: 24 February 2021

Publisher's Note: MDPI stays neutral with regard to jurisdictional claims in published maps and institutional affiliations.

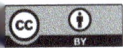

Copyright: © 2021 by the authors. Licensee MDPI, Basel, Switzerland. This article is an open access article distributed under the terms and conditions of the Creative Commons Attribution (CC BY) license (https://creativecommons.org/licenses/by/4.0/).

Abstract: In contrast-enhanced computed tomography, total body weight adapted contrast injection protocols have proven successful in achieving a homogeneous enhancement of vascular structures and liver parenchyma. However, because solid organs have greater perfusion than adipose tissue, the lean body weight (fat-free mass) rather than the total body weight is theorised to cause even more homogeneous enhancement. We included 102 consecutive patients who underwent a multiphase abdominal computed tomography between March 2016 and October 2019. Patients received contrast media (300 mgI/mL) according to bodyweight categories. Using regions of interest, we measured the Hounsfield unit (HU) increase in liver attenuation from unenhanced to contrast-enhanced computed tomography. Furthermore, subjective image quality was graded using a four-point Likert scale. An artificial intelligence algorithm automatically segmented and determined the body compositions and calculated the percentages of lean body weight. The hepatic enhancements were adjusted for iodine dose and iodine dose per total body weight, as well as percentage lean body weight. The associations between enhancement and total body weight, body mass index, and lean body weight were analysed using linear regression. Patients had a median age of 68 years (IQR: 58–74), a total body weight of 81 kg (IQR: 73–90), a body mass index of 26 kg/m^2 (SD: ±4.2), and a lean body weight percentage of 50% (IQR: 36–55). Mean liver enhancements in the portal venous phase were 61 ± 12 HU (≤70 kg), 53 ± 10 HU (70–90 kg), and 53 ± 7 HU (≥90 kg). The majority (93%) of scans were rated as good or excellent. Regression analysis showed significant correlations between liver enhancement corrected for injected total iodine and total body weight ($r = 0.53$; $p < 0.001$) and between liver enhancement corrected for lean body weight and the percentage of lean body weight ($r = 0.73$; $p < 0.001$). Most benefits from personalising iodine injection using %LBW additive to total body weight would be achieved in patients under 90 kg. Liver enhancement is more strongly associated with the percentage of lean body weight than with the total body weight or body mass index. The observed variation in liver enhancement might be reduced by a personalised injection based on the artificial-intelligence-determined percentage of lean body weight.

Keywords: computed tomography; artificial intelligence; contrast media; body composition

1. Introduction

Even if ultrasound represents the first-line technique for the assessment of liver structure and potential lesions [1], contrast-enhanced computed tomography (CT) is commonly used to detect and characterise liver lesions [2,3]. The majority of these lesions are hypovascular and are, therefore, better identifiable with portal venous contrast enhancement [4,5]. A minimum enhancement of liver tissue of 50 HU is considered essential to ensure appropriate detectability [6–8]. The degree of contrast enhancement in CT is dependent on different factors: CT scan parameters (e.g., tube voltage, scan delay), injection parameters (e.g., amount of injected iodine), and patient-related factors (e.g., height, weight, cardiac output) [9]. The most widespread practise is to administer iodine contrast in fixed-contrast media injection protocols. Fixed protocols result in varying enhancement levels because of differences in body size and composition [9]. Lowering the dose of contrast media decreases the sensitivity and specificity in the detection and characterisation of liver lesions [10]. Higher doses of contrast media are costly and might increase the risk of renal toxicity [11,12]. A personalised protocol for iodine dosing should be preferred to the standard fixed-contrast protocol [13]. In this respect, body-weight-adapted contrast injection protocols have proven successful in achieving a more homogeneous enhancement of vascular structures and liver parenchyma in patients [8,14–17]. However, total body weight (TBW) is not the only relevant body-size-related factor; lean body weight (LBW) and body mass index (BMI) might also be important. Solid organs have greater perfusion than adipose tissue [18]; consequently, using LBW (or the fat-free mass) as the basis for determining the amount of iodine is hypothesised to result in more uniform liver enhancement than using TBW or BMI [18,19].

Some previous studies concluded that injection protocols based on LBW rather than on TBW alone performed better in terms of liver enhancement [13,18–20]. However, we find these results not to be generalisable to our clinic because many of the aforementioned studies were performed in populations with smaller ranges in weight.

Furthermore, these studies did not use body composition on a per patient basis, but performed analysis on averaged body composition values [13,19] or estimated the body composition using empirically derived formulas [18,20].

We want to take personalised medicine a step further, using artificial intelligence as a way to determine body composition. We will use a tool that automatically segments clearly visible structures such as fat, muscle, and bone on scanned images and determines the body composition of a patient. The automated nature of this technique makes it possible to dose contrast material in real-time and in a personalised fashion, and may have wide implications.

In this study, we retrospectively evaluated the influence of TBW, BMI, and artificial-intelligence-derived LBW on liver enhancement in multiphase abdominal CT, showing that subjective image quality was related to liver enhancement.

2. Materials and Methods

2.1. Patients

We retrospectively included patients from the period of March 2016 to October 2019. We included the first CT scan of all patients who underwent a multiphase abdominal CT, including an unenhanced CT for suspicion of a kidney tumour, on a spectral CT scanner in the University Medical Center Utrecht. Inclusion criteria were an age of 18 years or older and known patient weight and height. Based on these criteria, we identified 122 patients. Exclusion criteria were patients with liver cirrhosis ($n = 2$), a fatty liver (<40 HU) ($n = 12$), numerous liver metastases ($n = 1$), a partial hepatectomy ($n = 2$), and technical problems during CT examination ($n = 1$), leaving a study population of 102 patients. The Dutch Law on Medical Research (WMO) did not apply to this retrospective cohort study according to the local medical ethical committee (METC, ref. 20-025/C). No informed consent was obtained given the anonymous research data handling.

2.2. Imaging Protocols

All included multiphase CTs were performed on a spectral CT scanner (IQon Spectral CT, Philips Healthcare, Best, The Netherlands). The scan range for the unenhanced and arterial phase was the upper abdomen. The scan range for the portal venous phase was set from approximately 1 cm cranial of the diaphragm to the lower pelvis. The scan range for the (possible) equilibrium phase was set from the kidneys to just caudal of the bladder.

Scans were performed with the following parameters: tube voltage 120 kV, 64 × 0.625 mm collimation, gantry rotation time of 0.27 s, and tube current was switched on with a quality reference tube current of 116 mAs. Image reconstruction was performed in the axial plane for the unenhanced and arterial phase, with 3 and 5 mm slice thicknesses and 2 and 4 mm increments. Image reconstruction was performed in the axial, coronal, and sagittal plane for the portal venous phase, with 5 mm slice thicknesses and 4mm increments. All images were reconstructed using a B (abdominal) kernel at iDose level 3.

All scans were performed with bolus tracking. A circular region of interest (ROI) was placed in the abdominal aorta with a threshold of 150 HU. The post-threshold delay before scanning was 20 s for the arterial phase and 90 s for the portal venous phase.

2.3. Contrast Material Injection and CT Protocols

All patients received an 18–20 G cannula in an antecubital vein before injection. Preheated iodinated contrast (Ultravist, Iopromide 300 mgI/mL; Bayer Healthcare, Berlin, Germany) was injected using a standard dual-head CT power injector (Stellant, Bayer Healthcare, Berlin, Germany). The contrast media was preheated to 37 °C to decrease viscosity [21].

In current clinical practice, body-weight-adapted protocols are used for the multiphase abdominal CT. Injection parameters were divided into three different weight groups: ≤70 kg, 70–90 kg, and ≥90 kg. The total injected volume, iodine, and flow rate were: 120 mL, 36.0 gI, 4 mL/s for group ≤70 kg; 150 mL, 45.0 gI, 4.5 mL/s for group 70–90 kg, and 185 mL, 55.5 gI, 5 mL/s for group ≥90 kg, respectively. A saline flush of 50 mL followed the contrast bolus at the same flow rate. In some cases, technicians adapted the amount of contrast media according to their experience, which was recorded in the scan protocol. In further analysis, we did not analyse weight groups, but instead used the weight of the patient; therefore, changes in scan protocol had no effect on analyses.

2.4. Quantitative Image Analysis

The body composition was calculated with the Quantib-U bod composition algorithm [22] on unenhanced images (Figure 1) [23]. Firstly, using a convolutional neural network, the method automatically detected the slice at the third lumbar vertebra from the CT data set (resampled to 5mm slices). Secondly, this slice was automatically segmented into visceral fat, subcutaneous fat, psoas muscle, abdominal muscle, and long spine muscle using a second convolutional neural network. Using the areas of these segmentations in proportion to those of the entire slice, percentages of body composition were calculated. To minimise the influence of the exact slice that was selected, the areas were computed by segmenting a total of five slices around the detected L3 level—two above and two below—and averaging the results. The %LBW (percentage of lean body weight) was defined as 100%—% total body fat (=subcutaneous fat % + visceral fat %). Total fat and LBW in kilograms were then calculated using TBW. Moreover, %LBW is an areal measure and LBW is in kilograms.

CT liver enhancement values (HU) were measured (M.K., who has seven years of experience in CT imaging) on the unenhanced and portal venous phase images using circular regions of interest (ROI) of 1–2 cm in diameter. ROIs were placed in three different liver segments (S2, S8, and S7) according to the Couinaud segmental classification and mean values were calculated (Figure 2). The degree of contrast enhancement in the liver was defined as the change in enhancement values (ΔHU) and was calculated by subtraction of the unenhanced values from post-contrast enhancement values.

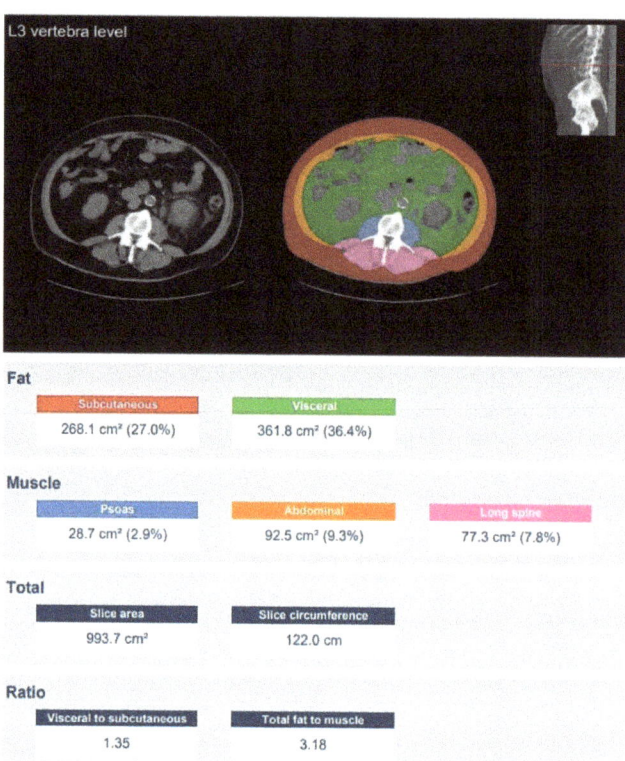

Figure 1. Fully automatic measurement of body composition at the lumbar 3 level [22]. Lean body weight (LBW) was defined as the difference between body weight and body fat weight, expressed in kilograms. In this example, LBW is 36.6% of the total body weight (100%—27.0% (subcutaneous fat)—36.4% (visceral fat) = 36.6% (LBW)).

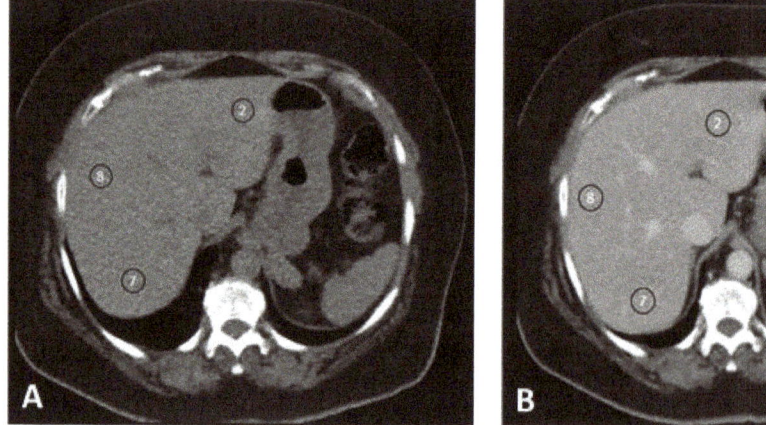

Figure 2. Region of interest (ROI) placement according to the Couinaud segmental classification to measure liver enhancement. ROIs were drawn in S2, S8, and S7 of the liver (when available) in unenhanced and enhanced images (portal venous phase). The degree of enhancement (ΔHU) was calculated by subtracting the unenhanced enhancement values (**A**) from enhanced enhancement values (**B**).

2.5. Qualitative Image Analysis

The quality of all scans was independently graded by two radiologists (F.W. and M.K., with eleven and four years of experience in abdominal radiology, respectively) who were blinded to the injection protocols. The timing of the scans and the subjective liver enhancement were scored. For scan timing, a five-point scale was used to evaluate enhancement of the common portal vein (1 = too early (non-diagnostic); 2 = early (moderate, but still diagnostic); 3 = portal venous phase (good); 4 = late (moderate, but still diagnostic); 5 = too late (non-diagnostic)). Liver enhancement was assessed using a four-point Likert scale (1 = excellent; 2 = good; 3 = moderate but still diagnostic; 4 = non-diagnostic). We arbitrarily defined enhancements of >70 HU and <40 HU as non-diagnostic.

2.6. Statistical Analysis

Statistical analyses were performed in SPSS version 26 (SPSS Inc., Chicago, IL, USA). Normality was checked using histograms and the Shapiro-Wilk test. Continuous variables were reported as the mean with standard deviation ($\pm$ SD) for normally distributed data and as the median with an interquartile range (IQR) for non-normal distributed data. Categorical variables were reported as proportions. Continuous variables with normal distributions were compared using the repeated measures ANOVA for dependent measures or a one-way ANOVA for independent measures. A Kruskal–Wallis test was used for non-parametric continuous variables. All tests were performed with post hoc comparison. The inter-rater variability was determined using Cohen's kappa. All p-values were 2-sided and a p-value of less than 0.05 was considered to be statistically significant.

Enhancement parameters of the liver obtained for further analyses were changed into enhancement values per gram of iodine ($\Delta HU/gI$). These enhancement values were subsequently adjusted for TBW or LBW in kilograms ($\Delta HU/(gI/TBW)$ and $\Delta HU/(gI/LBW)$), according to a method proposed by Heiken et al. [8] and Kondo et al. [19]. We used %LBW on a per-patient basis. Both single- and multivariable linear regressions between TBW, BMI, and %LBW and changes in enhancement values per gram of iodine ($\Delta HU/gI$) or the adjusted enhancement values $\Delta HU/(gI/TBW)$ and $\Delta HU/(gI/LBW)$ were evaluated (Table S1).

2.7. Simulation of Future Potential Clinical Applicability

Based on the formed regression formulas, we analysed the potential impacts for future patients by assessing the amount of contrast media needed to reach sufficient liver enhancement using our regression formulas for both %LBW and TBW. Our calculations for sufficient enhancement were based on an increase of 50 HU in the portal venous phase [6–8].

3. Results

3.1. Baseline Characteristics

The 102 patients (70.6% male) had a median age of 68 years (IQR: 57–74). Their median TBW was 81.0 kg (IQR: 72.8–90.0)—19.6% were below 70 kg and 19.6% were above 90 kg. The median %LBW was 49.8% (IQR: 35.8–55.3) and the mean BMI was 26.3 kg/m2 (SD: $\pm$4.18). Patients in the group $\leq$ 70 kg received a median of 36.0 g (IQR: 36.0–43.5) of iodine, the group 70–90 kg received 45.0 g (IQR: 39.0–45.0), and the group $\geq$ 90 kg 45.0 g (IQR: 45.0–45.7). Overall, the patients received 42.6 g (SD: $\pm$4.42) of iodine per scan (Table 1).

Table 1. Baseline characteristics. Normally distributed data are given as means with ±SDs and non-parametric data are given as medians with interquartile ranges (IQRs). TBW = total body weight; LBW = lean body weight in kilograms or percentage of lean body weight; BMI = body mass index.

Characteristic	Group ≤ 70 kg	Group 70–90 kg	Group ≥ 90 kg	Total
No participants	20	62	20	102
Sex male	45.0%	75.8%	80.0%	70.6%
Age (year)	70 (59–76)	69 (56–74)	64 (59–73)	68 (57–74)
TBW (kg)	62.5 (56.3–64.8)	81.0 (75.8–85.0)	101 (94.7–110)	81.0 (72.8–90.0)
LBW (kg)	40.8 (32.2–46.2)	40.8 (34.9–44.0)	41.4 (38.9–45.9)	41.1 (35.8–44.1)
%LBW	69.6 (55.3–73.8)	51.0 (43.8–53.7)	40.5 (37.5–44.5)	49.8 (42.1–55.3)
Height (cm)	168 (±13.1)	176 (±8.02)	180 (±10.9)	176 (±9.11)
BMI	21.3 (±2.01)	26.3 (±2.47)	31.5 (±4.10)	26.3 (±4.18)
Grams of iodine (mean)	38.7 (±3.88)	42.6 (±3.62)	46.3 (±3.96)	42.6 (±4.42)
Grams of iodine (median)	36.0 (36.0–43.5)	45.0 (39.0–45.0)	45.0 (45.0–45.7)	45.0 (39.0–45.0)
Grams of iodine/TBW	0.632 (±0.693)	0.530 (±0.534)	0.453 (±0.060)	0.532 (±0.081)
Grams of iodine/LBW	1.00 (±0.281)	1.07 (±0.176)	1.12 (±0.139)	1.07 (±0.196)
Mean (± SD) or Median (IQR)				

3.2. Quantitative Image Quality

Mean enhancement values in different liver segments were as follows: S2 54.3 HU (SD: ±5.83), S8 54.8 HU (SD: ±6.61), and S7 54.3 HU (SD: ±9.30). There was no significant difference in enhancement between the liver segments for all groups. The overall mean enhancement was 54.6 HU (SD: ±10.2; range: 25.0–93.3) and 28.4% did not reach the proposed enhancement of 50 HU or more. The mean enhancement value was for ≤70 kg 60.7 HU (SD: ±12.4), for 70-90 kg was 53.3 HU (SD: ±9.25), and for ≥90 kg was 52.4 HU (SD: ±7.45). The between-group difference reached significance ($p = 0.007$) and in post hoc analysis the ≤70 kg group was enhanced significantly more than the 70–90 kg group ($p = 0.019$) and ≥90 kg group ($p = 0.034$) (Table 2). The percentages of patients enhanced by <50 HU were 20%, 30%, 35% in the ≤70 kg, 80–90 kg, and ≥90 kg groups, respectively. The percentages of patients enhanced by >70 HU were 30%, 4.8%, 0.0% in the ≤70 kg, 80–90 kg, and ≥90 kg groups, respectively (Table S2).

3.3. Qualitative Image Quality

The inter-rater variability was good for scan timing ($k = 0.882$ (95% CI: 0.825–0.920)) and liver enhancement ($k = 0.921$ (95% CI: 0.833–0.946)). For timing, no scans were found to be non-diagnostic (Table S3). For liver enhancement, nearly all scans were of good (25.5%) or moderate (5.90%) quality, while one scan was non-diagnostic scored by only one of the observers (objective liver enhancement 25 HU) (Table S4). Most scans of moderate quality scored lower than 40 HU.

3.4. Regression Analysis

For the association between liver enhancement values per gram of iodine (ΔHU/gI) and body parameters, a correlation was observed with TBW ($r = 0.531$; $R2 = 0.282$; $p < 0.001$), while no significant values were observed for BMI ($p = 0.253$) or %LBW ($p = 0.493$) (Table S1). The formula for this relationship is: gI = ΔHU/(2.075-0.01 TBW), which can also be written as gI = ΔHU/(2.075-0.01 TBW) (Figure 3A). For the liver enhancement values additionally adjusted per gram of iodine per TBW (ΔHU/(gI/TBW)), no significant correlations were found (BMI; $p = 0.139$. TBW; $p = 0.302$. %LBW; $p = 0.628$) (Table S1). For the liver enhancement values additionally adjusted per gram of iodine per LBW (ΔHU/(gI/LBW)) the strongest association was observed with %LBW ($r = 0.733$; $R2 = 0.538$; $p < 0.001$), no significant correlations were observed for BMI ($p = 0.099$) or TBW ($p = 0.371$) (Figure 3B) (Table S1). The formula for this relationship is: ΔHU/(gI/LBW) = 10.3 + 0.823 %LBW or gI = ΔHU/(10.3/LBW + 82.3/TBW).

Table 2. Enhancement in liver segments for the weight groups.

Enhancement	Group ≤ 70 kg	Group 70–90 kg	Group ≥ 90 kg	Total	p-Value
S2 blanco	60.5 (±5.77)	56.7 (±5.02)	53.6 (±6.30)	56.8 (±5.83)	0.000
S2 PV	120.6 (±11.6)	109.8 (±11.7)	105.7 (±9.86)	111.1 (±12.3)	0.000
S2 SD	9.57 (±1.43)	11.1 (±1.89)	12.1 (±1.91)	11.0 (±1.92)	0.000
Δ S2	60.0 (±10.6)	53.1 (±10.7)	52.1 (±6.73)	54.3 (±10.3)	0.014
S8 blanco	60.7 (±5.24)	55.7 (±5.84)	51.0 (±6.61)	55.7 (±6.61)	0.000
S8 PV	120.9 (±14.2)	109.2 (±10.9)	104.4 (±9.52)	110.5 (±12.5)	0.000
S8 SD	9.19 (±0.981)	10.2 (±1.47)	11.2 (±2.18)	10.3 (±1.75)	0.000
Δ S8	60.1 (±12.6)	53.5 (±10.8)	53.4 (±8.18)	54.8 (±10.9)	0.043
S7 blanco	59.5 (±5.56)	54.5 (±5.35)	50.8 (±6.82)	54.7 (±6.32)	0.000
S7 PV	118.7 (±10.8)	107.8 (±10.1)	103.1 (±8.34)	109.0 (±11.1)	0.000
S7 SD	9.29 (±1.10)	10.6 (±1.70)	12.2 (±2.35)	10.7 (±2.09)	0.000
Δ S7	60.1 (±12.6)	53.3 (±9.25)	52.4 (±7.45)	54.3 (±9.30)	0.022
Δ S2 Δ S8 Δ S7	0.667	0.939	0.520	0.114	
Mean Δ	60.7 (±12.4)	53.3 (±9.75)	52.6 (±6.63)	54.6 (±10.2)	0.007 *
Mean (± SD)					

Enhancement values for the liver segments S2, S8, and S7 for the different weight groups. Values are given as means with ± SDs; p-values are calculated using a one-way ANOVA or repeated measures ANOVA. The blanco scans are non-enhanced scans, PV scans are scans made in the portal venous phase, the SD is given for the mean region of interest (ROI) SD, and lastly the mean enhancement is given; ΔS2 ΔS8 ΔS7 is the significance of enhancement between the three liver segments. The mean enhancement (mean ΔHU) is the average of ΔS2 ΔS8 ΔS7. Note: * Post hoc analysis showed a significant difference between ≤70 kg and 70–90 kg weight categories and between ≤70 kg and ≥90 kg weight categories.

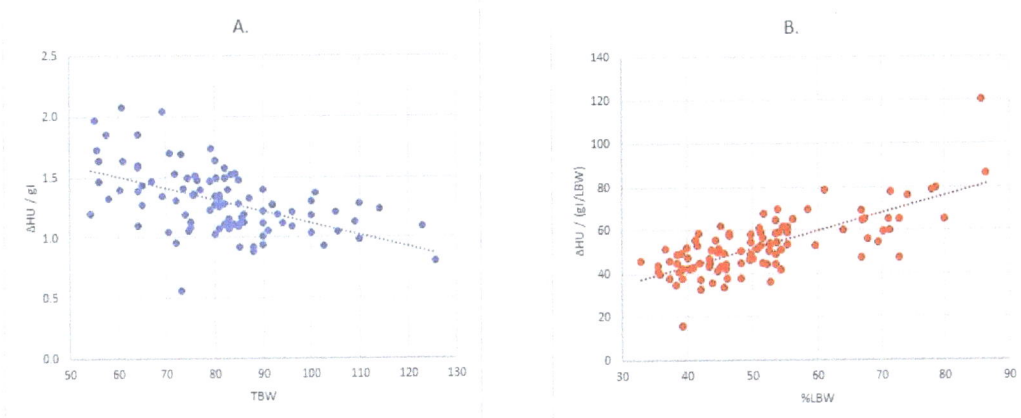

Figure 3. Regression analysis between enhancement and body size measures: (**A**) relationship between ΔHU/gI and TBW ($r = 0.531$; $R^2 = 0.282$; $p < 0.001$); (**B**) relationship between ΔHU/(gI/LBW) and %LBW ($r = 0.733$; $R^2 = 0.538$; $p < 0.001$). Note: TBW: total body weight; LBW: lean body weight.

3.5. Simulation of Future Potential Clinical Applicability

For the 102 included patients, we used an average of 42.6 g of iodine (SD: ±4.42; range: 36–55.5) per scan in the standard protocol, totaling approximately 4345 g of iodine and 14.5 litres of contrast for 102 patients. This is on average 0.532 g (SD: ±0.0811; range: 0.33–0.75) of iodine per kilogram TBW. For our regression formula based on %LBW, an estimated average of 39.4 g (SD: ±6.05; range: 27.6–57.5) of iodine per scan would be sufficient to achieve 50 HU for each patient in the study population. This would be on average 0.486 g (SD: ±0.0210; range: 0.44–0.53) of iodine per kilogram of TBW, which is 4019 g iodine and 13.4 litres of contrast for 102 patients (Figure 4). As an example, we would like to illustrate the added value of LBW for two patients weighing 80 kg with different %LBW values. The first patient had a %LWB of 35.5% and the expected amount of contrast to reach 50 HU was 35.9 g. The second patient had a %LWB of 78.5% and the expected amount of contrast to reach 50 HU was 41.9 g. Hence, there would be a difference of six grams of iodine for these patients who received 45 g of contrast and were enhanced by 63 HU and 57 HU, respectively.

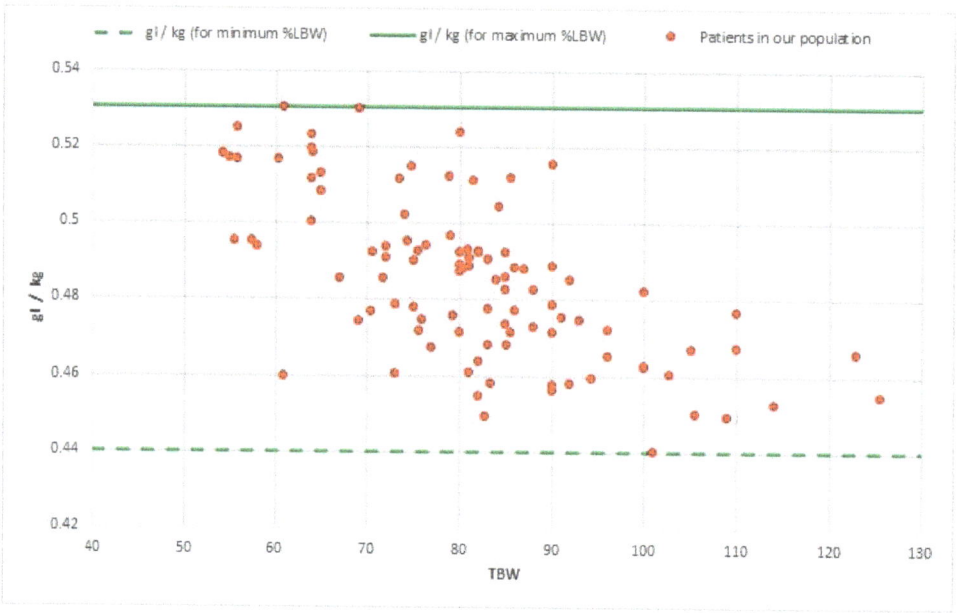

Figure 4. Analysis of future contrast applications: grams of iodine (gI) per kilogram (kg) TBW in the LBW formula; grams of iodine per kilogram of TBW (total body weight) in the LBW (lean body weight) formula for the population of our study. The grams of iodine per kilogram of TBW all lay between the patient with the maximum LBW (iodine (gr) maximum LBW/kg) and the patient with the lowest LBW (iodine (gr) minimum LBW/kg). Herein, the highest spreads were found in the ≤70 kg and 70–90 kg weight groups.

4. Discussion

Our results showed that the highest influence on liver enhancement was of %LBW, followed by TBW. Although the mean enhancement was >50 HU in all weight groups, the spread within groups was substantial; over one-quarter of patients did not reach the 50 HU liver enhancement threshold. Those who were enhanced by <40 HU were nearly all heavyweight patients of 90 kg or heavier, while patients enhanced by >70 HU were mostly patients weighing less than 70 kg. This indicates that our current protocol based on three weight categories overadministers contrast in lightweight patients and underadministers contrast in heavier patients. A more personalised protocol based on artificial-intelligence-determined body composition might both reduce overall contrast usage in our population and make liver enhancement more consistent between patients, but this requires prospective confirmation.

Several previous studies have investigated TBW- and LBW-adjusted contrast dosing protocols [8,18–20,24]. Heiken et al. [8] suggested the use of 0.521 g of iodine per kilogram of TBW for a 50 HU liver enhancement, while Kondo et al. [19] indicated that the use of LBW rather than TBW served better to achieve a consistent enhancement with reduced patient-to-patient variability. They suggested using an amount of 0.642 g of iodine per kilogram of LBW, based on a hepatic enhancement of 50 HU and a fixed average body fat percentage. Our finding supports the findings of Kondo et al. [19] and other studies [18,20,24]. However, both the studies of Kondo et al. [19] and Matsumoto et al. [24] concluded that LBW-based protocols best perform in the normal and high weight/BMI groups. In contrast, we found that LBW played the most important role in the weight groups ≤ 70 kg and 70–90 kg, wherein the spread of gI/TBW was the highest. For the group ≥ 90 kg, there was only a minor spread, and thus LBW played a less important role in this group in our study.

The differences between our results and the above-mentioned studies could be explained by the fact that the population in the study by Kondo et al. [19] was only partially comparable to our population. Our population represented a broader weight spectrum, with a range of 54–126 kg and with a median just above 80 kg, whereas in the study by Kondo et al. [19] the study population had a TBW range of 30–80 kg, with a mean just above 50 kg. Our study might, thus, have implications for a population with a wider range in weight. Reassuringly, we found the same results in the overlapping parts of the studies by Kondo et al. [19] and Matsumoto et al. [20]; LBW might be a better variable to determine the amount of iodine contrast used for light and average weight patients.

Contrast administration based on LBW might be economically effective. There was a difference of 3.2 g between the mean iodine dose per scan in the formula based on LBW and the mean iodine dose used in our current protocol. Based on the 600,000 yearly abdominal CT scans performed in the Netherlands, the new personalised method could save 1.8 tonnes of iodine a year [25], which is approximately €580,000 of yearly savings. Moreover, despite the conclusion that LBW performs better in personalising contrast application and the fact that the implementation of this finding might be beneficial if replicated prospectively, we conclude that the influence of LBW is minor. Similar to Kondo et al. [19], our equation is based on both TBW and LBW (the opposite of body fat percentage), and when dissecting the formula based on LBW (gI = ΔHU/(10.3/LBW + 82.3/TBW)) we find that TBW is still the most important factor and that LBW only has less influence.

In the study by Kondo et al. [19], an average body fat percentage of 23% was used for every patient to perform analysis, whilst some patients in their population had body fat percentages of up to 50%. We used per-patient calculated body composition for analysis. For the calculation of %LBW, we were able to use an artificial intelligence algorithm that automatically calculates body composition based on CT slices [22]. The tool proved useful for determining the body composition values for the large quantity of patients in our study, especially because this process was fully automated.

In the literature, several methods have been used to estimate the LBW (e.g., methods proposed by James [26], Boer [27], and Janmahasatian [28]), yet no consensus has been reached on a golden standard. Therefore, our artificial intelligence tool [22] may have wide implications in measuring LBW rather than in estimating LBW. In a clinical scenario, the tool can be used in protocols containing unenhanced or arterial phase scans. If the protocol does not contain unenhanced or arterial phase scans, the body composition can be determined in several ways: from earlier recorded scans or by performing one single slice through the abdomen before scanning (as done for bolus timing acquisitions). Furthermore, bolus tracking slices may be (re)used in the future when the algorithm is tested on such arterial slices. However, the latter still has to be evaluated in future research. Moreover, while this study addresses abdominal scans, the AI algorithm can segment neck, chest, pelvis, or lower extremity scans as well when acquired, to calculate the body composition without the use of the abdomen. Once validated, the benefit could extend to those regions as well.

The limitations of this study are that this is a retrospective study design using a limited number of patients. As we needed to calculate enhancement, regular abdominal CT could not be included. Secondly, there were two outliers with enhancement levels <40 HU. The low enhancement could be due to small contrast extravasation, although this was not recorded. Another explanation could be a poor cardiac output, which results in poor enhancement and image quality [17]. However, we used premonitoring for contrast timing in our scan protocol and no scans were found to be non-diagnostic based on the timing of the scan.

Future prospective studies could investigate the impact of personalised dosing on liver enhancement and diagnostic properties, which should also take tube voltage into account [14]. Many studies already investigated the potential of low kVp settings (e.g., 70, 80, and 100 kVp) [2,14,29–32] or virtual monochromatic imaging with low kV reconstruction [33–37] in combination with a reduced amount of injected iodine in a more lightweight population using CT angiography protocols, wherein only the signal during the first pass of contrast media is crucial [29]. However, this has not properly been investigated for abdominal protocols yet, which rely on longer contrast media boluses to provide homogeneous enhancement of parenchymal organs, such as the liver. With the newest CT technologies (e.g., automated kVp selection, monochromatic data reconstruction, and iterative reconstruction), it is expected that more CT scans will be performed using lower kVp settings in the future [38]. As lower kVp/kV settings result in higher attenuation values, there is an opportunity to save even more contrast media than the above-mentioned €580,000. We anticipate that personalised contrast dosing is at least partly additional to the above-mentioned technological innovations.

5. Conclusions

In summary, in this study, we investigated the relationship between body parameters, such as TBW, LBW, and BMI, on liver enhancement in CT. We found that contrast-enhanced CT values of 40 HU and higher were of diagnostic value when assessed visually. Our data suggest the use of an artificial intelligence body composition-based algorithm to determine LBW can reduce interpatient variability in liver enhancement whilst saving contrast media. The automated nature of the algorithm makes real-time personalisation of contrast dosing technically feasible. Further research should focus on how to integrate body-composition-based personalised contrast dosing with lower tube voltage settings or monochromatic imaging.

Supplementary Materials: The following are available online at https://www.mdpi.com/2075-4426/11/3/159/s1, Table S1: Correlations in regression. Table S2: Enhancement values per group. Table S3: Subjective phase classification per rater. Table S4: Subjective enhancement classification on the four-point Likert scale per rater.

Author Contributions: Conceptualisation, M.K., W.B.V., P.M., B.d.V. and D.J.d.J.; methodology, M.K. and D.J.d.J.; software, W.B.V., P.M. and B.d.V.; validation, M.K.; formal analysis, M.K. and D.J.d.J.; investigation, M.K. and F.J.W.; resources, P.M. and B.d.V.; writing—original draft preparation, M.K. and D.J.d.J.; writing—review and editing, W.B.V., P.M., B.d.V. and F.J.W.; supervision, M.K.; project administration, M.K. All authors have read and agreed to the published version of the manuscript.

Funding: This research received no external funding.

Institutional Review Board Statement: Ethical review and approval were waived for this study. The Dutch Law on Medical Research (WMO) did not apply to this retrospective cohort study according to the local medical ethical committee (METC, ref. 20-025/C).

Informed Consent Statement: Patient consent was waived due to the anonymous research data handling (METC, ref. 20-025/C).

Data Availability Statement: The data presented in this study are available on request from the corresponding author. The data are not publicly available due to ongoing unpublished research.

Acknowledgments: We would like to thank the radiology technicians of the UMC Utrecht for their work in collecting data. Moreover, we would like to thank A. Schilham for contributing useful advise. D. de Jong is a medical student participating in the Honours programme of the Faculty of Medicine, UMC Utrecht.

Conflicts of Interest: The scientific guarantor of this publication is M. Kok. The authors of this manuscript declare that the Department of Radiology of the UMC Utrecht receives research support form Philips Healthcare and some of the contributing authors declare having a relationship with Quantib-U (B. de Vos and P. Moeskops).

References

1. Tchelepi, H.; Ralls, P.W. Ultrasound of focal liver masses. *Ultrasound Q.* **2004**, *20*, 155–169. [CrossRef]
2. Robinson, E.; Babb, J.; Chandarana, H.; Macari, M. Dual Source Dual Energy MDCT: Comparison of 80 kVp and Weighted Average 120 kVp Data for Conspicuity of Hypo-Vascular Liver Metastases. *Investig. Radiol.* **2010**, *45*, 413–418. [CrossRef] [PubMed]
3. Haider, M.A.; Amitai, M.M.; Rappaport, D.C.; O'Malley, M.E.; Hanbidge, A.E.; Redston, M.; Lockwood, G.A.; Gallinger, S. Multi–Detector Row Helical CT in Preoperative Assessment of Small (≤1.5 cm) Liver Metastases: Is Thinner Collimation Better? *Radiology* **2002**, *225*, 137–142. [CrossRef]
4. Stevens, W.R.; Johnson, C.D.; Stephens, D.H.; Batts, K.P. CT findings in hepatocellular carcinoma: Correlation of tumor characteristics with causative factors, tumor size, and histologic tumor grade. *Radiology* **1994**, *191*, 531–537. [CrossRef] [PubMed]
5. Gore, R.M.; Thakrar, K.H.; Wenzke, D.R.; Newmark, G.M.; Mehta, U.K.; Berlin, J.W. That liver lesion on MDCT in the oncology patient:is it important? *Cancer Imaging* **2012**, *12*, 373–384. [CrossRef]
6. Brink, J.A.; Heiken, J.P.; Forman, H.P.; Sagel, S.S.; Molina, P.L.; Brown, P.C. Hepatic Spiral CT: Reduction of Dose of Intravenous Contrast Material. *Radiology* **1995**, *197*, 88–89. [CrossRef] [PubMed]
7. Patel, B.N.; Rosenberg, M.; Vernuccio, F.; Ramirez-Giraldo, J.C.; Nelson, R.; Farjat, A.; Marin, D. Characterization of Small Incidental Indeterminate Hypoattenuating Hepatic Lesions: Added Value of Single-Phase Contrast-Enhanced Dual-Energy CT Material Attenuation Analysis. *AJR Am. J. Roentgenol.* **2018**, *211*, 571–579. [CrossRef]
8. Heiken, J.P.; Brink, J.A.; McClennan, B.L.; Sagel, S.S.; Crowe, T.M.; Gaines, M.V. Dynamic incremental CT: Effect of volume and concentration of contrast material and patient weight on hepatic enhancement. *Radiology* **1995**, *195*, 353–357. [CrossRef]
9. Bae, K.T. Intravenous Contrast Medium Administration and Scan Timing at CT: Considerations and Approaches. *Radiology* **2010**, *256*, 32–61. [CrossRef]
10. Sica, G.T.; Ji, H.; Ros, P.R. CT and MR Imaging of Hepatic Metastases. *AJR Am. J. Roentgenol.* **2000**, *174*, 691–698. [CrossRef] [PubMed]
11. Gleeson, T.G.; Bulagahapitiya, S. Contrast-induced Nephropathy. *Review* **2004**, *183*, 1673–1689. [CrossRef]
12. Cohan, R.H.; Dunnick, N.R. Intravascular contrast media: Adverse reactions. *AJR Am. J. Roentgenol.* **1987**, *149*, 665–670. [CrossRef]
13. Kondo, H.; Kanematsu, M.; Goshima, S.; Tomita, Y.; Miyoshi, T.; Hatcho, A.; Moriyama, N.; Onozuka, M.; Shiratori, Y.; Bae, K.T. Abdominal Multidetector CT in Patients with Varying Body Fat Percentages: Estimation of Optimal Contrast Material Dose. *Radiology* **2008**, *249*, 872–877. [CrossRef]
14. Martens, B.; Hendriks, B.M.F.; Eijsvoogel, N.G.; Wildberger, J.E.; Mihl, C. Individually Body Weight–Adapted Contrast Media Application in Computed Tomography Imaging of the Liver at 90 kVp. *Investig. Radiol.* **2019**, *54*, 177–182. [CrossRef]
15. Mihl, C.; Kok, M.; Altintas, S.; Kietselaer, B.L.J.H.; Turek, J.; Wildberger, J.E.; Das, M. Evaluation of individually body weight adapted contrast media injection in coronary CT-angiography. *Eur. J. Radiol.* **2016**, *85*, 830–836. [CrossRef] [PubMed]
16. Hendriks, B.M.F.; Kok, M.; Mihl, C.; Bekkers, S.C.A.M.; Wildberger, J.E.; Das, M. Individually tailored contrast enhancement in CT pulmonary angiography. *Br. J. Radiol.* **2016**, *89*, 20150850. [CrossRef] [PubMed]
17. Bae, K.T.; Heiken, J.P.; Brink, J.A. Aortic and hepatic contrast medium enhancement at CT. Part I. Prediction with a computer model. *Radiology* **1998**, *207*, 647–655. [CrossRef]
18. Ho, L.M.; Nelson, R.C.; Delong, D.M. Determining Contrast Medium Dose and Rate on Basis of Lean Body Weight: Does This Strategy Improve Patient-to-Patient Uniformity of Hepatic Enhancement during Multi–Detector Row CT? *Radiology* **2007**, *243*, 431–437. [CrossRef]
19. Kondo, H.; Kanematsu, M.; Goshima, S.; Tomita, Y.; Kim, M.-J.; Moriyama, N.; Onozuka, M.; Shiratori, Y.; Bae, K.T. Body Size Indexes for Optimizing Iodine Dose for Aortic and Hepatic Enhancement at Multidetector CT: Comparison of Total Body Weight, Lean Body Weight, and Blood Volume. *Radiology* **2010**, *254*, 163–169. [CrossRef]
20. Matsumoto, Y.; Masuda, T.; Sato, T.; Arataki, K.; Nakamura, Y.; Tatsugami, F.; Awai, K. Contrast Material Injection Protocol with the Dose Determined According to Lean Body Weight at Hepatic Dynamic Computed Tomography: Comparison Among Patients with Different Body Mass Indices. *J. Comput. Assist. Tomogr.* **2019**, *43*, 736–740. [CrossRef] [PubMed]
21. Kok, M.; Mihl, C.; Mingels, A.A.; Kietselaer, B.L.; Mühlenbruch, G.; Seehofnerova, A.; Wildberger, J.E.; Das, M. Influence of contrast media viscosity and temperature on injection pressure in computed tomographic angiography: A phantom study. *Investig. Radiol.* **2014**, *49*, 217–223. [CrossRef] [PubMed]
22. Moeskops, P.; de Vos, B.; Veldhuis, W.B.; de Jong, P.A.; Išgum, I.; Leiner, T. Automatic quantification of body composition at L3 vertebra level with convolutional neural networks. *Eur. Congr. Radiol.* **2020**. [CrossRef]
23. Morsbach, F.; Zhang, Y.-H.Y.H.; Martin, L.; Lindqvist, C.; Brismar, T. Body composition evaluation with computed tomography: Contrast media and slice thickness cause methodological errors. *Nutrition* **2019**, *59*, 50–55. [CrossRef] [PubMed]
24. Awai, K.; Takada, K.; Onishi, H.; Hori, S. Aortic and Hepatic Enhancement and Tumor-to-Liver Contrast: Analysis of the Effect of Different Concentrations of Contrast Material at Multi-Detector Row Helical CT. *Radiology* **2002**, *242*, 757–763. [CrossRef]
25. RIVM Trends in het aantal CT-onderzoeken. Available online: https://www.rivm.nl/medische-stralingstoepassingen/trends-en-stand-van-zaken/diagnostiek/computer-tomografie/trends-in-aantal-ct-onderzoeken (accessed on 5 August 2020).
26. James, W.P.T.; Waterlow, J.C. *Research on Obesity: A Report of the DHSS/MRC Group*; Her Majesty's Stationery Office: London, UK, 1976.

27. Boer, P. Estimated lean body mass as an index for normalization of body fluid volumes in humans. *Am. J. Physiol. Ren. Fluid Electrolyte Physiol.* **1984**, *247*, F632–F636. [CrossRef]
28. Janmahasatian, S.; Duffull, S.B.; Ash, S.; Ward, L.C.; Byrne, N.M.; Green, B. Quantification of Lean Bodyweight. *Clin. Pharmacokinet.* **2005**, *44*, 1051–1065. [CrossRef]
29. Kok, M.; Turek, J.; Mihl, C.; Reinartz, S.D.; Gohmann, R.F.; Nijssen, E.C.; Kats, S.; van Ommen, V.G.; Kietselaer, B.L.J.H.; Wildberger, J.E. Low contrast media volume in pre-TAVI CT examinations. *Eur. Radiol.* **2016**, *26*, 2426–2435. [CrossRef] [PubMed]
30. Masuda, T.; Nakaura, T.; Funama, Y.; Sato, T.; Higaki, T.; Matsumoto, Y.; Yamashita, Y.; Imada, N.; Kiguchi, M.; Baba, Y. Contrast enhancement on 100-and 120 kVp hepatic CT scans at thin adults in a retrospective cohort study: Bayesian inference of the optimal enhancement probability. *Medicine (Baltimore).* **2019**, *98*. [CrossRef]
31. Nakamoto, A.; Yamamoto, K.; Sakane, M.; Nakai, G.; Higashiyama, A.; Juri, H.; Yoshikawa, S.; Narumi, Y. Reduction of the radiation dose and the amount of contrast material in hepatic dynamic CT using low tube voltage and adaptive iterative dose reduction 3-dimensional. *Medicine (Baltimore)* **2018**, *97*. [CrossRef]
32. Araki, K.; Yoshizako, T.; Yoshida, R.; Tada, K.; Kitagaki, H. Low-voltage (80-kVp) abdominopelvic computed tomography allows 60% contrast dose reduction in patients at risk of contrast-induced nephropathy. *Clin. Imaging* **2018**, *51*, 352–355. [CrossRef] [PubMed]
33. Leng, S.; Yu, L.; Fletcher, J.G.; McCollough, C.H. Maximizing iodine contrast-to-noise ratios in abdominal CT imaging through use of energy domain noise reduction and virtual monoenergetic dual-energy CT. *Radiology* **2015**, *276*, 562–570. [CrossRef] [PubMed]
34. Lu, X.; Lu, Z.; Yin, J.; Gao, Y.; Chen, X.; Guo, Q. Effects of radiation dose levels and spectral iterative reconstruction levels on the accuracy of iodine quantification and virtual monochromatic CT numbers in dual-layer spectral detector CT: An iodine phantom study. *Quant. Imaging Med. Surg.* **2019**, *9*, 188. [CrossRef] [PubMed]
35. D'Angelo, T.; Cicero, G.; Mazziotti, S.; Ascenti, G.; Albrecht, M.H.; Martin, S.S.; Othman, A.E.; Vogl, T.J.; Wichmann, J.L. Dual energy computed tomography virtual monoenergetic imaging: Technique and clinical applications. *Br. J. Radiol.* **2019**, *92*, 20180546. [CrossRef] [PubMed]
36. Kang, H.-J.; Lee, J.M.; Lee, S.M.; Yang, H.K.; Kim, R.H.; Nam, J.G.; Karnawat, A.; Han, J.K. Value of virtual monochromatic spectral image of dual-layer spectral detector CT with noise reduction algorithm for image quality improvement in obese simulated body phantom. *BMC Med. Imaging* **2019**, *19*, 76. [CrossRef]
37. Kawahara, D.; Ozawa, S.; Yokomachi, K.; Tanaka, S.; Higaki, T.; Fujioka, C.; Suzuki, T.; Tsuneda, M.; Nakashima, T.; Ohno, Y. Accuracy of the raw-data-based effective atomic numbers and monochromatic CT numbers for contrast medium with a dual-energy CT technique. *Br. J. Radiol.* **2018**, *91*, 20170524. [CrossRef]
38. Raman, S.P.; Johnson, P.T.; Deshmukh, S.; Mahesh, M.; Grant, K.L.; Fishman, E.K. CT dose reduction applications: Available tools on the latest generation of CT scanners. *J. Am. Coll. Radiol.* **2013**, *10*, 37–41. [CrossRef]

MDPI
St. Alban-Anlage 66
4052 Basel
Switzerland
Tel. +41 61 683 77 34
Fax +41 61 302 89 18
www.mdpi.com

Journal of Personalized Medicine Editorial Office
E-mail: jpm@mdpi.com
www.mdpi.com/journal/jpm

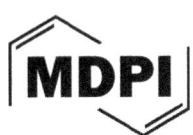

www.ingramcontent.com/pod-product-compliance
Lightning Source LLC
LaVergne TN
LVHW070649100526
838202LV00013B/921

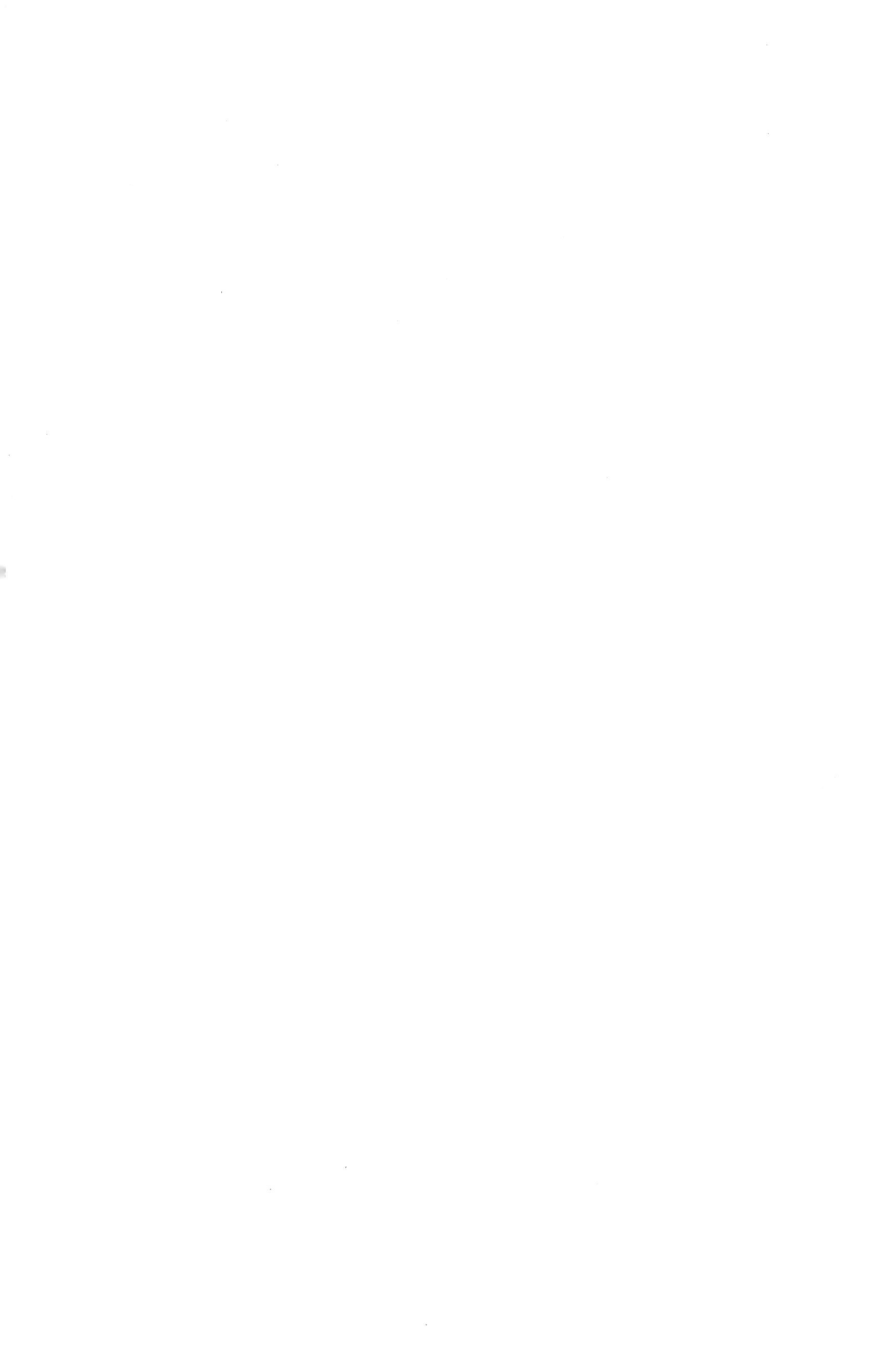